theclinics.com

CLINICS IN SPORTS MEDICINE

Imaging of Upper Extremities

GUEST EDITOR
Timothy G. Sanders, MD

CONSULTING EDITOR
Mark D. Miller, MD

July 2006 • Volume 25 • Number 3

SAUNDERS
An Imprint of Elsevier, Inc.
PHILADELPHIA LONDON TORONTO MONTREAL SYDNEY TOKYO

W.B. SAUNDERS COMPANY
A Division of Elsevier Inc.

1600 John F. Kennedy Blvd. • Suite 1800 • Philadelphia, Pennsylvania 19103

http://www.theclinics.com

CLINICS IN SPORTS MEDICINE
July 2006
Editor: Debora Dellapena

Volume 25, Number 3
ISSN 0278-5919
ISBN 1-4160-3798-5

Reprints: For copies of 100 or more, of articles in this publication, please contact the Commercial Reprints Department, Elsevier Inc., 360 Park Avenue South, New York, New York 10010-1710. Tel. (212) 633-3813; Fax: (212) 462-1935 e-mail: reprints@elsevier.com.

Clinics in Sports Medicine (ISSN 0278-5919) is published quarterly by W.B. Saunders, 360 Park Avenue South, New York, NY 10010-1710. Months of publication are January, April, July, and October. Business and Editorial offices: 1600 John F. Kennedy Blvd., Suite 1800, Philadelphia, PA 19103-2899. Accounting and Circulation Offices: 6277 Sea Harbor Drive, Orlando, FL 32887-4800. Periodicals postage paid at New York, NY, and additional mailing offices. Subscription prices are \$190.00 per year (US individuals), \$295.00 per year (US institutions), \$95.00 per year (US students), \$215.00 per year (Canadian individuals), \$350.00 per year (Canadian institutions), \$125.00 (Canadian students), \$245.00 per year (foreign individuals), \$350.00 per year (foreign institutions), and \$125.00 per year (foreign students). Foreign air speed delivery is included in all *Clinics* subscription prices. All prices are subject to change without notice. POSTMASTER: Send address changes to *Clinics in Sports Medicine*, Elsevier Periodicals Customer Service, 6277 Sea Harbor Drive, Orlando, FL 32887-4800. **Customer Service: 1-800-654-2452 (US). From outside of the US, call 1-407-345-4000.** E-mail: hhspcs@harcourt.com.

Clinics in Sports Medicine is covered in *Index Medicus, Current Contents/Clinical Medicine, Excerpta Medica, and ISI/Biomed.*

Printed in the United States of America.

ELSEVIER
SAUNDERS

CLINICS IN SPORTS MEDICINE

Imaging of Upper Extremities

CONSULTING EDITOR

MARK D. MILLER, MD, Professor, Department of Orthopaedic Surgery; Director, Division of Sports Medicine, University of Virginia Health System, Charlottesville, Virginia

GUEST EDITOR

TIMOTHY G. SANDERS, MD, Director of Research and Education, National Musculoskeletal Imaging, Weston, Florida; and Assistant Clinical Professor, Uniformed Services University, Bethesda, Maryland

CONTRIBUTORS

MARK W. ANDERSON, MD, Associate Professor of Radiology and Chief of Musculoskeletal Imaging, University of Virginia Health Sciences Center, Charlottesville, Virginia

LAURA W. BANCROFT, MD, Associate Professor of Radiology, Department of Radiology, Mayo Clinic, Jacksonville, Florida

JENNY T. BENCARDINO, MD, Department of Radiology, Huntington Hospital, North Shore Long Island Jewish Health System, Huntington, New York

LIDA CHAIPAT, MD, Musculoskeletal Imaging, Massachusetts General Hospital, Boston, Massachusetts

CLAIRE A. COGGINS, MD, Assistant Professor, Musculoskeletal Radiology, Department of Radiology, Virginia Commonwealth University, Richmond, Virginia

AARON COVEY, MD, Department of Orthopaedic Surgery and Rehabilitative Medicine, Yale University School of Medicine, New Haven, Connecticut

JOHN V. CRUES III, MD, Medical Director and Director of MRI Fellowship, RadNet, Los Angeles; Visiting Clinical Professor of Radiology, University of California, San Diego, California

ARTHUR A. DE SMET, MD, Professor of Radiology, Division of Musculoskeletal Radiology, Department of Radiology, University of Wisconsin Clinical Science Center, Madison, Wisconsin

DAVID M. DINES, MD, Professor of Orthopaedic Surgery, Albert Einstein College of Medicine at Long Island Jewish Medical Center; Chairman, Department of Orthopaedic Surgery, Long Island Jewish Medical Center, New Hyde Park, New York

KATHLEEN H. EMERY, MD, Clinical Associate Professor of Radiology and Pediatrics, Cincinnati Children's Hospital Medical Center; Section Chief Body MRI, University of Cincinnati Medical Center, Cincinnati, Ohio

SHAYA GHAZINOOR, MD, Musculoskeletal MRI Fellow, RadNet, Los Angeles, California

LEE D. KATZ, MD, Professor of Diagnostic Radiology and Orthopaedic Surgery and Rehabilitative Medicine, Yale University School of Medicine, New Haven, Connecticut

RICHARD KIJOWSKI, MD, Assistant Professor of Radiology, Division of Musculoskeletal Radiology, Department of Radiology, University of Wisconsin Clinical Science Center; and Musculoskeletal Radiologist, University of Wisconsin Hospital and Clinics, Madison, Wisconsin

THEODORE T. MILLER, MD, Associate Professor of Radiology, New York University School of Medicine, New York; Chief, Division of Musculoskeletal Imaging, Department of Radiology, North Shore University Hospital and Long Island Jewish Medical Center, Great Neck, New York

JOSH B. MOOSIKASUWAN, MD, Fellow, Department of Radiology, North Shore University Hospital, Great Neck, New York

WILLIAM E. PALMER, MD, Director, Musculoskeletal Imaging, Massachusetts General Hospital, Boston, Massachusetts

JEFFREY J. PETERSON, MD, Assistant Professor of Radiology, Department of Radiology, Mayo Clinic, Jacksonville, Florida

ZEHAVA SADKA ROSENBERG, MD, Department of Radiology, Hospital for Joint Diseases, New York University Medical Center, New York, New York

MICHAEL J. TUITE, MD, Professor of Radiology, University of Wisconsin Medical School; Director of Musculoskeletal Radiology, University of Wisconsin Hospital and Clinics, Madison, Wisconsin

JIM WU, MD, Instructor, Department of Diagnostic Radiology, Beth Israel Deaconess Medical Center, Boston, Massachusetts

ELSEVIER
SAUNDERS

CLINICS IN SPORTS MEDICINE

Imaging of Upper Extremities

CONTENTS VOLUME 25 • NUMBER 3 • JULY 2006

MRI provides excellent soft tissue contrast and allows for multiplanar imaging in anatomic planes. Because of these advantages MRI has become the study of choice for imaging of shoulder pathology. Some structures, such as the rotator cuff, humeral head contour, and glenoid shape, are evaluated well with conventional MRI. When more sensitive evaluation of the labrum, capsule, articular cartilage, and glenohumeral ligaments is required or when a partial-thickness rotator cuff tear is suspected, magnetic resonance arthrography with intra-articular contrast can be performed. For MR arthrography contrast is injected directly into the glenohumeral joint. This article reviews the appearances of normal anatomic structures in MRI of the shoulder and disorders involving the rotator cuff and glenoid labrum.

MRI is a valuable tool for evaluating the athlete with elbow pain, particularly in those with nonlocalizable pain. MRI also is helpful in sorting out the cause of pain in athletes who may have acute trauma superimposed on tendinopathy or other chronic injuries from repetitive microtrauma. Even in athletes in whom the cause of pain confidently can be diagnosed clinically, MRI can document the injury severity, which can be helpful for estimating recovery time or in preoperative planning. By contributing to an accurate early diagnosis, MRI also can help minimize the time that athletes are away from their sports. The authors describe their approach to the MRI interpretation of elbow injuries in athletes, including osteochondral lesions, epicondylitis, and tears of the medial collateral ligament.

Sports-related injuries to the wrist range from minor sprains to severe soft tissue disruption that can pose a risk to the normal function of the upper extremity. It is important to identify the specific nature of such injuries so as to establish an accurate diagnosis and deliver appropriate treatment. MRI of the wrist has greatly benefited from the use of dedicated surface coils, which allow fine depiction of soft tissue and cartilaginous structures. A review of the normal anatomy, MR interpretation pitfalls, and most common abnormalities of the tendons, ligaments, triangular fibrocartilage complex, and nerves of the wrist are presented.

A wide spectrum of abnormalities can affect the throwing shoulder. The injuries are often particular to a specific phase of the throw and are well demonstrated with MR imaging. In this article, the authors review the phases of the throw, MR imaging techniques, and the MR appearances of the injuries associated with particular phases.

Pain in the postoperative shoulder is difficult for all individuals involved. The patient has already undergone a surgical procedure and is presenting now with pain possibly relating to a complication of the procedure or reinjury. In addition, the patient typically has undergone a series of maneuvers, from physical therapy to cortisone injection, without relief of the symptoms. For the orthopaedic surgeon the possibility of a complication of the procedure is disheartening. Finally, for the radiologist the postoperative shoulder usually is more difficult to interpret because of a change in the normal anatomy, not knowing exactly what was accomplished at surgery or what techniques or types of equipment were used, and, more typically, the presence of artifact.

MRI is a useful diagnostic method for evaluating nerve disease at the shoulder and elbow. MRI can depict the normal anatomy of the nerves, confirm and identify the cause of the neuropathy, identify the site of entrapment based on muscle denervation patterns, and detect unsuspected

ELSEVIER
SAUNDERS

CLINICS IN SPORTS MEDICINE

FORTHCOMING ISSUES

October 2006

Imaging of Lower Extremities
Timothy G. Sanders, MD
Guest Editor

January 2007

Sports Nutrition
Leslie Bonci MPH, RD
Guest Editor

April 2007

Working as a Team Physician
Jeff G. Konin, PhD, ATC, PT

RECENT ISSUES

April 2006

Hip Injuries
Srino Bharam, MD
and Marc J. Philippon, MD
Guest Editors

January 2006

Stress Fractures
Christopher C. Kaeding, MD
Guest Editor

October 2005

The Interface Between Sport Psychiatry and Sports Medicine
Ian R. Tofler, MB, BS
and Eric D. Morse, MD
Guest Editors

Clin Sports Med 25 (2006) xi
CLINICS IN SPORTS MEDICINE

FOREWORD

Imaging of Upper Extremities

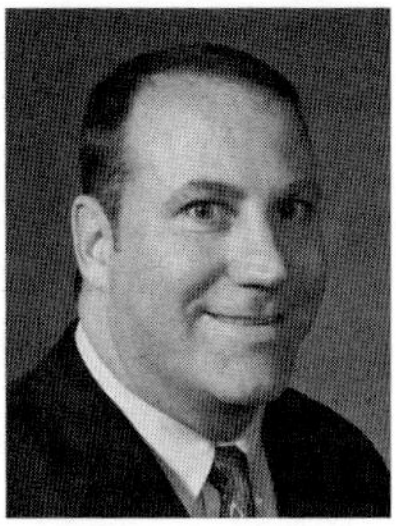

Mark D. Miller, MD
Consulting Editor

It is so much easier to see something if you know what you are looking for! That is the purpose of the next two issues of the *Clinics in Sports Medicine*. Dr. Tim Sanders, whom I have known and had the pleasure of working with over the last 10 years, has put together a pair of absolutely outstanding issues on musculoskeletal imaging. This first issue focuses on the upper extremity, and it will be followed by a lower extremity issue. Tim has already educated many of us with his excellent current concepts articles in the *American Journal of Sports Medicine* and his podium presentations, including his recent review at the Colorado Orthopaedic Review Course.

Dr. Sanders has assembled an "all star" panel of radiologists, who know what they are talking about and, more importantly, can teach even the most imaging-illiterate of us. From the fingers to the shoulder, from kids to adults, from radiographs to ultrasound to MRI, this issue covers it all. This is perhaps one issue that orthopaedic surgeons may enjoy even more than our nonoperative colleagues, because there are more pictures! Please enjoy this issue. I know I will!

Mark D. Miller, MD
University of Virginia
Department of Sports Medicine
McCue Center – 3rd Floor
Emmet St. & Massie Rd.
Charlottesville, VA 22903, USA

E-mail address: mdm3p@virginia.edu

0278-5919/06/$ – see front matter
doi:10.1016/j.csm.2006.04.001

sportsmed.theclinics.com

Clin Sports Med 25 (2006) xiii–xiv
CLINICS IN SPORTS MEDICINE

PREFACE

Imaging of Upper Extremities

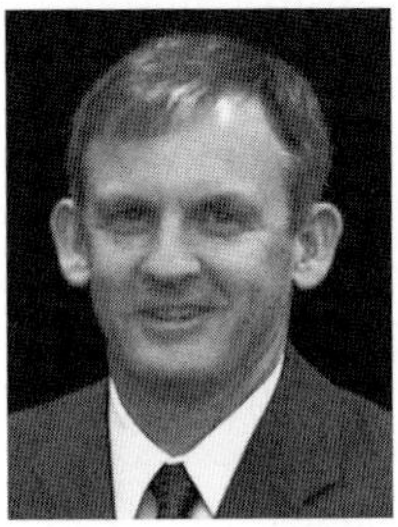

Timothy G. Sanders, MD
Guest Editor

The role of imaging in the evaluation of sports-related injuries of the upper extremities has evolved significantly over the past decade, with MRI becoming the imaging modality of choice for the evaluation of most soft-tissue injuries ranging from overuse injuries to acute traumatic injuries. Ultrasound has also emerged as a useful problem-solving tool that can be used in the targeted evaluation of certain upper-extremity injuries. To maximize the diagnostic value of these tools, the treating physician must possess a solid fund of knowledge regarding the roles of the various imaging modalities and an understanding of which studies are best suited for the evaluation of specific injuries.

This issue deals primarily with the more complex imaging modalities of MRI and ultrasound. First, excellent review articles provide a basic approach to the evaluation of an MR examination of the shoulder, elbow, and wrist. These articles provide a framework for the interpretation of these complex exams, reviewing the pertinent imaging anatomy as well as specific injury patterns that can be seen on MRI. Next, the role of MRI is discussed as it pertains to specific clinical problems that involve the shoulder, including an article on the MR evaluation of shoulder pain in the high-performance thrower and a review of the complexities of imaging the postoperative shoulder. Next, a review of the numerous nerve entrapment syndromes of the upper extremity specific to the athlete is provided, and the role of MRI in establishing these sometimes-elusive diagnoses is discussed. Stress fractures of the upper extremity are uncommon and often overlooked clinically. The various stress fractures of the upper extremity and their imaging appearance are comprehensively reviewed. The hand and wrist are at

0278-5919/06/$ – see front matter
doi:10.1016/j.csm.2006.02.004

sportsmed.theclinics.com

increased risk for injury in many sports, and imaging of the small anatomic soft-tissue structures of these areas can be challenging. Two articles discuss the role of complex imaging modalities in these anatomic areas. The first provides a comprehensive review of MRI of ulnar-sided wrist pain, and the second deals with the imaging of the fingers and thumb. Several unique upper-extremity injuries are seen in the pediatric age group, and these are mostly related to the immature and developing skeleton. Special imaging considerations of pediatric sports-related injuries are discussed in a separate article. The next article reviews the utility of ultrasound in the evaluation of upper-extremity injuries and provides a comparison of the sensitivity and specificity of ultrasound as it compares to MRI. Finally, in response to the proliferation of low-field-strength magnets, particularly in the outpatient setting, a thorough literature review is provided comparing the use of low-field- and high-field-strength MRI. This article discusses the benefits and drawbacks of the use of low-field-strength magnets.

I would like to thank the many authors who have contributed their time and expertise to make this issue a reality, and I would also like to thank Deb Dellapena of Elsevier for her support in putting this issue together. Finally, I hope that the readers find this issue helpful in furthering their understanding of the role of imaging as it pertains to the evaluation of sports-related injuries of the upper extremities.

Timothy G. Sanders, MD
National Musculoskeletal Imaging
1930 N. Commerce Parkway
Suite #5
Weston, FL 33326, USA

E-mail address: RADMANTGS@cs.com

Clin Sports Med 25 (2006) 371–386
CLINICS IN SPORTS MEDICINE

ELSEVIER
SAUNDERS

Shoulder Magnetic Resonance Imaging

Lida Chaipat, MD, William E. Palmer, MD*

Musculoskeletal Imaging, Massachusetts General Hospital, 55 Fruit Street, YAW 6030, Boston, MA 02114, USA

MRI provides excellent soft tissue contrast and allows for multiplanar imaging in anatomic planes. Because of these advantages MRI has become the study of choice for imaging of shoulder pathology. Some structures, such as the rotator cuff, humeral head contour, and glenoid shape, are evaluated well with conventional MRI. When more sensitive evaluation of the labrum, capsule, articular cartilage, and glenohumeral ligaments is required or when a partial-thickness rotator cuff tear is suspected, magnetic resonance (MR) arthrography with intra-articular contrast can be performed. For MR arthrography contrast is injected directly into the glenohumeral joint. This article reviews the appearances of normal anatomic structures in MRI of the shoulder and disorders involving the rotator cuff and glenoid labrum.

TECHNIQUE

Imaging is performed with the patient in the supine position, arm at the side, and the shoulder slightly externally rotated [1]. A dedicated surface coil is placed close around the shoulder to optimize signal-to-noise ratio. Imaging time usually is 1 hour or less.

Specific imaging protocols vary by institution. At our hospital the standard shoulder MRI protocol includes triplanar imaging. The following sequences are obtained: coronal oblique proton density (PD), coronal oblique T2 with fat saturation, sagittal oblique T2, sagittal oblique T1, and axial gradient echo.

Axial (transverse) images are obtained perpendicular to the long axis of the body. From an axial image through the supraspinatus muscle, the coronal oblique sequences are prescribed parallel to the supraspinatus tendon. Sagittal oblique sequences then are oriented perpendicular to the coronal images.

For MR arthrography gadolinium contrast is injected directly into the glenohumeral joint under fluoroscopic guidance. The injected solution distends the capsule, separates the glenohumeral ligaments, and outlines intra-articular structures.

*Corresponding author. *E-mail address*: palmer.william@mgh.harvard.edu (W.E. Palmer).

0278-5919/06/$ – see front matter
doi:10.1016/j.csm.2006.03.002

sportsmed.theclinics.com

At the authors' hospital a 22- or 20-gauge 3.5 in spinal needle is inserted into the glenohumeral joint and approximately 12 mL of a solution containing gadolinium, normal saline solution, iodinated contrast, and lidocaine is injected. (Solution is made by mixing 0.4 mL of gadopentate dimeglumine with 50 mL of normal saline. Then 10 mL of this solution is mixed with 5 mL of iodinated contrast and 5 mL of preservative-free lidocaine 1%.) MRI is initiated within 30 min before fluid in the joint can be resorbed [1].

Triplanar T1 sequences with or without fat suppression are obtained to take advantage of the contrast provided by the injected solution. A T2-weighted sequence is performed to evaluate the extra-articular structures for pathology, such as bursal surface partial-thickness rotator cuff tear, soft tissue mass, and bone marrow abnormality.

NORMAL ANATOMY

The shoulder is composed of two articulations: the glenohumeral joint and the acromioclavicular (AC) joint [2]. Glenohumeral articulation is maintained by the joint capsule, glenohumeral ligaments, rotator cuff musculature, and labrum. The labrum is a ring of fibrocartilage that is adherent to the glenoid rim. The intact labrum increases the concavity of the bony glenoid and the superior labrum serves as the anchor for the long head of the biceps tendon. The joint capsule may insert variably on the periphery of the labrum or on the neck of the scapula [3]. Distally, the capsule inserts on the anatomic neck of the humerus.

The glenohumeral ligaments are cordlike thickenings in the anterior and inferior joint capsule. They include the superior, middle, and inferior glenohumeral ligaments. The superior and middle glenohumeral ligaments attach to the anterior labrum. The inferior glenohumeral ligament has anterior and posterior bands that attach to the anterior inferior and posterior inferior labrum, respectively. The size of glenohumeral ligaments varies from patient to patient.

The rotator cuff is comprised of tendons from the supraspinatus, infraspinatus, teres minor, and subscapularis muscles. The supraspinatus, infraspinatus, and teres minor muscles arise from the posterior surface of the scapula, cross posterior to the humeral head, and insert on the greater tuberosity. The supraspinatus insertion is most superior and the teres minor insertion most inferior on the tuberosity. The infraspinatus and teres minor tendons may appear fused, and a separate teres minor tendon may not be seen [4].

The subscapularis muscle arises from the anterior surface of the scapula, crosses anterior to the humeral head, and inserts on the lesser tuberosity. The deep fibers of the subscapularis tendon blend with the transverse humeral ligament across the bicipital groove and help maintain the normal position of the biceps tendon.

The supraspinatus and teres minor muscles have single muscle bellies and tendons. The subscapularis and infraspinatus are made up of multiple muscle bellies and small tendons that coalesce to form common tendon insertions.

The rotator cuff interval is the space between the supraspinatus and subscapularis tendons along the anterior superior humeral head. Through this space run the intracapsular portion of the biceps tendon, coracohumeral ligament, and the superior glenohumeral ligament.

On their course to their insertion sites on the humeral head the rotator cuff tendons pass under the coracoacromial arch and AC joint. The coracoacromial arch is made up of the coracoid process, coracoacromial ligament and the acromion. Hypertrophic abnormalities of the AC joint or arch structures may cause mechanical impingement on the underlying rotator cuff muscle or tendon, particularly the supraspinatus tendon.

Interposed between the coracoacromial arch and supraspinatus tendon lies the subacromial-subdeltoid bursa, which normally does not contain fluid. Fluid may be seen within the bursa when there is bursitis or when fluid leaks into it from the glenohumeral joint through a full-thickness cuff tear.

Because of normal openings in the joint capsule, the glenohumeral joint is in communication with the subscapular recess (beneath the subscapularis muscle) and the long head of the biceps tendon sheath. When a joint effusion is present fluid often is seen in the recess or tendon sheath and does not have pathologic significance.

The AC joint is a synovial joint surrounded by a fibrous capsule. This capsule is reinforced by fibers of the AC ligament. The coracoacromial and coracoclavicular ligaments also are important in maintaining normal position of the clavicle and acromial process. Tearing of these ligaments results in various degrees of AC joint separation.

NORMAL MRI APPEARANCE

The fibrous structures in the shoulder are highly organized tissues with normally low signal on all pulse sequences. These structures include the joint capsule, glenohumeral ligaments, rotator cuff tendons, and the labrum. When there is disruption of the organization structure because of tendinopathy or tear, the signal intensity increases. Unfortunately, there are confounding factors that may cause artifactually increased signal intensity in the absence of pathology. These are discussed in more depth elsewhere in this article.

Articular cartilage is intermediate in signal intensity on T2 and spin echo sequences. Fluid appears as high in signal intensity on T2-weighted and short tau inversion recovery imaging, which is a fluid-sensitive sequence. Normal musculature is intermediate in signal intensity on all pulse sequences. Increased T1 signal may be seen with fatty atrophy and increased T2 signal may be seen with edema.

Normal cortical bone is dark on all pulse sequences because of the lack of mobile protons, whereas the marrow space usually is T1 hyperintense because of fat content. Heterogenous areas of low T1 signal may be seen with red marrow conversion. This finding is common particularly in patients who have systemic disease and increased red blood cell turnover. Examples include smokers and patients who have chronic obstructive pulmonary disease or renal insufficiency. The marrow of patients who have hematologic disorders, such as multiple myeloma, may have an identical appearance.

APPROACH TO ROTATOR CUFF EVALUATION

One approach to evaluating the rotator cuff on MRI is to begin by reviewing the coronal oblique PD images to get an overview of the anatomy (Fig. 1). Proton density images are weighted intermediately between T1 and T2 signal. They provide superior signal-to-noise ratio and spatial resolution, albeit at the expense of soft tissue contrast. Large cuff tears and distortions of the anatomy may be identified. Shoulder alignment may be evaluated also.

Occasionally because of improper positioning or patient motion the shoulder is imaged in internal rotation. This imaging leads to overlap of the supraspinatus and infraspinatus tendons on coronal oblique images [5]. The coronal oblique plane usually is the most useful plane for cuff evaluation because it parallels the course of the most commonly torn cuff tendons, the supraspinatus and infraspinatus [6]. The subscapularis often is seen well in the coronal oblique plane but is evaluated best on axial images. The teres minor tendon is seen best in the sagittal oblique plane but rarely is torn.

After a general overview of anatomy is obtained by reviewing the coronal oblique PD images, the T2-weighted images with fat suppression may be evaluated for abnormally increased signal in the tendons or bones (Fig. 2). The coronal and sagittal oblique fast spin echo (FSE) T2 fat-suppressed images are highly sensitive for pathology; however, they are prone to artifactually increased signal and artifact unless the time to echo (TE) is greater than 30 msec. Once a potential abnormality is identified on one of the fat-suppressed sequences the finding should be confirmed on orthogonal images.

Next, the axial images should be reviewed with particular attention to the subscapularis muscle. Finally, review of the sagittal T1 sequence is useful to evaluate for muscle atrophy and mechanical impingement of the rotator cuff by hypertrophic degenerative changes in the coracoacromial arch structures.

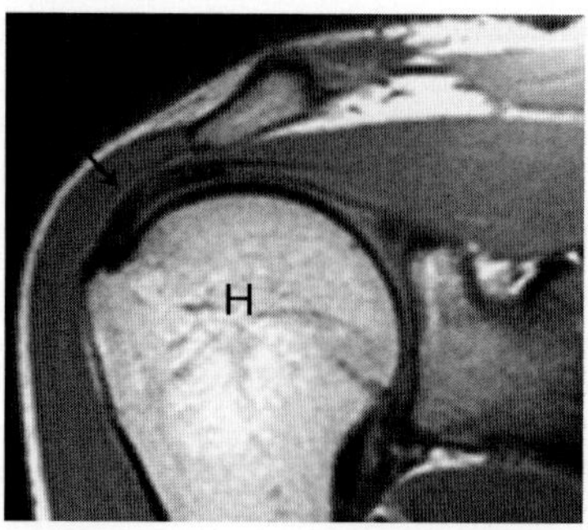

Fig. 1. Normal rotator cuff tendon. On PD oblique coronal image, the supraspinatus tendon (*arrow*) shows uniform thickness and signal intensity. The tendon is intact on the greater tuberosity without muscle atrophy or fatty change. H, humeral head.

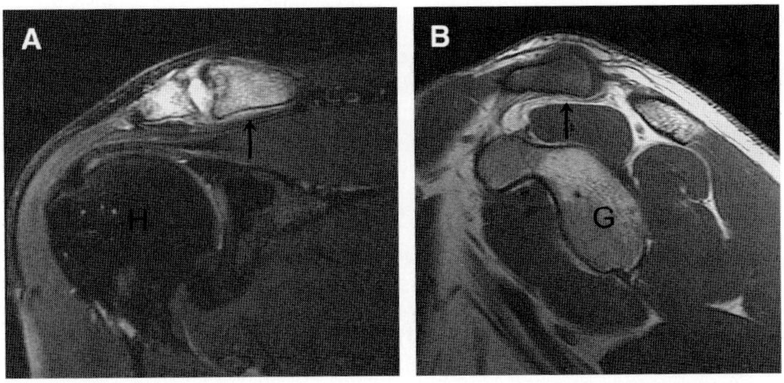

Fig. 2. Severe bone marrow edema in patient with suspected rotator cuff tear. Fat-suppressed T2-weighted oblique coronal image (*A*) shows high-signal bone marrow edema involving the distal clavicle (*arrow*) and adjacent acromion. On T1-weighted oblique sagittal image (*B*), the distal clavicular marrow edema (*arrow*) is low in signal intensity. The cuff tendon (*A*) and cuff muscles (*B*) are normal. G, glenoid; H, humeral head.

ROTATOR CUFF TEARS

The spectrum of rotator cuff pathology ranges from tendinopathy and fraying to partial- or full-thickness tearing. Partial-thickness tears may be classified further as occurring on the articular or bursal surface of the tendon. A third type of partial-thickness tear is the intrasubstance tear, which occurs within the substance of the tendon without extending to the tendon surface. This type of tear is uncommon but is important to identify on MRI because the tendon surface may appear normal at arthroscopy and the tear may be missed.

Tendinopathy is identified by increased signal within the tendon substance. The abnormally increased signal intensity remains below that of fluid on T2-weighted sequences [7]. Tendinopathy may be present with or without tendon thickening or thinning. [1]. Fraying is described when the normal linear dark signal at the margin of a tendon becomes indistinct, but no gap in the tendon fibers is identified.

The most specific sign of a cuff tear is discontinuity of the cuff fibers with fluid signal in the intervening gap (Figs. 3 and 4). Unfortunately, this gap may only be seen in fairly large tears that measure more than several millimeters. For smaller tears the signal on T2-weighted imaging and secondary signs of cuff tearing should be considered carefully. Secondary signs include fluid in the subacromial or subdeltoid bursa, tendon retraction, and muscular atrophy. The latter two signs may have implications for the type of surgical repair that is required and so should be evaluated routinely on every MRI obtained for rotator cuff evaluation. The appearance of the torn fibers also should be noted, because poor quality, diffusely torn tendon may not be suitable for repair (Fig. 5).

The myotendinous junction normally is located beneath the AC joint. When it is more proximal a full-thickness tear should be suspected. In cases of partial-thickness tearing only the torn fibers retract. Some partial- and full-thickness

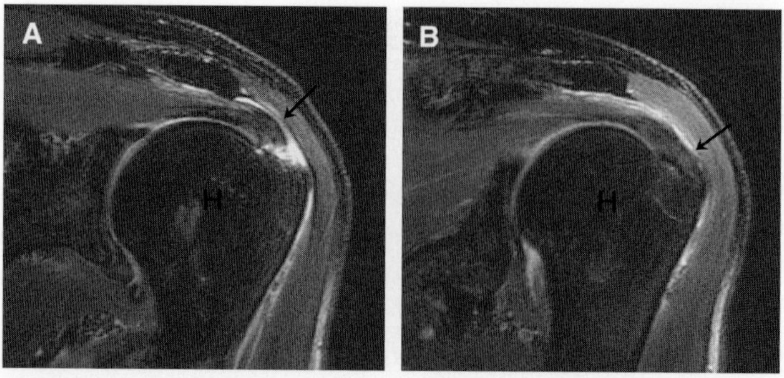

Fig. 3. Full-thickness rotator cuff tear in 54-year-old patient. On fat-suppressed T2-weighted oblique coronal image (*A*), distal supraspinatus tendon (*arrow*) is disrupted by focal high-signal fluid and is mildly retracted from the greater tuberosity. More posterior slice (*B*) shows intact infraspinatus tendon (*arrow*) and normal attachment to the greater tuberosity. H, humeral head.

cuff tears may have a delaminating component with the tear dissecting proximally between the deep and superficial tendon fibers. The torn fibers may demonstrate different degrees of retraction (Fig. 6). The degree of retraction of the cuff fibers should be measured because this has a direct relationship to prognosis. The anterior–posterior dimension of the tear also is important and is measured best on the sagittal sequences.

An intrasubstance tear is described when there is fluid intensity signal within the substance of the tendon that does not extend to either the articular or bursal surface.

In some chronic cuff tears and following rotator cuff repair, granulation tissue and fibrosis may fill the gap, resulting in isointense or dark signal. In these

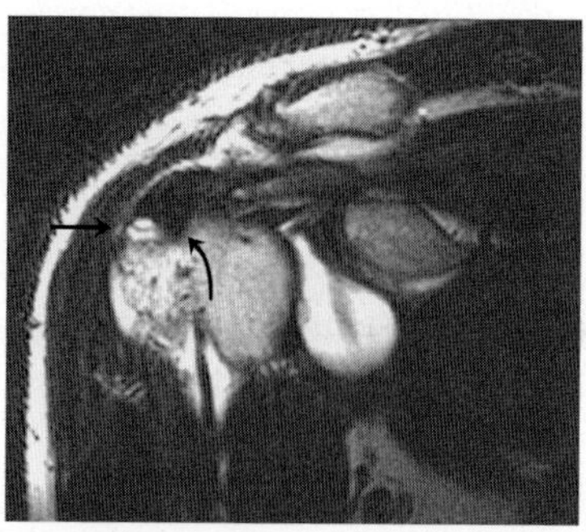

Fig. 4. Large partial-thickness bursal surface rotator cuff tear in 56-year-old patient. On T2-weighted oblique coronal image, distal supraspinatus tendon shows focal fluid (*straight arrow*) disrupting bursal fibers from greater tuberosity. Articular surface fibers (*curved arrow*) remain intact on greater tuberosity. H, humeral head.

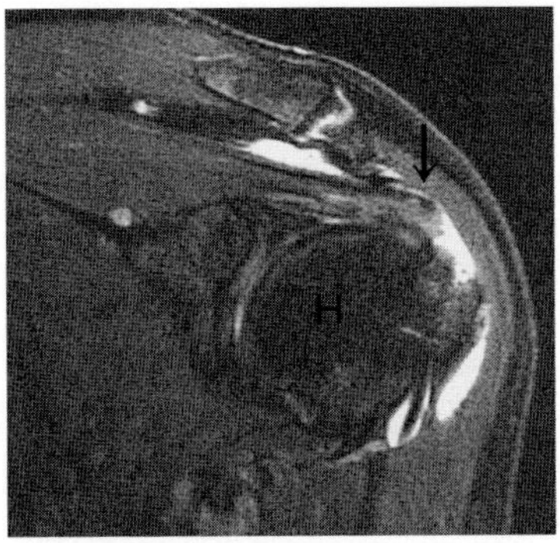

Fig. 5. Full-thickness rotator cuff tear and poor tendon quality in a 62-year-old patient. On fat-suppressed T2-weighted oblique coronal image, distal supraspinatus tendon (*arrow*) is moderately retracted from the greater tuberosity and shows increased signal intensity indicating severe degeneration. This tendon required extensive débridement at surgery. H, humeral head.

cases secondary signs of cuff tears again may be helpful. Occasionally MR arthrogram is necessary to diagnose these chronic tears.

Although some small partial- and full-thickness tears also are not visible on conventional MRI, overall diagnostic accuracy is good with sensitivity and specificity of approximately 90% for full-thickness tears in high-field MRI systems. In cases in which there is a high suspicion for an occult small full-thickness or partial-thickness articular surface tear, MR arthrogram may aid in the diagnosis because it has higher reported sensitivity and specificity. In one recent study of 76 patients, MR arthrography was compared with results at arthroscopy [8]. The study found the sensitivity of MR arthrogram to be 84% and the specificity to be 96%. This minimally invasive procedure may

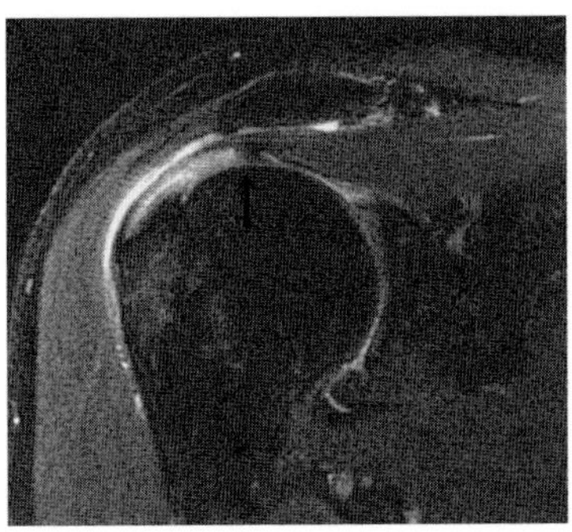

Fig. 6. Large partial-thickness undersurface rotator cuff tear in 45-year-old patient Fat-suppressed T2-weighted oblique coronal image shows broad-based partial-thickness tear with prominent retraction of undersurface fibers (*arrow*) indicating tendon delamination and poor tendon quality. This large tear involved supraspinatus and infraspinatus tendons.

be worthwhile in younger patients who have refractory shoulder pain, because studies have demonstrated that arthroscopic débridement of even shallow (25% thickness) articular surface tears can result in a significant decrease in pain [9]. In certain athletic populations with a high prevalence of cuff and labral tears it may be reasonable to proceed directly to MR arthrography without first obtaining a conventional MRI.

The main drawback of MR arthrography is patient discomfort following contrast injection. In the previously mentioned study [8] all 76 patients reported soreness above baseline symptoms for 24 to 48 hours after injection, although no serious complications, such as infection or nerve injury, occurred.

On MR arthrography a cuff tear is diagnosed when contrast leaks into the substance of the tendon (Figs. 7 and 8). A full-thickness tear is described when contrast from the glenohumeral joint leaks though the tendon into the subacromial or subdeltoid bursa. When contrast is seen in the subscapularis muscle some caution must be taken before diagnosis of a tear, because extra-articular injection of contrast during the fluoroscopic portion of the examination may occur. Bursal surface partial tears do not communicate with the joint space and thus are not seen better with arthrography compared with conventional MRI.

The supraspinatus is the most commonly torn tendon, often because of impingement by subacromial spurs or hypertrophic degenerative changes at the AC joint. The supraspinatus also may be torn in cases of internal impingement syndrome in which the posterior superior humeral head contacts the posterior glenoid during abduction with external rotation (Fig. 9).

The infraspinatus is the next most commonly torn tendon, often because of extension of tears from the supraspinatus. The subscapularis may become torn after massive rotator cuff tears of the supraspinatus and infraspinatus. It also may be torn in isolation after acute traumatic anterior shoulder dislocation

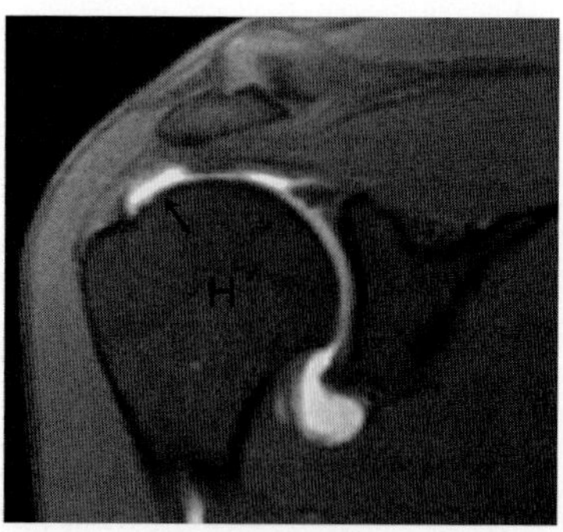

Fig. 7. Partial-thickness undersurface rotator cuff tear in 42-year-old patient. Following intra-articular injection of contrast material, fat-suppressed T1-weighted oblique coronal image demonstrates focal high-signal contrast collection (*arrow*) at articular surface of supraspinatus. There is no contrast in the subacromial-subdeltoid space. H, humeral head.

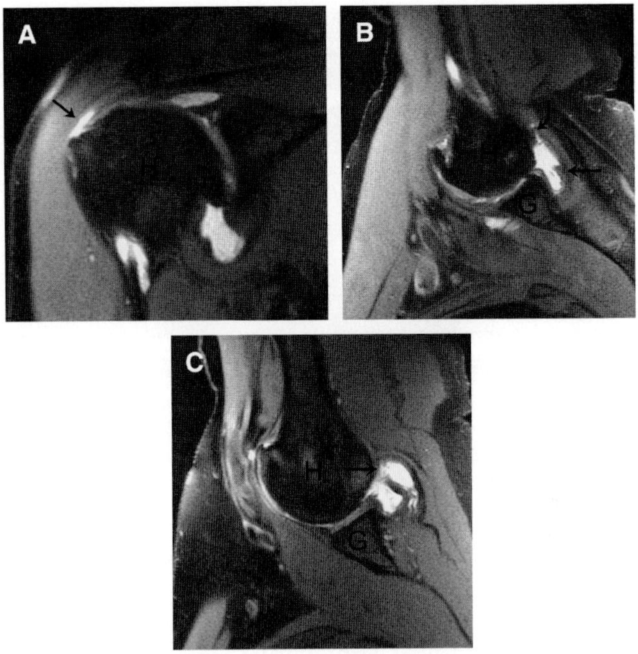

Fig. 8. Subtotal rotator cuff tear with severe tendon delamination in 49-year-old patient. On fat-suppressed T1-weighted oblique coronal MR arthrographic image (*A*) contrast extends to the bursal surface fibers of supraspinatus tendon (*arrow*) without leak into the subacromial-subdeltoid space. H, humeral head. Fat-suppressed T1-weighted abducted externally rotated (ABER) image (*B*) shows intact bursal surface fibers on the greater tuberosity (*curved arrow*) and retracted articular surface fibers (*straight arrow*). G, glenoid; H, humeral head. More posteriorly, ABER image (*C*) demonstrates contrast solution (*arrow*) within the infraspinatus tendon because of intrasubstance fiber delamination. G, glenoid; H, humerus.

or less commonly because of subcoracoid impingement. Subcoracoid impingement in turn occurs in patients who have congenitally narrow coracohumeral intervals because of unusually long coracoid processes.

PITFALLS IN ROTATOR CUFF IMAGING

Intermediate or inhomogeneous signal in the cuff tendons are causes of diagnostic difficulty. Although the signal may be because of tendinopathy or partial tearing, artifacts such as magic angle phenomenon, inhomogeneous fat suppression, and partial volume averaging also may cause an increase in signal.

Magic angle phenomenon occurs on short TE sequences, such as PD sequences. Artifactually increased signal may be seen where the fibers of the cuff tendons are aligned at a 55-degree angle to the main magnetic field. At that angle there is T2 lengthening that results in focally increased signal. This artifact is recognized by its characteristic location where the tendon begins to slope downwards. The artifact is confirmed by comparison to T2 images that have a long TE and so do not show the artifact [1].

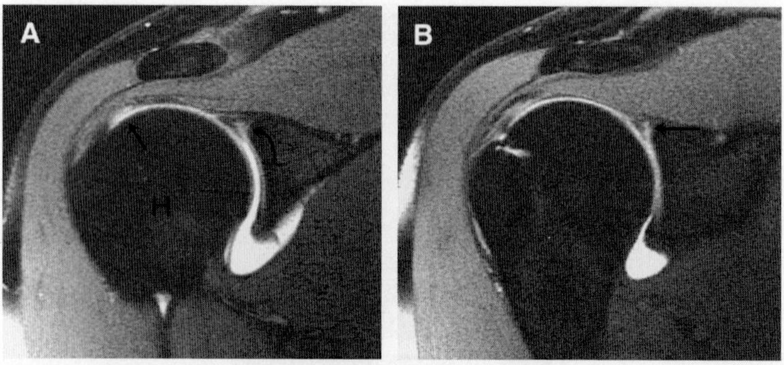

Fig. 9. Internal impingement in 28-year-old patient. Following intra-articular injection of contrast material, fat-suppressed T1-weighted oblique coronal image (*A*) demonstrates small partial-thickness articular surface tear (*straight arrow*) of supraspinatus tendon and tear of superior labrum (*curved arrow*). More posteriorly (*B*), high-signal contrast material leaks under the superior glenoid labrum, indicating type 2 superior labrum, anterior-to-posterior (SLAP) lesion (*arrow*). At arthroscopy, internal impingement was confirmed, and the tendon and labral lesions were débrided. H, humeral head.

The appearance of calcium on MRI can be deceptive. Calcifications in the cuff may appear dark or bright and may be misinterpreted as subacromial spurs or as tears. The presence of calcific tendinopathy is excluded easily by obtaining radiographs. In addition, bony changes associated with impingement, such as subacromial enthesophytes and sclerosis, and remodeling of the greater tuberosity, are appreciated more easily on radiographs than on MRI [10]. Whenever possible MRI studies should be read in conjunction with comparison radiographs.

INSTABILITY

Two main categories of instability include multidirectional atraumatic instability and traumatic instability [11]. Multidirectional instability usually is seen in young patients, is often bilateral, and is believed to be because of capsular laxity, which is not evaluated well with MRI. These patients typically are not sent for imaging [12].

Traumatic instability most commonly occurs after a shoulder dislocation and is usually unidirectional. Because anterior shoulder dislocation is much more common than posterior dislocation, recurrent anterior instability is more common than posterior instability. Traumatic anterior dislocation often results in tearing of the anterior inferior labrum (Bankart lesion) and in other cases there may be fracture of the anterior inferior glenoid rim (Bankart fracture) (Fig. 10). The inferior glenohumeral ligament is the main passive stabilizer of the glenohumeral joint and its anterior band attaches to the anterior inferior labrum (Fig. 11). Tears of the anterior inferior labrum or fracture of the glenoid rim at this site destabilizes the glenohumeral ligament anchor. The inferior glenohumeral ligament becomes incompetent and the shoulder becomes unstable

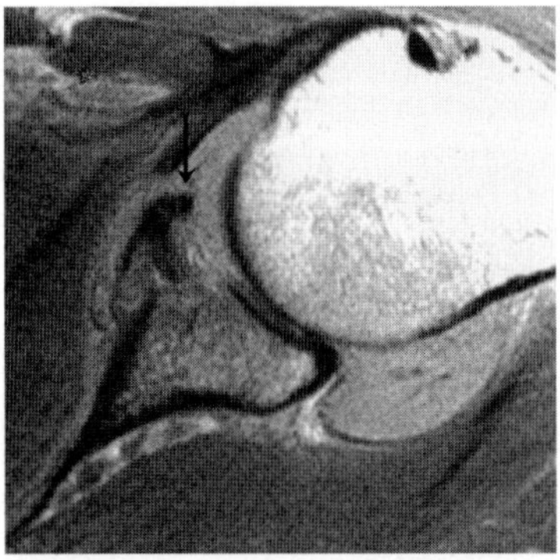

Fig. 10. Glenoid rim fracture following dislocation in 46-year-old patient. On PD axial image, the anteroinferior glenoid shows cortical discontinuity and medial displacement indicating fracture. The labrum (*arrow*) remains attached to the glenoid rim.

(Fig. 12). A similar situation may occur after posterior dislocation with rupture of the posterior band of the inferior glenohumeral ligament, posterior labral tear, and recurrent posterior instability.

Rarely, the inferior glenohumeral labral-ligamentous complex may rupture at a site other than the labrum or glenoid. One example of this situation is humeral avulsion of the inferior glenohumeral ligament (HAGL lesion) (Fig. 13). Although uncommon, a HAGL lesion is identified best in the acute setting before resolution of edema and hemorrhage. It may be important to identify on MRI because it may be difficult to see during arthroscopy and can cause significant shoulder instability.

Tears also may occur in the superior labrum. Typically these superior labral tears do not cause physical signs of instability; however, patients may have pain

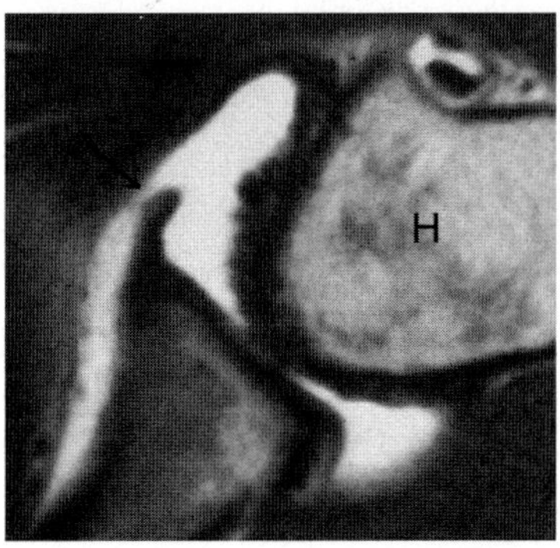

Fig. 11. Normal inferior labral-ligamentous complex. T1-weighted arthrographic MR axial image shows the inferior glenohumeral ligament (*arrow*) at its attachment site to the anteroinferior glenoid labrum. Labral tear in this location is closely associated with anterior instability because of incompetence of the inferior glenohumeral ligament. H, humerus.

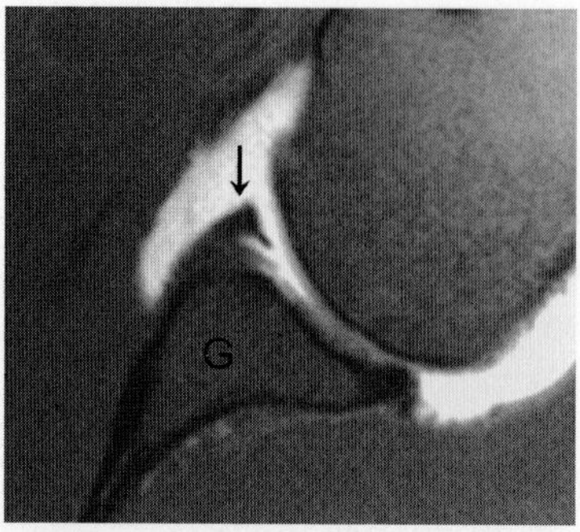

Fig. 12. Anteroinferior glenoid labral tear in 20-year-old patient with anterior instability. Following intra-articular injection of contrast material, fat-suppressed T1-weighted axial image shows contrast material partially undercutting the anteroinferior glenoid labrum (*arrow*), which is mildly displaced from the glenoid rim. Contrast also undercuts adjacent articular cartilage indicating delamination and flap formation. G, glenoid.

and a subjective feeling of instability. Superior labral tears may extend into the biceps anchor or may be caused by avulsion because of stress on the biceps tendon. This latter scenario often is seen in overhead-throwing athletes, swimmers, and tennis players. Repetitive overhead motions in these athletes causes traction on the biceps tendon, which is anchored on the superior labrum. The chronic stress on this bicipital-labral complex ultimately leads to tearing of the biceps anchor. A superior labral tear that involves the biceps anchor is more likely to be considered for surgical repair [13].

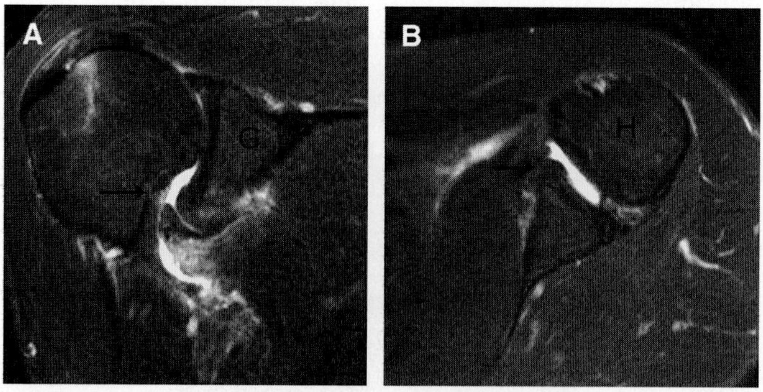

Fig. 13. Humeral avulsion of the inferior glenohumeral ligament following anterior dislocation in a 38-year-old patient. Fat-suppressed T2-weighted oblique coronal image (*A*) shows edema or hemorrhage distal to the axillary pouch and inferior glenohumeral ligament, which is discontinuous at its expected attachment site to the humerus (*arrow*). On fat-suppressed T2-weighted axial image (*B*), the anteroinferior labral-ligamentous complex remains attached normally to glenoid rim (*arrow*). G, glenoid; H, humerus.

LABRUM ON MRI

The superior and inferior labra are visualized best on coronal oblique images, whereas the anterior and posterior labra are seen best on axial images (Figs. 14 and 15). A labral tear is diagnosed when an irregular line of fluid or intra-articular contrast tracks into the labral substance or between the labrum and the glenoid articular cartilage (Fig. 16). When a labral tear extends through the joint capsule, a paralabral cyst may develop in an extra-articular location. The cyst may be the most apparent sign of a labral tear, and is a highly specific finding. Most often these cysts develop along the posterosuperior glenoid rim [14]. Displacement of the labrum away from the glenoid is another sign of a tear. When the labrum is displaced there may be stripping of the attached periosteum along the medial glenoid neck resulting in an anterior labral-ligamentous periosteal sleeve avulsion lesion (Fig. 16B).

Unfortunately, the size, shape, and signal intensity of the normal labrum show variations that decrease accuracy in the diagnostic evaluation of labral injury on conventional MRI [15,16]. Most commonly the superior and anterior labra are triangular in shape whereas the posterior and inferior portions are rounded [13]. The superior labrum usually is larger than the inferior labrum and the posterior labrum usually is larger than the anterior labrum [4]. In the study by Zanetti and colleagues [16], arthroscopic findings were compared with findings on MR arthrograms in 55 patients. Only 50% of the arthroscopically proven normal labral parts had the expected low signal intensity and triangular contour on MR images. In the same study, 31% of the arthroscopically normal labral parts had linear or globular high signal on MR arthrographic images, possibly because of myxoid changes of the labral substance [17]. Normal variants, such as attenuation, complete separation, and complete absence of the labrum, also contributed to diagnostic difficulty.

Because of the wide variation in labral appearance, caution must be used when diagnosing a labral tear on conventional MRI. This is true especially

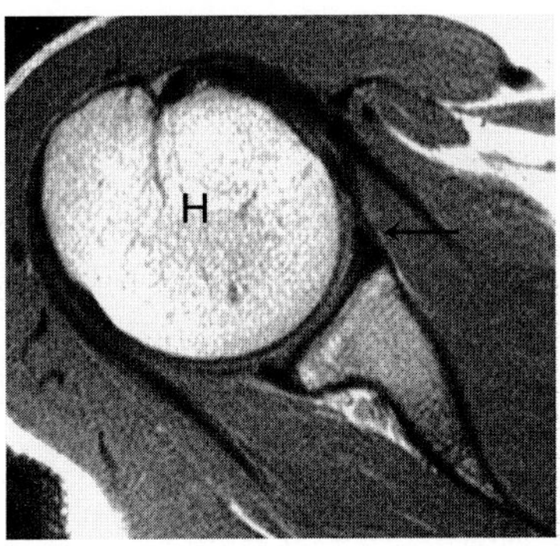

Fig. 14. Normal anterior, posterior glenoid labrum. On PD axial image, both anterior (*arrow*) and posterior labra show normal contours and locations overlying the glenoid rim. The labrum is partially undercut by articular cartilage. H, humeral head.

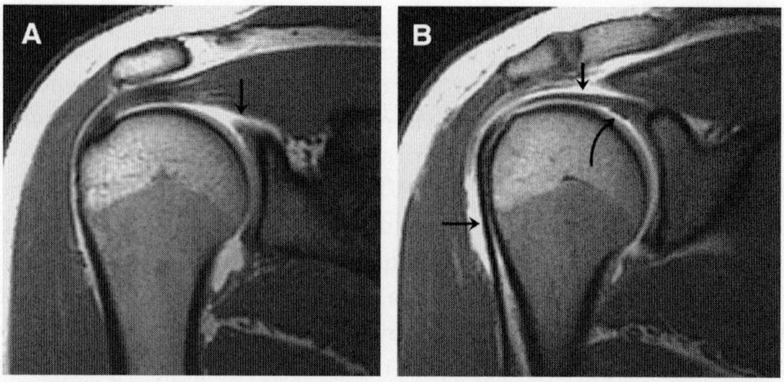

Fig. 15. Normal superior labrum, labral-bicipital complex. Following intra-articular injection of contrast material, T1-weighted oblique coronal image (*A*) shows normal contour of superior (*arrow*) and inferior glenoid labra without sublabral leak of contrast material. More anteriorly (*B*), the superior labrum (*curved arrow*) shows normal relationship to biceps tendon (*straight arrows*).

of the anterior and anterior superior portions of the labrum where the most common normal variants occur. These variants include sublabral recess, sublabral foramen, and congenital absence of the superior labrum.

A sublabral recess is diagnosed when a thin, smooth line of high signal is present between the articular cartilage and the superior labrum. The line of high signal should follow the contour of the glenoid and it should not extend posterior to the biceps anchor. If it is seen posterior to the biceps anchor a superior labral tear should be suspected [18].

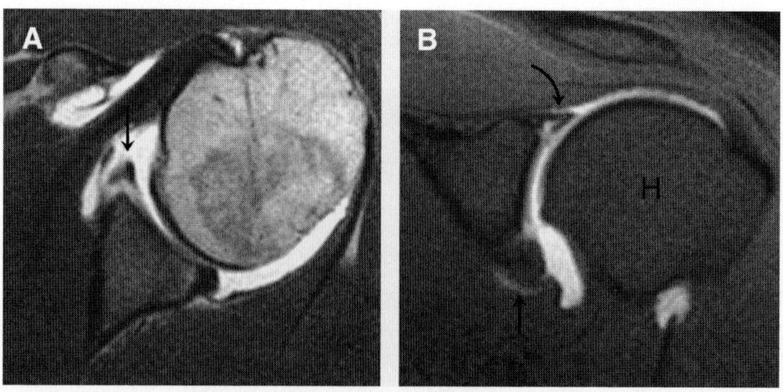

Fig. 16. Bankart lesion and superior tear extension in 34-year-old patient with anterior instability. Following intra-articular injection of contrast material, T1-weighted axial image (*A*) shows contrast material completely undercutting the anterior glenoid labrum (*arrow*). On fat-suppressed T1-weighted oblique coronal image (*B*), the inferior labral-ligamentous complex (*straight arrow*) is thickened with mild medial displacement suggesting periosteal sleeve avulsion. The tear extends into the superior labrum (*curved arrow*). H, humeral head.

Absence of the anterior superior labrum occurs in 2% of patients. When it is associated with a thickened middle glenohumeral ligament (MGHL) it is called a Buford complex [16]. Another variant that occurs in the anterior superior labrum is a sublabral foramen, a normal detachment of the labrum from the anterior superior glenoid. It is found in approximately 11% of patients and mimics a labral tear on MR images [4].

MR arthrography can overcome some of these diagnostic problems because it provides distention and separation of intra-articular structures and fills labral tears. The diagnostic accuracy of MR arthrography in diagnosing anterior inferior labral tears is greater than 90%. Additional imaging with the shoulder in abduction and external rotation (ABER position) can further improve anterior inferior labral evaluation [19–21]. In this position the anterior band of the inferior glenohumeral ligament is pulled taut and creates traction on the anterior inferior labrum [19]. If an anterior labral tear is present, the partially detached labrum is pulled away from the glenoid and contrast material fills the defect. The ABER position is achieved by flexing the elbow and placing the patient's hand behind the head [19]. Axial oblique imaging then is performed parallel to the long axis of the humerus.

OSSEOUS INJURIES

When there is a clinical suspicion for osseous injury some surgeons prefer CT arthrography for evaluation because fractures of the glenoid are depicted better on CT compared with MRI [16,22]. These inferior glenoid fractures can contribute to recurrent instability and glenoid reconstruction may be necessary.

When the posterior lateral humeral head impacts on the inferior glenoid during an anterior dislocation a fracture of the superior humeral head may occur, called a Hill-Sachs fracture. The presence of a Hill-Sachs fracture is appreciated best on the most superior axial images through the humeral head. Below that level there is a normal flattening of the posterior inferior humeral head contour. Because of that normal flattening a Hill-Sachs lesion should not be diagnosed if it is seen below the level of the coracoid process.

SUMMARY

MRI has become the preferred imaging modality for evaluating internal shoulder derangement. Injuries to the rotator cuff, labrum, glenohumeral ligaments, or osseous structures all may lead to symptoms of pain, weakness, and instability. These injuries are well depicted by MRI. Care must be taken, however, to recognize normal anatomic variations and MRI artifacts.

References

[1] Kassarjian A, Bencardino JT, Palmer WE. MR imaging of the rotator cuff. Magn Reson Imaging Clin N Am 2004;12(1):39–60.

[2] Greenway GD, Danzig LA, Resnick D, et al. The painful shoulder. Med Radiogr Photogr 1982;58(2):21–67.

[3] Resnick D. Arthrography, tenography, and bursography. In: Resnick D, editor. Diagnosis in bone and joint disorders, vol . 1. Philadelphia: Saunders; 1995. p. 277–409.
[4] De Maeseneer M, Van Roy P, Shahabpour M. Normal MR imaging anatomy of the rotator cuff tendons, glenoid fossa, labrum and ligaments of the shoulder. Magn Reson Imaging Clin N Am 2004;12(1):1–10.
[5] Davis SJ, Teresi LM, Bradley WG, et al. Effects of arm rotation on MR imaging of the rotator cuff. Radiology 1991;181:265–8.
[6] Tsai JC, Zlatkin MB. Magnetic resonance imaging of the shoulder. Radiol Clin North Am 1990;28(2):279–91.
[7] Kjellin I, Ho CP, Cervilla V, et al. Alterations in the supraspinatus tendon at MR imaging: correlation with histopathological findings in cadavers. Radiology 1991;181(3):837–41.
[8] Meister K, Thesing J, Montgomery WJ, et al. MR arthrography of partial thickness tears of the undersurface of the rotator cuff: an arthroscopic correlation. Skeletal Radiol 2004;33(3):136–41.
[9] Payne LZ, Altchek DW, Craig EV, et al. Arthroscopic treatment of partial rotator cuff tears in young athletes: a preliminary report. Am J Sports Med 1997;25:299–305.
[10] Recht MP, Resnick D. Magnetic resonance-imaging studies of the shoulder: diagnosis of lesions of the rotator cuff. J Bone Joint Surg Am 1993;75(8):1244–53.
[11] Cleeman E, Flatlow EL. Shoulder dislocations in the young patient. Orthop Clin North Am 2000;31(2):217–29.
[12] McCauley TR, Pope CF, Jokl P. Normal and abnormal glenoid labrum: assessment with multiplanar gradient echo MRI imaging. Radiology 1992;183(1):35–7.
[13] Resnick D, Kransdorf MJ. Internal joint derangements. In: Resnick D, Kransdorf MJ, editors. Bone and joint imaging. 3rd edition. Philadelphia: Elsevier Saunders; 2005. p 352.
[14] Tirman PFJ, Feller JF, Janzen DL, et al. Association of glenoid labral cysts with labral tears and glenohumeral instability: radiologic findings and clinical significance. Radiology 1994;190:653–8.
[15] Kaplan PA, Bryans KC, Davick JP, et al. MR imaging of the normal shoulder: variants and pitfalls. Radiology 1992;184(2):519–24.
[16] Zanetti M, Thorsten C, Dominik W, et al. MR arthrographic variability of the arthroscopically normal glenoid labrum: qualitative and quantitative assessment. Eur J Radiol 2001;11(4): 559–66.
[17] Loredo R, Longo C, Salonen D, et al. Glenoid labrum: MR imaging with histologic correlation. Radiology 1995;196(1):33–41.
[18] Smith DK, Chopp TM, Aufdemorte TB, et al. Sublabral recess of the superior glenoid labrum: study of cadavers with conventional nonenhanced MRI imaging, MR arthrography, anatomic dissection, and limited histological examination. Radiology 1996;201:251–6.
[19] Cvitanic O, Tirman PF, Feller JF, et al. Using abduction and external rotation of the shoulder to increase the sensitivity of MR arthrography in revealing tears of the anterior glenoid labrum. AJR Am J Roentgenol 1997;169(3):837–44.
[20] Kwak SM, Brown RR, Trudell D, et al. Glenohumeral joint: comparison of shoulder positions at MR arthrography. Radiology 1998;208:375–80.
[21] Tirman PF, Bost FW, Steinbach LS, et al. MR arthrographic depiction of tears of the rotator cuff: benefit of abduction and external rotation of the arm. Radiology 1994;192:851–6.
[22] Kreitner KF, Runkel M, Grebe P, et al. MR tomography versus CT arthrography in glenohumeral instabilities. Fortschr Geb Rontgenstr Nuklearmed 1992;157(1):37–42.

Clin Sports Med 25 (2006) 387–408

CLINICS IN SPORTS MEDICINE

ELSEVIER SAUNDERS

Sports-Related Injuries of the Elbow: An Approach to MRI Interpretation

Michael J. Tuite, MD[a,b,*], Richard Kijowski, MD[a,b]

[a]University of Wisconsin Medical School, 750 Highland Avenue, Madison, WI, 53705 USA
[b]Department of Radiology, University of Wisconsin Hospital and Clinics, E3/311, 600 Highland Avenue, Madison, WI 53792, USA

MRI is a valuable tool for evaluating the athlete with elbow pain, particularly in those with nonlocalizable pain. MRI also is helpful in sorting out the cause of pain in athletes who may have acute trauma superimposed on tendinopathy or other chronic injuries from repetitive microtrauma. Even in athletes in whom the cause of pain confidently can be diagnosed clinically, MRI can document the injury severity, which can be helpful for estimating recovery time or in preoperative planning. By contributing to an accurate early diagnosis, MRI also can help minimize the time that athletes are away from their sports.

There are some sports injuries in which the only imaging of the elbow that is necessary is a radiograph or CT. For many elbow injuries, however, MRI is preferred because of the superior soft tissue detail. Adding intra-articular contrast provides even better detail of the hyaline cartilage and of the undersurface partial tears of the medial collateral ligament (MCL). In this article the authors describe their approach to MRI interxpretation of elbow injuries in athletes, including osteochondral lesions, ligament and tendon tears, and nerve entrapment.

TECHNIQUE

There are multiple imaging planes and pulse sequences that have been recommended for imaging the elbow. Because the authors prefer to use thin sections yet keep overall scan times short enough so that the patient does not become too uncomfortable, we use slightly different protocols depending on the orthopedist's clinical

*Corresponding author. Department of Radiology, University of Wisconsin Hospital and Clinics, E3/311, 600 Highland Avenue, Madison, WI 53792. *E-mail address:* mjtuite@wisc.edu (M.J. Tuite).

0278-5919/06/$ – see front matter
doi:10.1016/j.csm.2006.02.002

sportsmed.theclinics.com

concern [1]. Most sports-related elbow injuries are imaged well with noncontrasted MRI images. The MRI sequences that the authors use are:

MRI protocol for elbow sports injuries

- Localizer
- Axial fat-suppressed T2-weighted images
- Sagittal fat-suppressed T2-weighted images
- Coronal fat-suppressed proton density weighted images

In addition, for loose body, capitellum osteochondritis dissecans (OCD), nerve impingement, biceps and triceps tear:

- Axial T1-weighted images
- Sagittal T1-weighted images

For MCL tear or epicondylitis:

- Axial fat-suppressed proton density weighted images
- Coronal T1-weighted images
- Coronal inversion recovery (STIR) images

MRI arthrography can be helpful in the athlete with a suspected partial tear of the MCL or a loose body [2]. Our standard elbow MRI arthrography protocol is:

MRI arthrography protocol for elbow sports injuries

Localizer
Axial T1-weighted images
Sagittal fat-suppressed T1-weighted images
Coronal fat-suppressed T1-weighted images
Sagittal fat-suppressed T2-weighted images
Coronal fat-suppressed T2-weighted images

OSSEOUS AND CHONDRAL LESIONS

Normal Variants

There are several normal osseous features of the elbow that are important to recognize because they may be more striking on MRI images than at arthroscopy. One of the most common is the pseudodefect of the capitellum, a normal anatomic feature that mimics an osteochondral lesion on MRI images [3]. The pseudodefect of the capitellum occurs posterolaterally where the normal articular surface of the capitellum ends abruptly giving a stepoff at the interface with the nonarticular portion of the distal humerus (Fig. 1). On MRI images with the elbow in full extension, the radial head is located at the posterior edge of the capitellar articular surface, just anterior to this nonarticular portion of the lateral condyle. Fortunately, pathologic osteochondral lesions of the capitellum typically occur in the anterior capitellum.

Two other normal anatomic variants occur in the trochlear groove at the junction of the olecranon and coronoid processes. In this location some

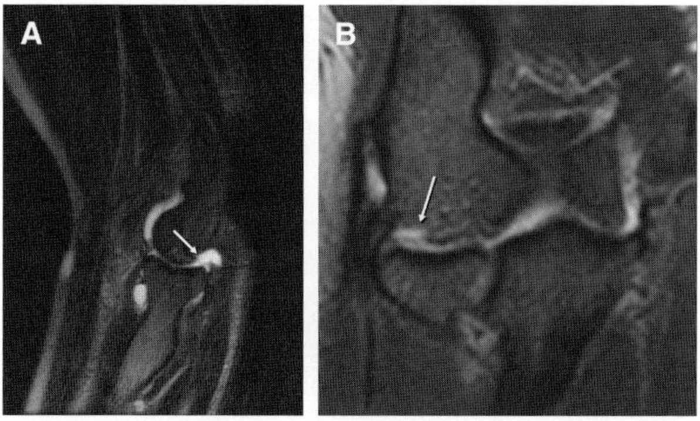

Fig. 1. Pseudodefect of the capitellum. (*A*) Sagittal T2-weighted image with the elbow in extension shows the normal nonarticular flat posterior aspect of the lateral condyle (*arrow*). (*B*) On a coronal T2-weighted image through the dorsal part of the radial head, the nonarticular portion of the lateral condyle (*arrow*) is adjacent to the articular surface of the radius simulating an osteochondral lesion.

individuals have either a small focal absence of the articular cartilage, called a mid-trochlear notch, or a thin transverse line of ossification of the hyaline cartilage called a mid-trochlear ridge [4]. The mid-trochlear notch appears as a focal defect in the hyaline cartilage seen best on sagittal images, and is often filled with fluid mimicking a focal chondral defect (Fig. 2). It is most prominent at the medial and lateral margins of the trochlear groove. The transverse mid-trochlear ridge occurs more centrally in the trochlear groove at the junction of the olecranon and coronoid processes. This ridge is usually only 2 to 3 mm high and does not extend above the thickness of the adjacent hyaline cartilage (Fig. 3).

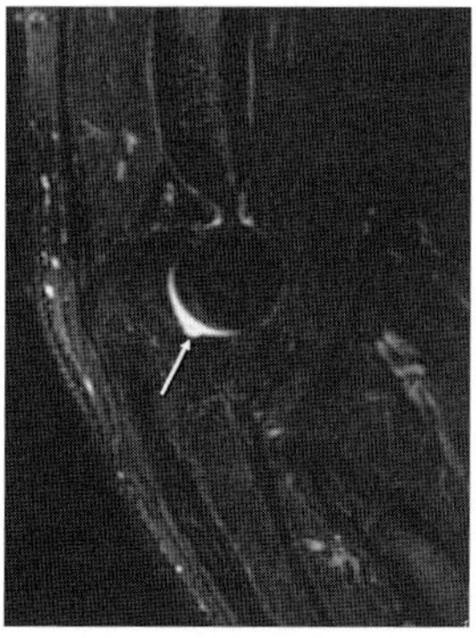

Fig. 2. Mid-trochlear notch. Sagittal T2-weighted image shows a small focal absence of cartilage (*arrow*) in the midportion of the trochlear groove consistent with the normal variant notch.

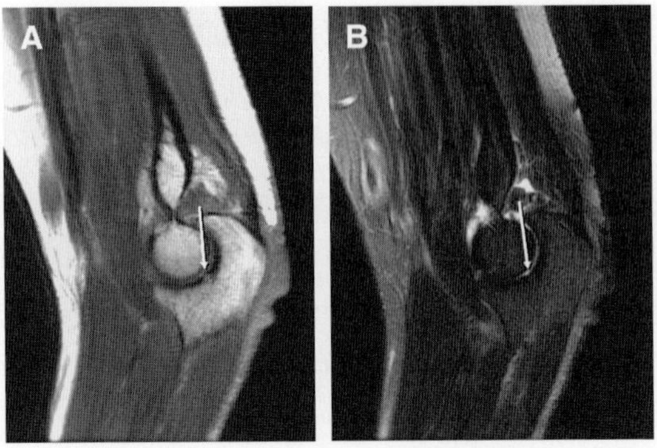

Fig. 3. Mid-trochlear ridge. (*A*) Sagittal T1-weighted image shows a small bump in the subchondral bone (*arrow*). (*B*) Sagittal T2-weighted image shows that the contour of the articular cartilage remains smooth over the ridge (*arrow*).

Osteochondral Lesions of the Capitellum

Osteochondral lesions of the capitellum usually are seen in young baseball pitchers, racket sports athletes, and gymnasts [5]. The same valgus stress that in the adult throwing athlete produces MCL tears can give an impaction osteochondral lesion in the child or adolescent. When the lesion is seen in children less than 12 years old with open physes, it is called Panner osteochondrosis. When it occurs in adolescents, it is called OCD. Although there is some controversy, many authors believe that the two conditions share the same cause [1]. Typical Panner osteochondrosis lesions in which there is only minimal flattening of the capitellar subchondral bone plate typically resolve without sequelae [6]. Older adolescents with an OCD lesion, especially if the physes are fusing and there is a discrete osteochondral fragment, may develop chronic sequelae, such as long-term pain, premature osteoarthritis, loss of terminal extension, and chronic instability of the radial head [7,8].

Osteochondral lesions of the capitellum can have several appearances on MRI images. Early or small lesions appear as a crescentic subchondral area of signal abnormality in the anterolateral capitellum [9]. They are usually low to intermediate signal on T1-weighted images and high signal on T2-weighted images and may have some flattening of the subchondral bone plate (Fig. 4). The adjacent articular cartilage may be irregular. More severe or advanced lesions have a bone fragment with a linear area of high or low signal at its interface with the adjacent bone marrow.

MRI is helpful for several reasons in the patient with suspected osteochondritis dissecans. First, lesions can be diagnosed on MRI before they are seen radiographically [9]. In small osteochondral lesions early treatment may prevent chronic symptoms [7]. Second, MRI can help with preoperative planning by showing accurately the size of the lesion, the integrity of the cartilage, and if there are associated loose bodies, particularly chondral bodies. Third, MRI can show accurately the size and viability of an osteochondral fragment and

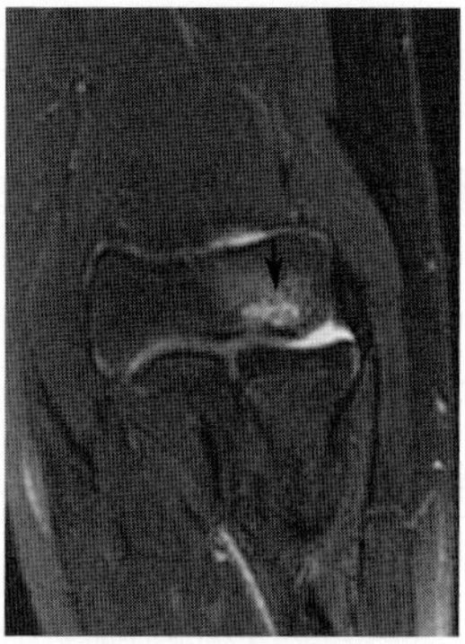

Fig. 4. OCD lesion in a 16-year-old male. Coronal T2-weighted image shows a focal area of high signal (*arrow*) in the capitellum. (*From* Kijowski R, De Smet A. Radiography of the elbow for evaluation of patients with osteochondritis dissecans of the capitellum. Skeletal Radiol 2005;34:266–71; with permission.)

whether it is unstable [10]. The most common finding of an unstable OCD fragment on MRI is linear high signal on T2-weighted images along most of the interface between the fragment and the capitellum [10]. This high signal represents either fluid or granulation tissue, both of which occur in unstable OCD lesions. OCD fragments that are stable do not have this high signal along the interface.

Some authors advocate performing an MRI arthrogram for patients with a suspected OCD of the capitellum. If contrast extends into a linear defect at the margins of the fragment, the fragment usually is mobile and unstable (Fig. 5) [11].

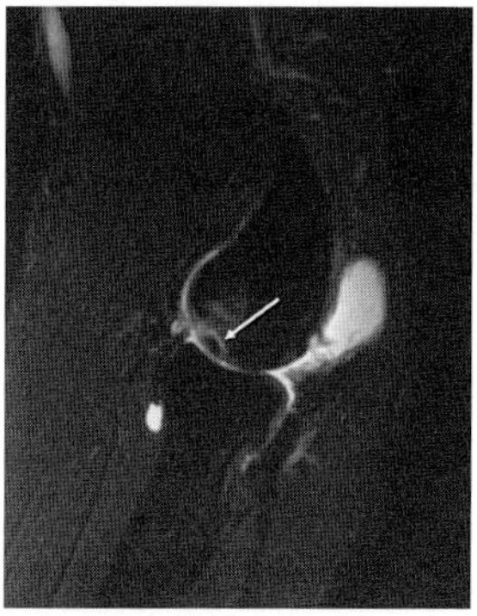

Fig. 5. Unstable OCD lesion in a 17-year-old male. Sagittal fat-suppressed T1-weighted image shows linear high signal (*arrow*) gadolinium contrast surrounding the OCD fragment.

Nondisplaced Fractures

MRI can be helpful in recognizing or characterizing nondisplaced fractures, and the imaging information may alter treatment. There are several types of fractures in which MRI can play a role. One is in identifying an otherwise radiographically occult fracture, such as a small radial head fracture (Fig. 6). MRI also can be helpful in avulsion fractures of the sublime tubercle in which it can help determine if the MCL is intact or if there is fibrous nonunion or a pseudarthrosis [12]. Another fracture that can be seen on MRI images before radiographic changes are apparent is Little Leaguer's elbow, a repetitive stress injury of the physis at the medial epicondyle apophysis (Fig. 7) [13]. Finally, fatigue fractures can occur in athletes who generate high forces on the bones around the elbow. For example, throwers who work up to full activity too quickly can develop stress fractures of the olecranon process. Like stress fractures elsewhere in the body, they are not only easier to identify on MRI images but can be staged, which may be helpful in predicting time to recovery.

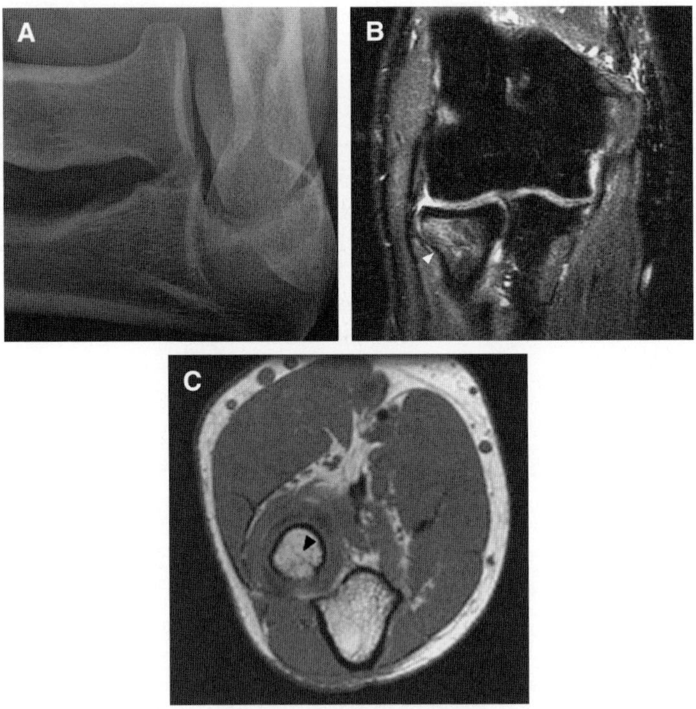

Fig. 6. Radiographically occult radial head fracture in a 30-year-old man. (*A*) Radial head view is normal. (*B*) Coronal T2-weighted image shows bone marrow edema in the radial head and neck (*arrowhead*). (*C*) Axial T1-weighted image shows the fracture line (*arrowhead*) in the radial neck. (*From* Kijowski R, Tuite M, Sanford M. Magnetic resonance imaging of the elbow. Part I: Normal anatomy, imaging technique, and osseous abnormalities. Skeletal Radiol 2005;33:685–97; with permission.)

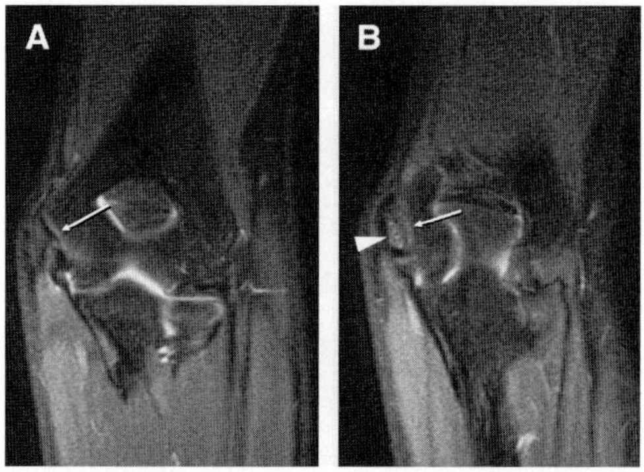

Fig. 7. (*A,B*) Little Leaguer's elbow in a 12-year-old girl. Adjacent T2-weighted images show high signal marrow edema adjacent to the medial epicondyle physis (*arrows*) and within the medial apophysis (*arrowhead*).

Loose Bodies

Intra-articular bodies sometimes can be difficult to diagnose on radiographs. Some of these bodies are composed of only cartilage, whereas others are ossified but are located deep in the olecranon or coronoid fossa and therefore obscured by superimposed bone structures. CT scans are excellent at showing ossified bodies, but intra-articular contrast (a CT arthrogram) often is necessary for seeing chondral bodies by CT.

Conventional MRI images can show even chondral intra-articular bodies [14], although in patients with only a small amount of fluid in the joint they may be identified only after carefully inspecting the two large humeral fossae. The advantage of MRI over CT is that it also can show marrow edema and extra-articular ligament injury. In some patients, however, even with a well-performed MRI scan it can be difficult to identify a loose body or determine if it is definitely intra-articular. In addition, osteophytes or focal areas of synovial hypertrophy can simulate an intra-articular body on conventional MRI images [14]. If a patient has osteophytes or other issues that may cause difficulty interpreting the MRI, but MRI is preferred over CT because of the superior soft tissue detail, an MRI arthrogram often is able to definitively demonstrate intra-articular bodies (Fig. 8) [15]. In all cases, cross-sectional imaging can provide a roadmap that may be helpful to the surgeon at arthroscopy.

Osteophytes

Athletes can develop osteophytes around the elbow, which may cause pain or reduced range of motion. One example is seen in throwers with posteromedial impingement who develop an osteophyte on the olecranon process, occasionally with adjacent chondromalacia or spur formation of the humerus in the adjacent olecranon fossa [16]. These osteophytes sometimes can be difficult to identify on radiographs, but are shown well on MRI cross-sectional images [17].

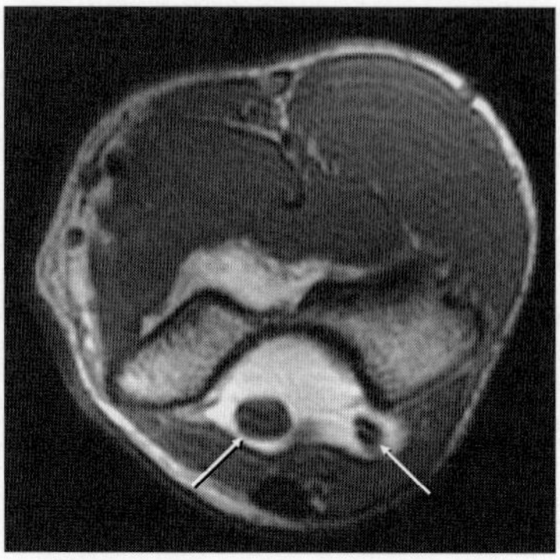

Fig. 8. Intra-articular loose bodies. Axial T1-weighted MRI arthrogram image shows two intra-articular loose bodies (*arrows*) surrounded by joint fluid near the superior olecranon fossa.

LIGAMENTOUS ABNORMALITIES

Ulnar Collateral Ligament Tears

Tears of the ulnar collateral ligament may occur following acute valgus stress injury to the elbow or following acute traumatic elbow dislocation [18,19].Ulnar collateral ligament tears are caused more commonly, however, by chronic repetitive stress to the elbow elicited by sports activities involving overhead throwing [20–23]. Most tears of the ulnar collateral ligament are full-thickness tears that involve the anterior bundle. The vast majority of these full-thickness tears occur in the midsubstance of the ligament. Complete soft tissue avulsions of the ulnar attachment and less commonly the humeral attachment of the anterior bundle can also occur [24,25]. Avulsion fractures of the sublime tubercle of the proximal ulna are rare but have been reported [26]. Partial-thickness tears of the ulnar collateral ligament also may occur. These partial-thickness tears, which involve the deep intracapsular layer of the anterior bundle, are especially common in baseball pitchers [27].

MRI of the elbow may be useful in evaluating the ulnar collateral ligament. The ulnar collateral ligament is visualized best on coronal T1-weighted and proton density weighted MRI images. The anterior bundle appears as a thin band of low signal intensity that extends along the medial joint line of the elbow (Fig. 9). The posterior and transverse bundles are difficult to visualize as discrete structures on MRI images [28,29].

The MRI findings of a torn ulnar collateral ligament include redundancy, irregularity, and poor definition of the ligament and abnormal signal intensity within and adjacent to the ligament. The abnormal morphology and signal intensity of the torn ulnar collateral ligament is believed to be because of the presence of edema and hemorrhage within the injured ligament. MRI has a sensitivity of 100% and a specificity of 100% for detecting full-thickness tears of the anterior bundle of the ulnar collateral ligament (Fig. 10) [28,29]. MRI has

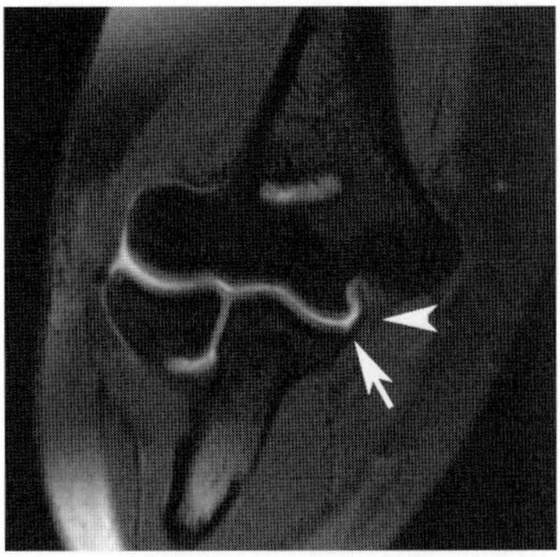

Fig. 9. Normal ulnar collateral ligament. Coronal fat-suppressed T1-weighted spin-echo image of the elbow shows the normal low signal intensity anterior band of the ulnar collateral ligament (*arrowhead*) extending from the medial epicondyle to the medial aspect of the base of the coronoid process. Note that the distal insertion of the ulnar collateral ligament attaches within 1 mm of the articular margin of the coronoid process (*arrow*).

a sensitivity of only 57% for detecting partial-thickness ligament tears, however (Fig. 11) [30].

MR arthrography of the elbow using saline or gadolinium intra-articular contrast also has been used to evaluate the ulnar collateral ligament. The presence of intra-articular contrast allows better delineation of the entire undersurface of the anterior bundle of the ulnar collateral ligament. On MR arthrography, intra-articular contrast can be seen filling the ulnar collateral recess of the elbow joint. This recess is a potential space beneath the medial epicondyle that is located between the undersurface of the proximal portion of the anterior bundle

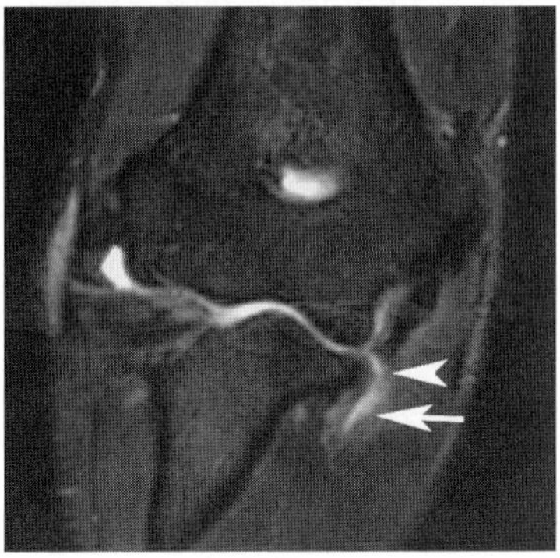

Fig. 10. Full-thickness tear of the ulnar collateral ligament in a 21-year-old male baseball pitcher with medial elbow pain. Coronal fat-suppressed T2-weighted fast spin-echo image of the elbow shows complete disruption of the distal fibers of the anterior bundle of the ulnar collateral ligament (*arrowhead*) with surrounding periligamentous edema (*arrow*).

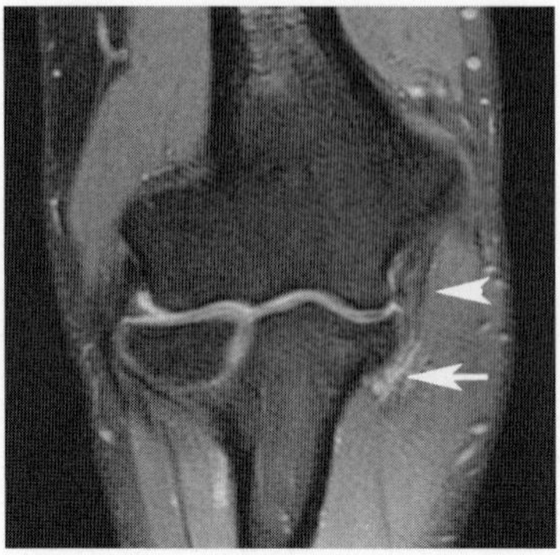

Fig. 11. Partial-thickness tear of the ulnar collateral ligament in a 19-year-old male baseball pitcher with medial elbow pain. Coronal fat-suppressed T2-weighted fast spin-echo image of the elbow shows thickening and irregularity of and intermediate signal intensity within the intact anterior bundle of the ulnar collateral ligament (*arrowhead*) with surrounding periligamentous edema (*arrow*).

of the ulnar collateral ligament and the medial aspect of the trochlea. The distal insertion of the anterior bundle of the ulnar collateral ligament attaches within 1 mm of the articular margin of the coronoid process of the ulna (Fig. 9) [31]. Any intra-articular contrast extending below the attachment of the anterior bundle to the base of the coronoid process is abnormal and indicates a tear of the ulnar collateral ligament (Fig. 12). The presence of intra-articular contrast improves the sensitivity of MR imaging for detecting partial-thickness tears of the anterior bundle of the ulnar collateral ligament [32].

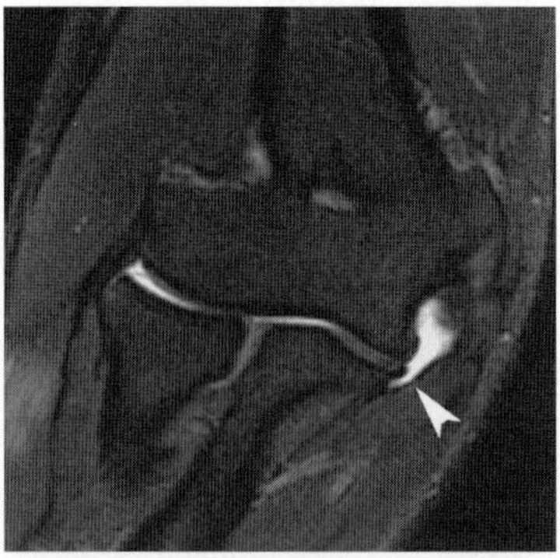

Fig. 12. Partial-thickness tear of the ulnar collateral ligament on MR arthrography in a 25-year-old male baseball pitcher with medial elbow pain. Coronal fat-suppressed T2-weighted spin-echo image of the elbow shows partial avulsion of the distal attachment of the anterior band of the ulnar collateral ligament from the medial aspect of the base of the coronoid process (*arrowhead*). Note that no contrast is seen extravasating into the periligamentous soft tissue indicating that only the deep fibers of the distal ulnar collateral ligament are torn.

Lateral collateral ligament tears

Tears of the lateral collateral ligament lead to a condition referred to as posterolateral rotatory instability of the elbow [33,34]. Tears of the lateral collateral ligament in young individuals usually are the result of an elbow dislocation. Tears of the lateral collateral ligament in adults most commonly are caused by a varus extension stress injury to the elbow that does not result in elbow dislocation [34]. Most tears of the lateral collateral ligament are full-thickness tears that involve the proximal attachment of the ulnar band to the lateral epicondyle [33,35]. Disruption of the ulnar band of the lateral collateral ligament also can occur following overaggressive release of the common extensor tendon origin for treatment of lateral epicondylitis [33–35].

MRI of the elbow may be useful in evaluating the lateral collateral ligament. The lateral collateral ligament is visualized best on coronal T1-weighted and proton density weighted MRI images. The ulnar band of the lateral collateral ligament appears as a thin band of low signal intensity that extends along the lateral joint line of the elbow and then crosses posterior to the radial head to insert onto the proximal ulna (Fig. 13). Only one study has described the MRI findings in patients with tears of the lateral collateral ligament. All patients showed abnormal signal intensity at the proximal attachment of the ulnar band of the lateral collateral ligament to the lateral epicondyle (Fig. 14) [35].

TENDINOUS ABNORMALITIES

Lateral Epicondylitis

Lateral epicondylitis is a pathologic condition of the common extensor tendon at its origin from the lateral epicondyle. Lateral epicondylitis also is known as tennis elbow because more than 50% of tennis players develop the condition at some time or another [36]. Lateral epicondylitis is far more common in

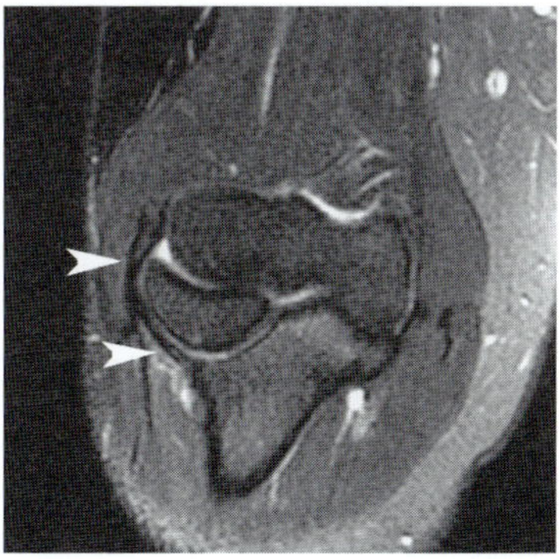

Fig. 13. Normal ulnar band of the lateral collateral ligament. Coronal fat-suppressed T2-weighted fast spin-echo image of the elbow shows the normal low signal intensity ulnar band of the lateral collateral ligament (*arrowheads*) extending from the lateral epicondyle to the lateral aspect of the proximal ulna.

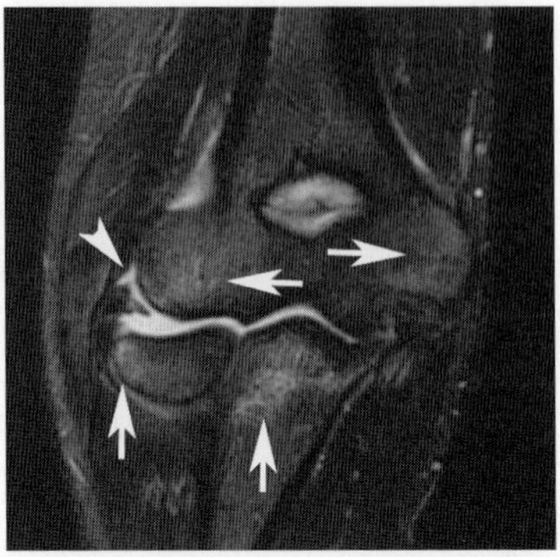

Fig. 14. Full-thickness tear of the ulnar band of the lateral collateral ligament in a 40-year-old male with lateral elbow pain following trauma. Coronal fat-suppressed T2-weighted fast spin-echo image of the elbow shows complete absence of the proximal fibers of the ulnar band of the lateral collateral ligament that normally attach to the lateral epicondyle (*arrowhead*). Note the associated posttraumatic bone marrow edema within the distal humerus, proximal ulna, and radial head (*arrows*).

nonathletes, however. Lateral epicondylitis is believed to represent an incomplete healing response to an initial microscopic or macroscopic avulsion injury of the common extensor tendon. The pathologic condition usually involves the origin of the extensor carpi radialis brevis tendon from the lateral epicondyle of the humerus. The origins of the extensor digitorum communis and extensor carpi radialis longus tendon occasionally are involved also [36–40].

MRI may be useful in evaluating the common extensor tendon origin in patients with lateral epicondylitis. MRI rarely is needed, however, because most patients are diagnosed easily by clinical history and physical examination. In individuals who do not respond to conservative treatment MRI may be helpful to determine the extent of tissue damage to the common extensor tendon origin and to exclude other causes of lateral elbow pain [41].

The common extensor tendon origin in patients with lateral epicondylitis usually is thickened and shows increased signal intensity on T1-weighted and T2-weighted images (Fig. 15). The areas of increased signal intensity within the diseased tendon correspond to areas of mucoid degeneration and neovascularization on histopathologic analysis. In many individuals with lateral epicondylitis, the common extensor tendon origin is thinned and shows areas of intense fluid-like signal intensity on T2-weighted images (Fig. 16). These areas of high T2 signal intensity usually correspond to areas of significant disruption of collagen fibers. Occasionally, however, they may represent areas of mucoid degeneration and neovascularization without disruption of the normal parallel orientation of collagen fibers [41,42]. Additional MRI findings in patients with lateral epicondylitis include bone marrow edema and periostitis of the lateral epicondyle, anconeus muscle edema, and fluid within the radial head bursa [43–46].

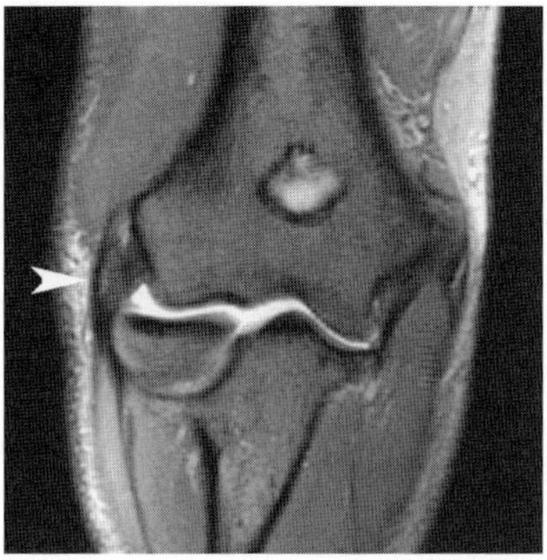

Fig. 15. Lateral epicondylitis in a 57-year-old male with chronic lateral elbow pain. Coronal T2-weighted fast spin-echo image of the elbow shows thickening and abnormal intermediate signal intensity within the common extensor tendon origin (*arrowhead*).

The normal common extensor tendon origin usually shows homogenous low signal intensity on T1-weighted and T2-weighted MRI images. Focal areas of increased T1 signal intensity within the origin of the common extensor tendon may be seen in asymptomatic individuals, however. In addition, increased T1 and T2 signal intensity within a thickened common extensor tendon origin has been described in asymptomatic high-performance athletes [42]. Furthermore, increased T2 signal intensity may be seen within and around the common extensor tendon for as long as one month following the injection of corticosteroid for treatment of lateral epicondylitis [47].

The MRI images of individuals with suspected lateral epicondylitis should be evaluated carefully for associated injuries to the lateral collateral ligament. One

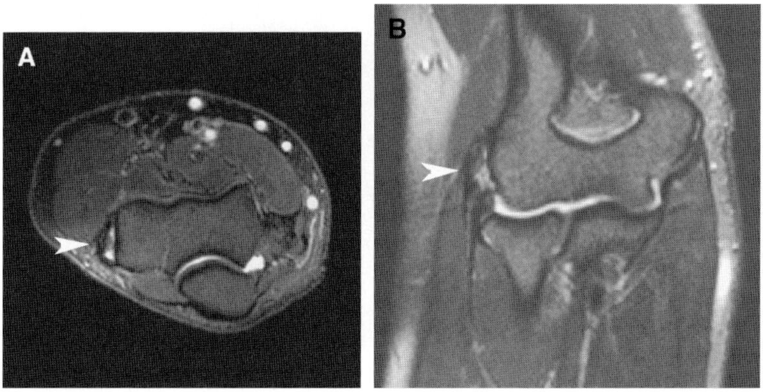

Fig. 16. Lateral epicondylitis in a 53-year-old female with chronic lateral elbow pain. Axial fat-suppressed T2-weighted fast spin-echo image (*A*) and coronal fat-suppressed T2-weighted fast spin-echo image (*B*) of the elbow shows thinning and abnormal fluid-like signal intensity within the common extensor tendon origin (*white arrowheads*).

study evaluated the ulnar band of the lateral collateral ligament in 35 consecutive patients who were referred for MR imaging of the elbow to rule out lateral epicondylitis. The vast majority of individuals with moderate to severe lateral epicondylitis were found to have associated partial-thickness and full-thickness tears of the ulnar band of the lateral collateral ligament [48]. If the lateral collateral ligament tears and the associated posterolateral rotatory instability of the elbow are not recognized, these individuals may be surgically treated for lateral epicondylitis with debridement of the common extensor tendon origin. This surgical procedure may destabilize the elbow further and worsen symptoms in these patients [49].

Medial Epicondylitis

Medial epicondylitis is a pathologic condition of the common flexor tendon at its origin from the medial epicondyle. Medial epicondylitis is much less common than lateral epicondylitis. Unlike lateral epicondylitis, medial epicondylitis is seen mainly in athletes. Most individuals with medial epicondylitis are involved in sports activities that generate repetitive valgus and flexion forces at the elbow. Medial epicondylitis is believed to represent an incomplete healing response to an initial microscopic or macroscopic avulsion injury of the common flexor tendon. The pathologic condition most commonly involves the tendon origins of the flexor carpi radialis muscle and pronator teres muscle [50,51].

MRI may be useful in evaluating the common flexor tendon origin in patients with medial epicondylitis. The origin of the common flexor tendon in these patients usually is thickened and shows increased signal intensity on T1-weighted and T2-weighted images. In many individuals, however, the common flexor tendon origin is thinned and shows areas of intense fluid-like signal intensity on T2-weighted images (Fig. 17). In contrast, the normal common

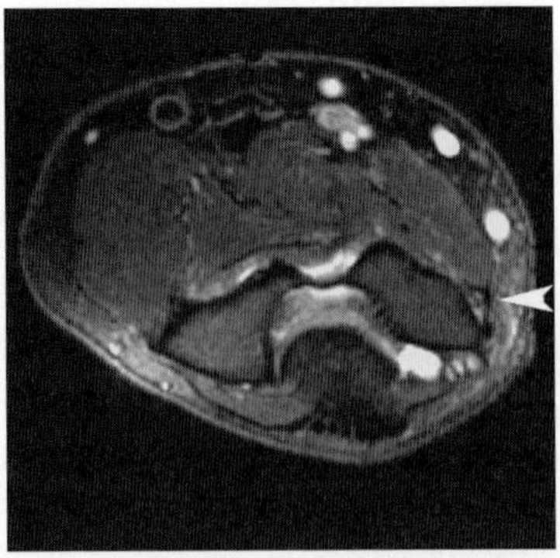

Fig. 17. Medial epicondylitis in a 47-year-old male racquetball player with chronic medial elbow pain. Axial fat-suppressed T2-weighted fast spin-echo image of the elbow shows thinning and abnormal fluid-like signal intensity within the common flexor tendon origin (*arrowhead*). (*From* Kijowski R, De Smet A. Magnetic resonance imaging findings in patients with medial epicondylitis. Skeletal Radiol 2005;34:196–202; with permission.)

flexor tendon origin usually shows homogenous low signal on T1-weighted and T2-weighted MRI images [42,52].

Biceps Tendon Injuries

Distal biceps tendon rupture most commonly occurs in the dominant extremity of males between 40 and 60 years of age. Rupture of the distal biceps tendon may be partial or complete. Rupture of the distal biceps tendon almost always is the result of a single traumatic event in which a sudden extension force is applied to the arm with the elbow flexed 90 degrees. Most tears of the distal biceps tendon occur at the insertion site of the tendon into the radial tuberosity. Intrasubstance tears and tears at the musculotendinous junction of the distal biceps tendon have been reported but are rare. The bicipital aponeurosis may or may not tear during rupture of the distal biceps tendon. If the bicipital aponeurosis is torn, the ruptured distal biceps tendon retracts proximally into the arm [53–59].

MRI can be used to evaluate individuals with distal biceps tendon injuries. Although a completely torn and retracted distal biceps tendon is recognized easily on physical examination, a partially torn or completely torn but nonretracted distal biceps tendon may be difficult to diagnose clinically. MRI has been shown to be helpful at confirming the presence of a distal biceps tendon injury and distinguishing between partial and complete biceps tendon rupture [60,61].

The distal biceps tendon is evaluated best on axial MRI images. Complete tendon rupture is characterized by the absence of the low signal intensity distal biceps tendon at its insertion site on the radial tuberosity and by the presence of soft tissue edema within the antecubital fossa. A variable amount of retraction of the distal biceps tendon usually is noted on sagittal images. (Fig. 18) [58,59]. Partial tendon rupture is characterized by the presence of increased signal intensity within an abnormally thickened or thinned distal biceps tendon [50–52]. It often is difficult to distinguish between tendinopathy and partial rupture of the distal biceps tendon on MRI [59,62]. Secondary findings of a partially torn distal biceps tendon include the presence of bone marrow edema within the radial tuberosity and the presence of fluid within the bicipitoradial bursa [44].

Triceps Tendon Injury

Rupture of the triceps tendon is a rare injury. Triceps tendon rupture occurs in both males and females and in individuals of all ages. Rupture of the triceps tendon is almost always the result of a single traumatic event. The mechanism of injury usually is a fall on an outstretched hand. Less common mechanisms of injury include a direct blow to the posterior elbow and a forceful eccentric contraction of the triceps muscle with the elbow flexed. Most tears of the triceps tendon occur at the insertion site of the tendon into the olecranon process of the proximal ulna. Intrasubstance tears and tears at the musculotendinous junction of the triceps tendon have been reported but are rare [63–70].

MRI can be used to evaluate individuals with triceps tendon rupture. MRI can distinguish between partial and complete rupture of the triceps tendon and can determine the amount of retraction of a completely torn tendon.

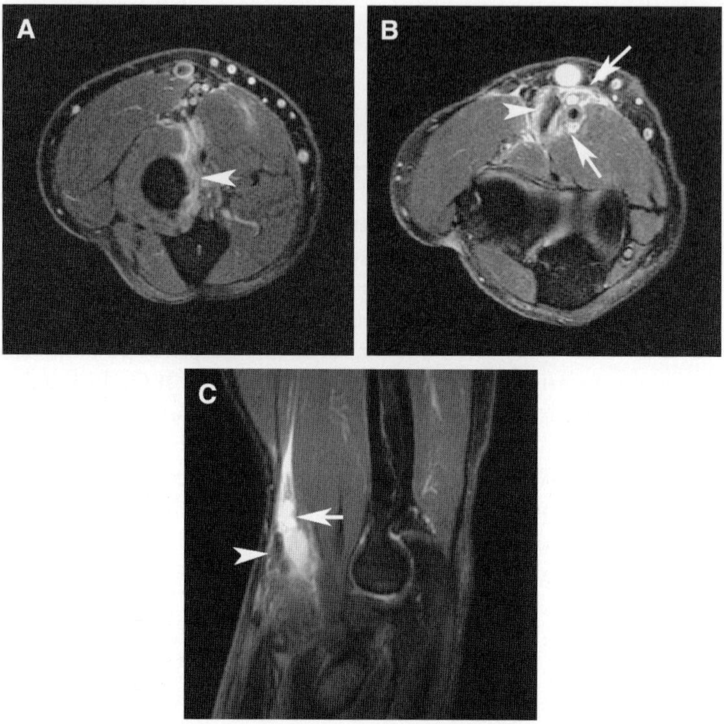

Fig. 18. Complete biceps tendon rupture in a 52-year-old male with anterior elbow pain following trauma. (*A*) Axial fat-suppressed T2-weighted fast spin-echo image of the elbow shows absence of the distal biceps tendon and fluid adjacent to the radial tuberosity (*arrowhead*). (*B*) Axial fat-suppressed T2-weighted fast spin-echo image of the elbow proximal to the previous image shows the retracted completely torn biceps tendon (*arrowhead*) with surrounding soft tissue edema within the antecubital fossa (*arrows*). (*C*) Sagittal fat-suppressed T2-weighted fast spin-echo image of the elbow better visualizes the extent of retraction of the completely torn biceps tendon (*arrowhead*) and the degree of soft tissue edema within the antecubital fossa (*arrow*).

The triceps tendon is visualized best on sagittal MRI images. Partial tendon rupture is characterized by a small fluid-filled defect within the distal triceps tendon and edema within the surrounding subcutaneous tissue. Complete rupture of the triceps tendon is characterized by a large fluid-filled gap between the distal triceps tendon and the olecranon process and a large amount of edema within the surrounding subcutaneous tissue. A variable amount of retraction of the completely torn distal triceps tendon usually is present (Fig. 19) [71,72].

NERVE ABNORMALITIES

MRI may be useful in evaluating patients with nerve disorders at the elbow. Inflammatory changes within a nerve caused by long-standing compression may alter its morphology and signal characteristics on MRI. Normal nerves

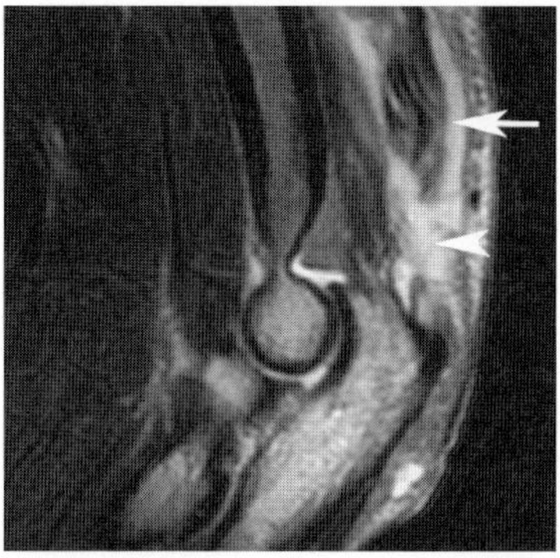

Fig. 19. Complete triceps tendon rupture in a 57-year-old male with posterior elbow pain following trauma. Sagittal T2-weighted spin-echo image of the elbow shows a large fluid-filled gap (*arrowhead*) between the completely torn and retracted distal triceps tendon (*arrow*) and the olecranon process.

are of intermediate to low signal intensity on all pulse sequences. They have the same signal intensity as adjacent muscle on T1-weighted images. On T2-weighted images, they may have slightly increased signal intensity when compared with adjacent muscle. Inflammation may cause increased signal intensity within the compressed nerve. This increased signal intensity is appreciated best on short tau inversion recovery or fat-suppressed T2-weighted images (Fig. 20). Inflammation also may lead to focal or diffuse thickening of the compressed

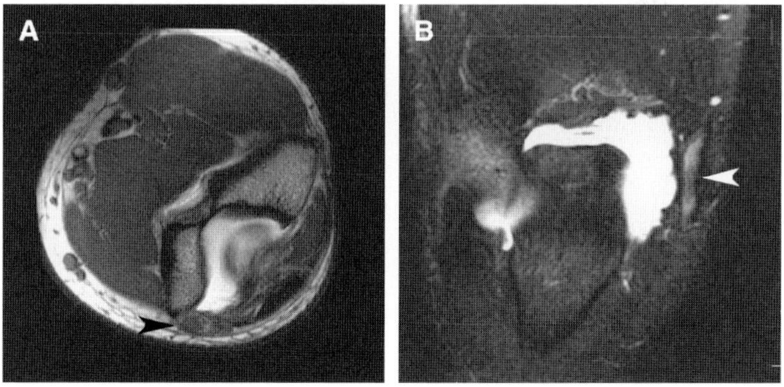

Fig. 20. Cubital tunnel syndrome in a 19-year-old baseball pitcher with medial elbow pain and evidence of ulnar neuropathy. (*A*) Axial T1-weighted spin-echo image of the elbow shows an enlarged ulnar nerve (*arrowhead*) within the cubital tunnel. (*B*) Coronal fat-suppressed T2-weighted spin-echo image of the elbow shows the thickened, edematous ulnar nerve (*arrowhead*) as it passes posterior to the medial epicondyle. (*From* Kijowski R, Tuite M, Sanford M. Magnetic resonance imaging of the elbow. Part II: Abnormalities of the ligaments, tendons, and nerves. Skeletal Radiol 2005;34:1–18; with permission.)

nerve. Nerve thickening may be present proximal to and at the site of compression [73,74].

When evaluating patients who have nerve disorders at the elbow, it is important to evaluate the muscles of the upper extremity. Changes in the morphologic and signal intensity of a muscle group may be the only imaging manifestations of an abnormality of the nerve that innervates the muscles. MRI is not reliable at detecting acute denervation of muscle. After a period of approximately one month, however, denervated muscle shows increased signal intensity on short tau inversion recovery images. Chronically denervated muscle demonstrates significant atrophy, variable signal intensity on short tau inversion recovery images, and conspicuous fatty infiltration on T1-weighted images [75].

MRI is most useful at evaluating patients with ulnar neuropathy at the elbow. The ulnar nerve is in a superficial location at the elbow and is surrounded by abundant fat. For this reason it is easy to identify the ulnar nerve at the elbow and to detect subtle changes in its morphology and signal intensity secondary to long-standing compression. MRI has been shown to be helpful at detecting a variety of disease processes related to cubital tunnel syndrome. Compression of the ulnar nerve within the cubital tunnel caused by osteoarthritis, posttraumatic deformities, and accessory muscles has been detected using MR imaging (Fig. 21) [73,74].

MRI is less useful at evaluating patients with median and radial neuropathy at the elbow. The median nerve and radial nerve are much more difficult to visualize at the elbow than the ulnar nerve. For this reason inflammatory

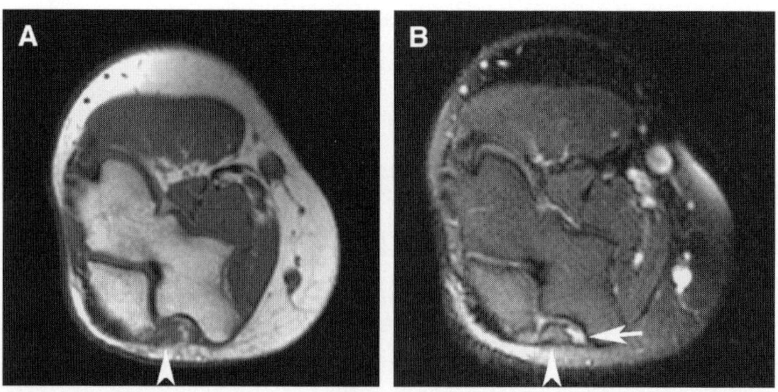

Fig. 21. Cubital tunnel syndrome in a 30-year-old female with medial elbow pain and evidence of ulnar neuropathy. (*A*) Axial T1-weighted spin-echo image of the elbow shows replacement of cubital tunnel retinaculum with an anconeus epitrochlearis muscle (*arrowhead*). (*B*) Axial fat-suppressed T2-weighted spin-echo images of the elbow in the same location shows the anconeus epitrochlearis muscle (*arrowhead*) and the adjacent edematous ulnar nerve (*arrow*) within the cubital tunnel. (*From* Kijowski R, Tuite M, Sanford M. Magnetic resonance imaging of the elbow. Part II: Abnormalities of the ligaments, tendons, and nerves. Skeletal Radiol 2005;34:1–18; with permission.)

changes within these nerves secondary to long-standing compression often are difficult to identify. Nevertheless, MRI may be useful at detecting space-occupying lesions that cause compression of the median nerve and radial nerve at the elbow [73,74,76,77].

SUMMARY

MRI is helpful in identifying the specific structures that are injured and the severity of the injury for many athletic injuries to the elbow. MRI should be the imaging modality of choice for the patient with complex sports-related elbow pain.

References

[1] Sonin AH, Fitzgerald SW. MR imaging of sports injuries in the adult elbow: a tailored approach. AJR Am J Roentgenol 1996;167:325–31.
[2] Steinbach LS, Palmer WE, Schweitzer ME. Special focus session. MR arthrography. Radiographics 2002;22:1223–46.
[3] Rosenberg ZS, Beltran J, Cheung YY. Pseudodefect of the capitellum: potential MR imaging pitfall. Radiology 1994;191:821–3.
[4] Rosenberg ZS, Beltran J, Cheung YY, et al. MR imaging of the elbow: normal variant and potential diagnostic pitfalls of the trochlear groove and cubital tunnel. AJR Am J Roentgenol 1995;164:415–8.
[5] Frostick SP, Mohammad M, Ritchie DA. Sports injuries of the elbow. Br J Sports Med 1999;33:301–11.
[6] Omer G. Primary articular osteochondroses. Clin Orthop Relat Res 1981;158:33–40.
[7] Takahara M, Ogino T, Fukushima S, et al. Nonoperative treatment of osteochondritis dissecans of the humeral capitellum. Am J Sports Med 1999;27:728–32.
[8] Klekamp J, Green NE, Mencio GA. Osteochondritis dissecans as a cause of developmental dislocation of the radial head. Clin Orthop 1997;338:36–41.
[9] Kijowski R, De Smet AA. Radiography of the elbow for evaluation of patients with osteochondritis dissecans of the capitellum. Skeletal Radiol 2005;34:266–71.
[10] Kijowski R, Tuite MJ, Sanford M. Magnetic resononce imaging of the elbow. Part 1: normal anatomy, imaging technique, and osseous abnormalities. Skeletal Radiol 2004;33: 685–97.
[11] Kramer J, Stiglbauer R, Engel A. MR contrast in osteochondritis dissecans. J Comput Assist Tomogr 1992;16:254–60.
[12] Glajchen N, Schwartz ML, Andrews JR, et al. Avulsion fracture of the sublime tubercle of the ulna: a newly recognized injury in the throwing athlete. AJR Am J Roentgenol 1998;170: 627–8.
[13] Hang DW, Chao CM, Hang YS. A clinical and roentgenographic study of little league elbow. Am J Sports Med 2004;21:79–84.
[14] Quinn SF, Haberman JJ, Fitzgerald SW, et al. Evaluation of loose bodies in the elbow with MR imaging. J Magn Reson Imaging 1994;4:169–72.
[15] Steinbach LS, Schwartz ML. Elbow arthrography. Radiol Clin North Am 1998;36:635–49.
[16] Wilson FD, Andrews JR, Blackburn TA, et al. Valgus extension overload in the pitching elbow. Am J Sports Med 1983;11:83–7.
[17] Gaary EA, Potter HG, Altcheck DW. Medial elbow pain in the throwing athlete: MR imaging evaluation. AJR 1997;168:795–800.
[18] Bennett J, Green M, Tullos H. Surgical management of chronic medial elbow instability. Clin Orthop 1992;278:62–8.
[19] Jobe F, Nuber G. Throwing injuries of the elbow. Clin Sports Med 1986;5:621–36.
[20] Jobe F, Stark H, Lombardo S. Reconstruction of the ulnar collateral ligament in athletes. J Bone Joint Surg 1986;68A:1158–63.

[21] Tullos HS, Erwin W, Woods G, et al. Unusual lesions of the pitching arm. Clin Orthop 1972;88:169–82.
[22] Ciccotti M, Jobe F. Medial collateral ligament instability and ulnar neuritis in the athlete's elbow. American Academy of Orthopaedic Surgeons Instructional Course Lectures 1999; 48:383–91.
[23] Conway J, Jobe F, Glousman R. Medial instability of the elbow in throwing athletes: treatment by repair or reconstruction of the ulnar collateral ligament. J Bone Joint Surg 1992;74A:67–83.
[24] Azar F, Andrews J, Wilk K. Operative treatment of ulnar collateral ligament injuries of the elbow in athletes. Am J Sports Med 2000;28:16–23.
[25] Salvo J, Rizio L, Zvijac J, et al. Avulsion fractures of the ulnar sublime tubercle in overhead throwing athletes. Am J Sports Med 2002;30:426–31.
[26] Timmerman L, Andrews J. Undersurface tears of the ulnar collateral ligament in baseball players. Am J Sports Med 1994;22:33–6.
[27] Mirowitz S, London S. Ulnar collateral ligament injury in baseball pitchers: MR imaging evaluation. Radiology 1992;185:573–8.
[28] Murphy Brian. MR imaging of the elbow. Radiology 1992;184:525–9.
[29] Timmerman L, Schwartz M, Andrews J. Preoperative evaluation of the ulnar collateral ligament by magnetic resonance imaging and computed tomography. Am J Sports Med 1994;22(1):26–31.
[30] Cotton A, Jacobson J, Brossman J, et al. MR arthrography of the elbow: normal anatomy and diagnostic pitfalls. J Comput Assist Tomogr 1997;21:516–22.
[31] Schwartz M, Al-Zahrani S, Morwessel R, et al. Ulnar collateral ligament injury in the throwing athlete: evaluation with saline-enhanced MR arthrography. Radiology 1995;197:297–9.
[32] O'Driscoll S, Bell D, Morrey B. Posterolateral rotatory instability of the elbow. J Bone Joint Surg 1991;73A:440–6.
[33] Nestor B, O'Driscoll S, Morrey B. Ligamentous reconstruction for posterolateral rotatory instability of the elbow. J Bone Joint Surg 1992;74A:1235–40.
[34] Potter H, Weiland A, Schatz J, et al. Posterolateral rotatory instability of the elbow: usefulness of MR imaging in diagnosis. Radiology 1997;204:185–9.
[35] Maylack F. Epidemiology of tennis, squash, and racquetball injuries. Clin Sports Med 1988;7:233–8.
[36] Coonrad R, Hooper R. Tennis elbow: its course, natural history, conservative and surgical management. J Bone Joint Surg 1973;55A:1177–82.
[37] Boyd H, Mcleod A. Tennis elbow. J Bone Joint Surg 1973;55A:1183–7.
[38] Regan W, Wold L, Coonrad R, et al. Microscopic histopathology of chronic refractory lateral epicondylitis. Am J Sports Med 1992;26:746–9.
[39] Doran A, Gresham G, Rushton N, et al. Tennis elbow: a clinicopathologic study of 22 cases followed for 2 years. Acta Orthop Scand 1990;61:535–8.
[40] Potter H, Hannafin J, Morwessel R, et al. Lateral epicondylitis; correlation of MR imaging, surgical, and histopathologic findings. Radiology 1995;196:43–6.
[41] Martin C, Schweitzer M. MR imaging of epicondylitis. Skeletal Radiol 1998;27:133–8.
[42] Ho CP. Sports and occupational injuries of the elbow: MR imaging findings. AJR Am J Roentgenol 1995;164:1465–71.
[43] Patten PM. Overuse syndromes and injuries involving the elbow: MR imaging findings. AJR Am J Roentgenol 1995;164:1205–11.
[44] Golimbu C. Elbow. In: Firooznia H, Golimbu C, Raffi M, et al, editors. MRI and CT of the Musculoskeletal System. St Louis: Mosby Books; 1992. p. 564–93.
[45] Coel M, Yamada C, Ko J. MR imaging of patients with lateral epicondylitis of the elbow: importance of increased signal intensity of the anconeus muscle. AJR Am J Roentgenol 1993;161:1019–21.
[46] Resendes M, Helms C, Fritz R, et al. MR appearance of intramuscular injections. AJR Am J Roentengenol 1992;158:1293–4.

[47] Bredella M, Tirman P, Fritz R, et al. MR imaging findings of lateral ulnar collateral ligament abnormalities in patients with lateral epicondylitis. AJR Am J Roentgenol 1999;173: 1379–82.

[48] Morrey B. Re-operation for failed tennis elbow surgery. J Shoulder Elbow Surg 1992; 1:47–9.

[49] Ollivierre C, Nirschl R, Pettrone F. Resection and repair for medial tennis elbow. Am J Sports Med 1995;23:214–21.

[50] Vangsness T, Jobe F. Surgical treatment of medial epicondylitis. J Bone Joint Surg 1991;73B: 409–11.

[51] Kijowski R, De Smet A. Magnetic resonance imaging findings in patients with medial epicondylitis. Skeletal Radiol 2005;34:196–202.

[52] Meherin J, Kilmore E. The treatment of ruptures of the distal biceps tendon. Am J Surg 1960;99:636–40.

[53] Boucher PR, Morton KS. Rupture of the distal biceps tendon. J Trauma 1967;7: 626–32.

[54] Friedmann E. Rupture of the distal biceps tendon: report on 13 cases. JAMA 1963;1184: 60–3.

[55] Agins H, Chess J, Hoekstra D, et al. Rupture of the distal insertion of the biceps tendon. Clin Orthop 1988;234:34–8.

[56] Bourne M, Morrey B. Partial rupture of the distal biceps tendon. Clin Orthop 1991;271: 143–8.

[57] Durr H, Stabler A, Pfahler M, et al. Partial rupture of the distal biceps tendon. Clin Orthop 2000;374:195–200.

[58] Rokito A, McLaughlin J, Gallagher M, et al. Partial rupture of the distal biceps tendon. J Shoulder Elbow Surg 1996;5:73–5.

[59] Fitzgerald S, Curry D, Erickson S, et al. Distal biceps tendon injury: MR imaging diagnosis. Radiology 1994;191:203–6.

[60] Falchook F, Zlatkin M, Erbacher G, et al. Rupture of the distal biceps tendon: evaluation with MR imaging. Radiology 1994;190:659–63.

[61] Williams B, Schweitzer M, Weishaupt D, et al. Partial tears of the distal biceps tendon: MR appearance and associated clinical findings. Skeletal Radiol 2001;30:560–4.

[62] Bennett BS. Triceps tendon rupture. J Bone Joint Surg 1962;44A:741–4.

[63] Farrer E, Lippert F. Avulsion of the triceps tendon. Clin Orthop 1981;161:242–6.

[64] Tarnmey F. Rupture and avulsion of the triceps. Clin Orthop 1972;83:177–83.

[65] Sollender J, Reyan G, Barden G. Triceps tendon rupture in weightlifter. J Shoulder Elbow Surg 1998;7:149–53.

[66] Bach B, Warren R, Wickiewicz T. Triceps rupture: a case report and literature review. Am J Sports Med 1987;15:285–9.

[67] Gilcrest EL. Rupture of the triceps tendon. JAMA 1925;84:1819.

[68] Seafoss R, Tripi J, Bowers W. Triceps brachii rupture: a case report. J Trauma 1976;16: 244–6.

[69] Sherman O, Snyder S, Fox J. Triceps tendon avulsion in a professional body builder. Am J Sports Med 1984;12:328–9.

[70] Gaines S, Durbin R, Marsalka D. The use of magnetic resonance imaging in the diagnosis of triceps tendon rupture. Contemp Orthop 1990;20:607–10.

[71] Tiger E, Mayer D, Glazer R. Complete avulsion of the triceps tendon: MRI diagnosis. Comput Med Imaging Graph 1993;17:51–4.

[72] Beltran J, Rosenberg Z. Diagnosis of compressive and entrapment neuropathies at the elbow: value of MR imaging. AJR Am J Roentgenol 1994;163:525–31.

[73] Rosenberg Z, Beltran J, Cheung Y. The elbow: MR features of nerve disorders. Radiology 1993;188:235–40.

[74] Fleckenstein J, Watumull D, Conner K, et al. Denervated human skeletal muscle: MR imaging evaluation. Radiology 1993;187:213–8.

[75] Ogino T, Minami A, Kato H. Diagnosis of radial nerve palsy caused by ganglion with use of different imaging techniques. J Hand Surg [Am] 1991;16A:230–5.
[76] Yamamoto T, Mizuno K, Soejima T, et al. Bicipitoradial bursitis: CT and MR appearance. Comput Med Imaging Graph 2001;25:531–3.
[77] Skaf A, Boutin R, Dantas R, et al. Bicipitoradial bursitis: MR imaging findings in eight patients and anatomic data from contrast material opacification of bursae followed by routine radiography and MR imaging of cadavers. Radiology 1999;212:111–6.

ELSEVIER
SAUNDERS

Clin Sports Med 25 (2006) 409–432

CLINICS IN SPORTS MEDICINE

Sports-Related Injuries of the Wrist: An Approach to MRI Interpretation

Jenny T. Bencardino, MD[a,*], Zehava Sadka Rosenberg, MD[b]

[a]Department of Radiology, Huntington Hospital, North Shore Long Island Jewish Health System, 270 Park Avenue, Huntington, NY 11747, USA

[b]Department of Radiology, Hospital for Joint Diseases, New York University Medical Center, 305 East 17th Street, New York, NY 10003, USA

Sports-related injuries to the wrist range from minor sprains to severe soft tissue disruption that can pose a risk to the normal functioning of the upper extremity. It is important to identify the specific nature of such injuries to establish an accurate diagnosis and deliver appropriate treatment. Superb, noninvasive depiction of the wrist's intricate anatomy may be obtained by using MRI. T1-weighted and high-resolution proton density images provide high anatomic detail, whereas T2-weighted images are useful for evaluating the alterations in water content characteristic of most pathologic conditions. Fluid-sensitive sequences, namely short tau inversion-recovery and fat-suppressed T2-weighted imaging, may be used to highlight the contrast differences between the low-signal tendons, ligaments, and triangular fibrocartilage and the abnormal free water. MRI of the wrist should be obtained in the axial, sagittal, and coronal planes. The axial and sagittal planes provide most of the information necessary to assess the tendons, extrinsic ligaments, and nerves at the wrist. The coronal and sagittal images are most helpful for evaluating the intrinsic ligaments and the triangular fibrocartilage.

NORMAL ANATOMY

Tendons

Flexor tendons

Understanding the normal anatomy of the flexor tendons may be simplified by classifying them according to their location within and outside the carpal tunnel. The flexor tendons contained within the carpal tunnel, deep to the flexor retinaculum, include the flexor digitorum superficialis, flexor digitorum profundus, and flexor pollicis longus tendons (Fig. 1). A common tendon sheath surrounds the long flexor tendons of the digits, whereas the flexor pollicis longus traverses within its own tendon sheath [1].

*Corresponding author. *E-mail address:* jennybencardino@yahoo.com (J.T. Bencardino).

0278-5919/06/$ – see front matter
doi:10.1016/j.csm.2006.02.007

sportsmed.theclinics.com

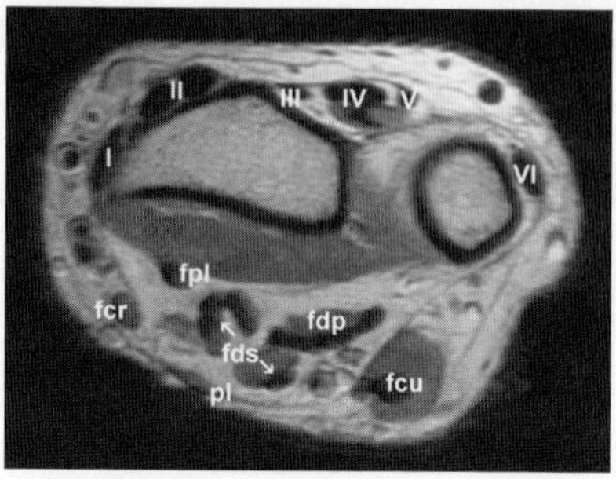

Fig. 1. Normal anatomy of the tendons. Axial proton-density weighted image at the level of the distal forearm demonstrating the flexor tendons and extensor compartments (I–VI). fcr, flexor carpi radialis; fcu, flexor carpi ulnaris; fdp, flexor digitorum profundus; fds, flexor digitorum superficialis; fpl, flexor pollicis longus; pl, palmaris longus.

The main flexors of the wrist, the flexor carpi radialis, flexor carpi ulnaris, and palmaris longus tendons, all travel outside the carpal tunnel (see Fig. 1). The flexor carpi radialis (FCR) travels within a fibro-osseous tunnel formed by a reflection of the flexor retinaculum just proximal to the trapezium. Within the tunnel, the FCR traverses along a groove on the trapezium. The FCR inserts via terminal slips into the trapezial tuberosity and into the bases of the second and third metacarpals.

The flexor carpi ulnaris (FCU) tendon, along with the pisiform bone, forms the ulnar boundary of Guyon's canal. The FCU tendon protects the ulnar nerve and artery at the wrist level. It also provides a clinical reference point when a local nerve block of the ulnar nerve is performed. The distal attachment sites of the FCU tendon include the palmar surface of the pisiform, hamate, and base of the fifth metacarpal.

Paratenon rather than a synovial sheath surrounds the palmaris longus tendon. The tendon has a straight course as it inserts into the flexor retinaculum and palmar aponeurosis. It is the most commonly used tendon for grafting during hand surgery. The palmaris longus is highly variable and ranges in size from a thin slip to a wide, flat tendon [2]. It is absent in 25% of the population. Occasionally the muscle belly of the tendon extends to the wrist level, forming the so-called "reversed palmaris longus muscle." This variant may cause mechanical compression of the median nerve [3–5].

Extensor tendons

The extensor retinaculum, along with vertical septae, divides the extensor tendons into six separate compartments delineated laterally and medially by the distal radius and ulna, respectively (see Fig. 1). Although each extensor compartment contains a single tendon sheath, it may be traversed by as many as three tendons. The extensor compartments are numbered from one to six from the radial to the ulnar surface. The extensor pollicis brevis tendon and the abductor pollicis longus tendon compose the first compartment. The second compartment is traversed by the extensor carpi radialis longus and extensor carpi radialis brevis tendons. The extensor pollicis longus tendon occupies the third compartment proximal to the radioulnar joint; distal to the joint the tendon joins the second compartment tendons. The third and fourth compartments are separated by Lister's tubercle of the distal radius. The fourth compartment holds the extensor digitorum and extensor indicis tendons, whereas the fifth compartment contains the extensor digiti minimi tendon, typically made up of two slips. The sixth compartment contains the extensor carpi ulnaris tendon.

Ligaments

Extrinsic ligaments

The extrinsic ligaments are capsular ligaments that tie the radius and ulna to the carpal bones and traverse the radiocarpal joint, midcarpal joint, or both. The extrinsic ligaments may be divided into volar and dorsal components. The volar radiocarpal ligaments are stronger and thicker than the dorsal ligaments and are the major stabilizers of wrist motion. Significant variations have appeared in the descriptive anatomy and nomenclature of these ligaments [6–9], resulting in some confusion in the literature.

The volar extrinsic ligaments are subdivided into the radiocarpal and ulnocarpal ligaments. The most important extrinsic volar stabilizer of the wrist, the radioscaphocapitate ligament, is the most radial of the major volar ligaments. It connects the radius to the distal carpal row and plays a major role in preventing rotatory subluxation of the scaphoid. The ligament arises from the volar aspect of the styloid process of the radius, crosses the waist of the scaphoid, and inserts into the head of the capitate, coalescing ulnarly with the ulnocapitate ligament to form the arcuate or deltoid ligament. It should be noted, however, that some authors believe the deltoid ligament is an intrinsic ligament with a capitotriquetral (ulnar arm) and a capitoscaphoid (radial arm) component.

The radiolunotriquetral ligament is the second strongest volar ligament. It originates at the radial styloid process, adjacent to the radioscaphocapitate ligament, and extends ulnarly to attach to the volar aspect of the triquetrum. This ligament functions as a sling to the lunate bone. The radioscapholunate, or ligament of Testut, is a small volar ligament, which arises from the volar aspect of the distal portion of the radius and inserts into the proximal volar surfaces of the scapholunate interval. This structure plays less of a role in stabilizing the wrist, but its importance may be related to the neurovascular structures that lie within the ligament.

The volar ulnocarpal ligaments include the ulnolunate and ulnotriquetral ligaments extending from the ulnar styloid process and triangular fibrocartilage to the lunate and triquetrum, respectively. The volar extrinsic ligaments are typically hypointense on MR images, although they may display a striated appearance on three-dimensional images [10,11]. They may be best evaluated on transverse and oblique sagittal images [11] but are frequently seen, at least in part, on coronal images.

The dorsal extrinsic ligaments are deep to the extensor retinaculum and extensor tendons. These ligaments are not as important functionally as the volar ligaments. The dorsal radiocarpal ligament originates from the distal radius at Lister's tubercle, attaching distally to the dorsal horn of the lunate and dorsal triquetrum. The dorsal intercarpal ligament, the most prominent of the dorsal ligaments, arises in the triquetrum, coursing radially as it fans out to insert on the dorsal ridge of the scaphoid, the trapezium, and the trapezoid. The interval located distal to the dorsal radiocarpal ligament and proximal to the dorsal intercarpal ligament is used as a dorsal surgical approach.

The dorsal extrinsic ligaments may be consistently visualized using high-resolution thin-slice sequences, such as those obtained with three-dimensional Fourier transform and MR arthrography [10–13]. The ligaments may be seen on coronal images but are better assessed on transverse and sagittal images. Not infrequently, and in a similar fashion to the volar ligaments, the dorsal ligaments display a striated appearance that should not be mistaken for tears.

Intrinsic ligaments

The intrinsic or interosseous ligaments are intracapsular structures, which originate and insert on the carpal bones [6,7]. The two most important interosseous ligaments are the scapholunate and lunotriquetral ligaments (Fig. 2). They link the carpal bones in the proximal row, precluding communication of the radiocarpal with the midcarpal joints. The scapholunate and lunotriquetral ligaments are both C-shaped structures with dorsal and volar components and a central, thinner, intramembranous portion [8].

The scapholunate ligament is composed of thick dorsal collagen bundles, rendering its dorsal component the most important for carpal stability [7,8]. Volarly, the scapholunate ligament is looser, so it can accommodate the various articulating curvatures of the scaphoid and lunate [14].

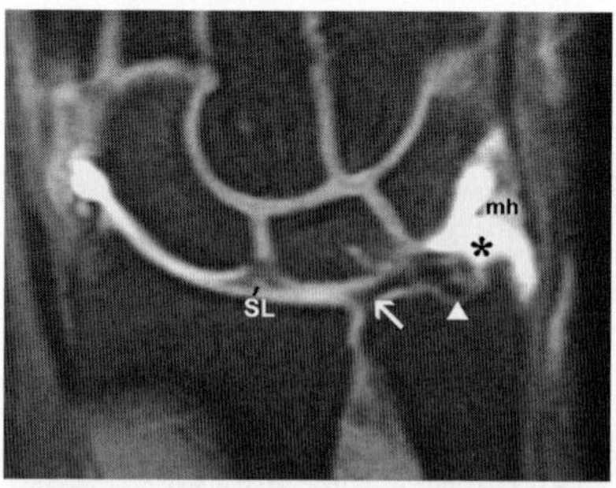

Fig. 2. Normal anatomy—prestyloid recess and meniscus homologue. Oblique coronal MR-arthrographic image demonstrates a focal collection of contrast at the level of the prestyloid recess (*asterisk*) outlining the meniscus homologue (mh). The radial (*arrow*) and ulnar (*arrowhead*) insertions of the triangular fibrocartilage are also seen. SL, scapholunate ligament.

The lunotriquetral ligament links the lunate and triquetral bones. It is a smaller and more taut ligament than the scapholunate ligament. Its stronger and thicker volar component blends with the triangular fibrocartilage.

The Triangular Fibrocartilage Complex

The triangular fibrocartilage complex (TFCC) is the primary stabilizer of the distal radioulnar joint (DRUJ). It also absorbs stress during axial loading of the wrist and limits lateral deviation of the carpus. The main components of the TFCC are the triangular fibrocartilage, the dorsal and volar radioulnar ligaments, the volar ulnolunate and ulnotriquetral ligaments, the meniscus homologue, the ulnar collateral ligament, and the extensor carpi ulnaris tendon sheath [15–19]. The complex anatomy of the TFCC has been studied with high-resolution MRI using microscopy coils [19], virtual MR arthroscopy [20], and recently 3-Tesla MRI (3TMR) imaging [21].

The head of the ulna and the sigmoid notch of the radius form the proximal osseous boundary of the TFCC. The distal osseous border is composed of the triquetrum and medial portion of the lunate. The triangular fibrocartilage inserts into the ulnar aspect of the lunate fossa of the radius and, through the upper and lower lamina of the ligament, into the ulnar styloid and into the fovea at the base of the ulnar styloid (Fig. 3; see Fig. 2). Occasionally, the ulnar insertion may span the entire length of the ulnar styloid process without distinct separation into bands [22,23]. Distally, the TFCC inserts into the hamate, triquetrum, and base of the fifth metacarpal and blends with fibers of the ulnar collateral ligament [15]. Volarly, the TFCC is attached to the triquetrum and lunate by the ulnotriquetral and ulnolunate ligaments, respectively. Dorsally, the TFCC is incorporated into the sheath of the extensor carpi ulnaris tendon [15].

The meniscus homologue is a complex fibrous structure that resides between the ulna and triquetrum (see Fig. 2). It has a common origin with the dorsal radioulnar ligament and inserts into the ulnar border of the triquetrum.

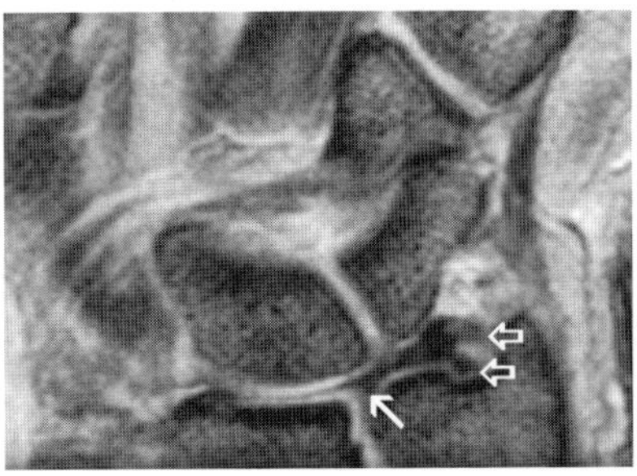

Fig. 3. Normal anatomy—triangular fibrocartilage. Oblique coronal gradient echo T2*-weighted image shows the radial (*arrow*) and ulnar (*open arrows*) insertions of the triangular fibrocartilage. Note cartilage undercutting at the radial attachment of the ligament and not the frequently encountered heterogeneity at the insertion to the ulnar styloid.

Nerves

Median nerve

Proximal to the wrist joint the median nerve travels between the flexor digitorum superficialis and FCR muscles. It then courses through the carpal tunnel along with the flexor tendons of the fingers and thumb. The carpal tunnel is a fibro-osseous canal bordered volarly by the flexor retinaculum, medially by the pisiform and the hook of the hamate, laterally by the scaphoid and trapezium, and dorsally by the carpal bones.

The flexor retinaculum is composed of three parts: the antebrachial fascia proximal to the wrist bones (see Fig. 4A), the transverse carpal ligament proper, extending from the scaphoid and trapezium to the pisiform and the hook of the hamate (see Fig. 4B), and, more distally, the palmar aponeurosis between the thenar and hypothenar muscles (see Fig. 4C) [24]. The carpal tunnel is narrowest at the level of the hook of hamate and trapezium.

The carpal tunnel contains synovium, the median nerve, and the nine extrinsic flexor tendons of the thumb and fingers, including the flexor pollicis longus tendon, the four flexor digitorum superficialis tendons, and the four flexor

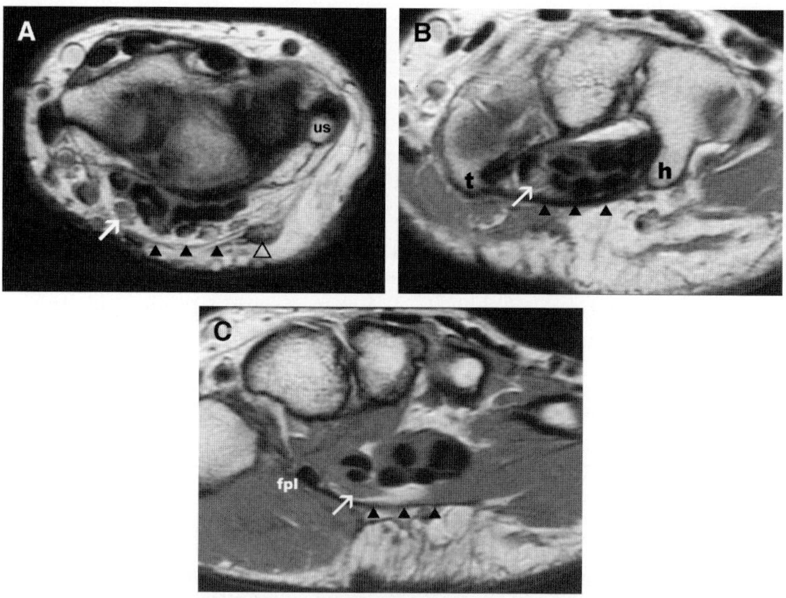

Fig. 4. Normal anatomy—carpal tunnel. (*A*) Axial proton-density weighted image at the level of the proximal carpus demonstrates the median nerve (*arrow*) underneath the antebrachial fascia (*arrowheads*). Flexor carpi ulnaris indicated by open arrowhead. us, ulnar styloid. (*B*) Axial image at the level of the transverse carpal ligament proper (*arrowheads*). Median nerve indicated by arrow. t, trapezium; h, hook of the hamate. (*C*) Axial image at the level of the metacarpals demonstrates the palmar aponeurosis (*arrowheads*) extending between the thenar and hypothenar muscles. Median nerve indicated by arrow. fpl, flexor pollicis longus tendon.

digitorum profundus tendons. Intratunnel bursae are located along the radial aspect of the flexor pollicis longus and ulnar aspect of the flexor digitorum superficialis and profundus to the third and fourth digits.

At the wrist the median nerve supplies the thenar eminence muscles: the abductor pollicis brevis, opponens pollicis, and the superficial head of the flexor pollicis brevis. It also supplies the first and second lumbricals and provides sensation to the palmar and distal dorsal aspects of the radial three and a half fingers.

Ulnar nerve

At the wrist the ulnar nerve, accompanied by the more lateral ulnar artery, traverses superficial to the flexor retinaculum within Guyon's canal, also known as the "pisohamate tunnel" or the "distal ulnar tunnel" [25]. The triangular fibro-osseous tunnel is bordered by the pisiform medially, the hook of the hamate laterally, and the palmar carpal ligament volarly (Fig. 5). The tendons of the flexor digitorum profundus, the transverse carpal ligament, the pisohamate and pisometacarpal ligaments, and the opponens digiti minimi muscle form the floor of the canal.

The ulnar nerve supplies sensory branches to the dorsal ulnar hand and a palmar branch to the skin over the hypothenar eminence proximal to Guyon's canal. Within the canal, the ulnar nerve gives off superficial and deep terminal branches. The superficial branch supplies a branch to the palmaris brevis muscle and provides sensation to the fifth finger and ulnar half of the fourth finger. The deep motor branch takes an acute lateral turn at the hook of the hamate and enters the pisohamate hiatus. This is the most vulnerable site for compression of the deep motor branch of the ulnar nerve. The deep motor branch innervates the hypothenar muscles, including the abductor digiti minimi, flexor digiti minimi, and opponens digiti minimi, as well as the adductor pollicis, the third and fourth lumbricals, and all the interossei muscles.

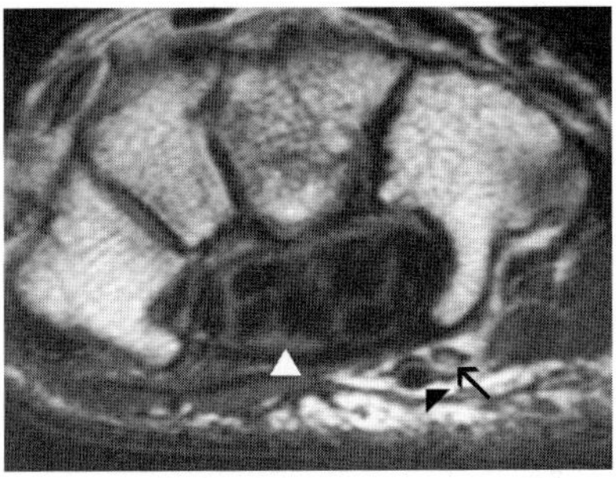

Fig. 5. Normal anatomy—ulnar nerve. Axial proton-density image demonstrates the ulnar nerve (*arrow*) within Guyon's canal. The ulnar nerve travels closer to the hook of the hamate than the adjacent artery and vein (*black arrowhead*). Median nerve indicated by white arrowhead.

NORMAL MR ANATOMY, VARIANTS, AND INTERPRETATION PITFALLS

Tendons

Magic angle effect is not uncommon in the wrist tendons, most frequently observed in the flexor pollicis longus tendon as it courses in the distal aspect of the carpal tunnel and in the palm [26]. Magic angle phenomenon has also been reported in the extensor pollicis longus and extensor carpi ulnaris tendons [27]. The absence of additional pathologic features and the presence of high signal on short TE images without signal alteration on other pulse sequences are highly suggestive of magic angle effect.

A minimal amount of physiologic fluid, often seen within the synovial sheaths, may also cause T2 prolongation around the extensor tendons, not indicative of tenosynovitis [27]. Striations and heterogeneous signal may be noted in the abductor pollicis longus tendon owing to the presence of multiple slips that can simulate longitudinal tears [27]. This appearance can be due to fat interposed between the tendinous fascicles and should not be misinterpreted as a pathologic condition. The positioning of the wrist at the time of MR examination, whether in neutral position, pronation, or supination, will influence the alignment of the extensor carpi ulnaris tendon within its ulnar styloid groove. Pfirrmann and colleagues [28] noted that the tendon is centered in its groove in the neutral position and pronation, whereas subluxation was seen in supination.

Ligaments

The intrinsic ligaments are best assessed on sequential thin-slice coronal MR images. Axial images can also aid in assessing tears, particularly of the scapholunate ligament. The volar and dorsal components of the ligaments extend along most of the proximal to distal margins of the bones, whereas the central components are usually thinner and more proximally located.

The scapholunate ligament often demonstrates a triangular configuration, especially at its central component, and less commonly exhibits a linear configuration [29]. The smaller lunotriquetral ligament is more difficult to visualize and most commonly exhibits a delta shape [30]. Linear or amorphous configurations can also be seen. Although most ligaments display a homogeneous low signal on all pulse-sequences, central or linear vertical intermediate signal may be seen within the scapholunate and lunotriquetral ligaments or at the ligament bone interfaces [29,30]. This intermediate signal should not be misinterpreted as a tear unless fluid signal is seen traversing the ligament or its interface.

The Triangular Fibrocartilage Complex

The triangular fibrocartilage (TFC) thickness is inversely proportional to the length of the ulna. Positive ulnar variance results in a thinner TFC, which may predispose it to tear [31]. Fenestration of the TFC can be seen, especially in older individuals [32,33]. On oblique coronal images, the TFC is triangular, with its apex attaching to the hyaline cartilage of the radius. The cartilaginous increased signal at the interface should not be misconstrued as a tear [18]. The ulnar insertion of the TFC may also have heterogeneous signal [23]. Striation of the dorsal and volar radioulnar ligaments is not uncommon [11]. Finally, fluid or contrast within the prestyloid recess between the TFC and meniscus homologue should not be misconstrued as a ligament tear (see Fig. 2) [23].

Nerves

The median nerve and ulnar nerve are best seen on axial MR images; both display intermediate signal on T1-weighted images and mild increased signal on fluid-sensitive images. The median nerve is round to oval proximal to the carpal tunnel and flat within the tunnel. The division of the nerve into its branches is usually identified at the level of the metacarpals.

Because of its smaller size, variations in the size and signal of the ulnar nerve can be difficult to assess. The nerve is highlighted by fat within Guyon's canal. It abuts the bones bordering the tunnel, a position that can aid in distinguishing it from its accompanying vessels. The ulnar nerve's position varies with wrist motion: it is located ulnar to the hook of hamate in wrist flexion and radial to the hook in wrist extension.

Numerous anatomic variants have been found at both the carpal tunnel (41%) and Guyon's canal (21%) [25,34]. Median nerve variations include alterations in the course of the thenar branch, accessory branches proximal to or at the distal carpal tunnel, bifid median nerve, and high division of the distal median nerve (Fig. 6) [35]. Furthermore, the motor branch may arise in the forearm or may be split by a persistent median artery or an aberrant muscle [35]. Many anomalous muscles have also been described in the carpal tunnel region, such as the reversed palmaris longus muscle, the accessory palmaris profundus, the accessory flexor digitorum superficialis, and aberrant origins of the thenar and lumbrical muscles [35–37].

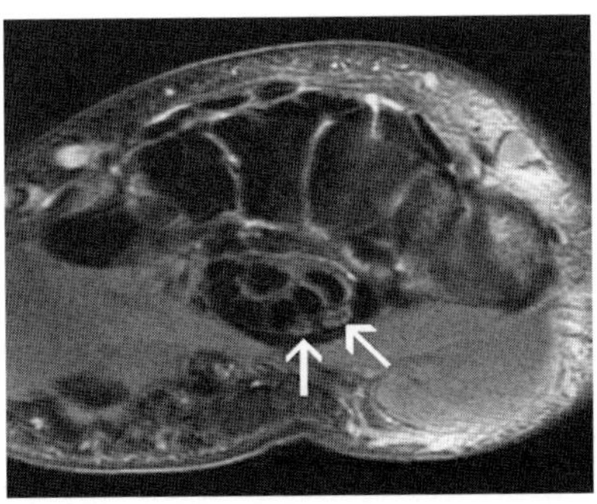

Fig. 6. Bifid median nerve. Axial fat-suppressed T2-weighted image shows high bifurcation of the median nerve (*arrows*) within the distal carpal tunnel.

PATHOLOGY

Tendons

Flexor tendons

Digital flexor tendon injuries in the wrist include lacerations and, less commonly, closed ruptures (Fig. 7) [38]. The latter are usually associated with a variety of underlying chronic conditions that weaken the tendons, such as rheumatoid arthritis, osteoarthritis, scaphoid nonunion [39], Kienbock disease, hook of the hamate fractures, nonhealed distal radial fractures [40], and carpal dislocations. Sudden hyperextension of a flexed finger, most frequently seen in football or rugby players and less commonly following an electrical injury, can also lead to acute closed ruptures [41].

In a series by Drape and colleagues [38], MRI proved useful in displaying the zone of rupture, assessing the edges of the proximal and distal tendons, and accurately measuring the gap between the retracted tendon ends. Gap size is considered an important factor in treatment decision making, because a gap greater than 30 mm necessitates a tendon graft rather than a primary tendon repair [42]. Assessment of integrity of the adjacent tendons before tendon graft may also be accomplished with MRI. MRI can also aid in locating the proximally retracted edge of the tendon, which in some cases may dislocate in between the adjacent tendons or even curl up in the palm [43,44].

In cases of volar carpal subluxation, rupture of the flexor pollicis longus tendon (FPL) may develop from chronic attrition against the volarly displaced scaphoid. Clinically, there is loss of active thumb flexion at the interphalangeal joint. The proximally displaced tendon edge may fold over itself at the entrance of the carpal tunnel, producing carpal tunnel symptoms. Surgical exploration of the volar aspect of the wrist should be performed to look for bony spicules that could have disrupted the FPL.

Tenosynovitis of the FCR is often traumatic in origin and may be secondary to either direct injury or chronic repetitive trauma. The tenosynovitis, however, may also develop insidiously, unrelated to trauma. Clinically, there is pain and crepitus over the FCR tendon in the region just proximal to the flexor creases of the wrist. MR findings include tendon sheath thickening with

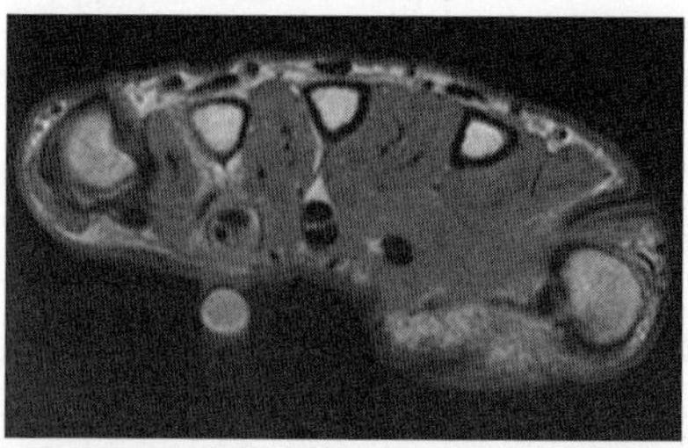

Fig. 7. Flexor tendon laceration. Axial proton-density–weighted image at the level of the metacarpals demonstrates a partial tear of the ring finger superficial flexor tendon (deep to marker) secondary to open laceration.

associated hyperintensity on T2-weighted images (Fig. 8). Inflammatory changes of the scapho-trapezial joint have also been described [45]. Because of its close proximity to the FCR, concomitant median nerve irritation may occur. MRI can be useful in approaching this entity, because the clinical diagnosis can be difficult, and it may be mistaken for scapho-trapezial joint disease, soft tissue ganglion, distal scaphoid fracture, distal radial fracture, and the Linburg syndrome [46].

Extensor tendons

De Quervain's disease is noted commonly in middle-aged women and may be bilateral in as many as 30% of patients. It is characterized by tendinopathy and stenosing tenosynovitis of the first extensor compartment, including the abductor pollicis longus and the extensor pollicis brevis tendons [47]. The condition is most often idiopathic [48]. A septum separating the first extensor compartment tendons has been described in as many as 70% of cases requiring surgical release for de Quervain's tenosynovitis [49]. Other predisposing factors include inflammatory conditions such as rheumatoid arthritis, acute trauma, and chronic repetitive microtrauma from radial and ulnar deviation of the wrist [50].

Typically, de Quervain's syndrome occurs at the level of the radial styloid or slightly proximal to it. The differential diagnosis includes infectious tenosynovitis of the first extensor compartment, first carpometacarpal joint osteoarthritis, FCR tenosynovitis, intersection syndrome, and isolated neuritis of the superficial radial nerve, also called "Wartenberg's syndrome." MRI characteristics are fairly typical and include thickening and heterogeneity of the first compartment tendons and sheath, tenosynovial effusion and surrounding loss of fat planes due to soft tissue edema, and low-signal scar tissue (Fig. 9)

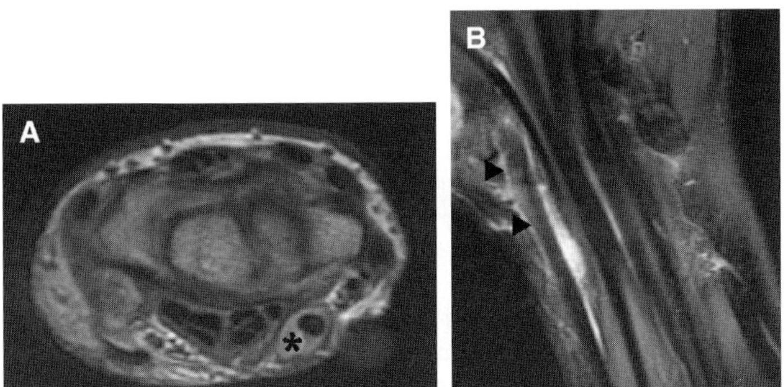

Fig. 8. Flexor carpi radialis longus tenosynovitis and partial rupture. Axial proton-density (*A*) and coronal fat-suppressed (*B*) T2-weighted images show fluid distending the FCR tendon sheath (*asterisk*) associated with intrasubstance tearing (*arrowheads*) at the level of the scaphoid-trapezial joint.

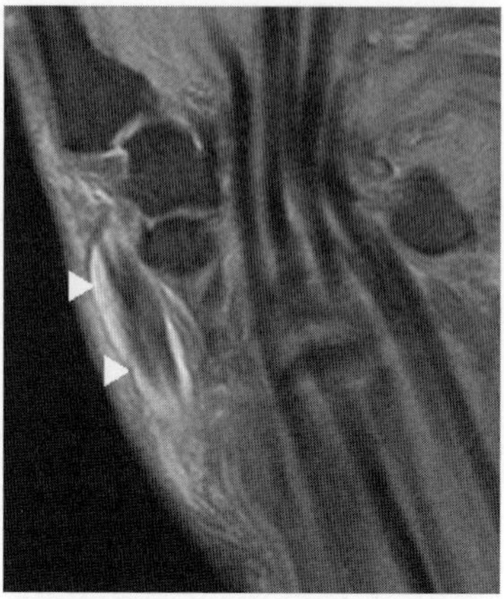

Fig. 9. De Quervain's tenosynovitis. Coronal fat-suppressed T2-weighted image demonstrates tendon sheath effusion, peritendinous edema, and tendon thickening of the first extensor compartment (*arrowheads*).

[47]. MRI can be useful in mapping the course of the superficial radial nerve before surgery and also in identifying causes for postsurgical failure.

The intersection syndrome is characterized by pain and swelling approximately 4 to 8 cm proximal to Lister's tubercle of the radius where the first extensor compartment tendons cross over the second extensor compartment tendons [51]. It is a peritendinosis of the second extensor compartment tendons that is most likely secondary to chronic overuse and friction and is commonly associated with sports-related activities, such as rowing, canoeing, playing racket sports, horseback riding, and skiing [52]. Tendon sheath stenosis can also cause entrapment of the extensor carpi radialis longus and extensor carpi radialis brevis tendons.

Intersection syndrome may be overlooked clinically, so MRI can play a significant role in its diagnosis [53,54]. MR findings reflect peritendinosis and include thickening and interstitial fluid concentrically surrounding the second and the first extensor compartment tendons and tendon sheaths, beginning at the point of crossover and extending proximally. Fluid-sensitive sequences are most useful to demonstrate these changes. Associated reactive tenosynovial effusion can be observed [51].

Chronic friction at Lister's tubercle can produce extensor pollicis longus tenosynovitis and rupture (Fig. 10). Predisposing factors include degenerative or posttraumatic spurring of Lister's tubercle, synovitis associated with rheumatoid arthritis, and systemic lupus erythematosus. Anatomic variants such as an accessory extensor pollicis longus muscle within the third extensor compartment [55] can also predispose to the condition. Nondisplaced or minimally displaced distal radial fractures can produce tears of the extensor pollicis longus (EPL) tendon, typically distal to the extensor retinaculum [56,57] where the

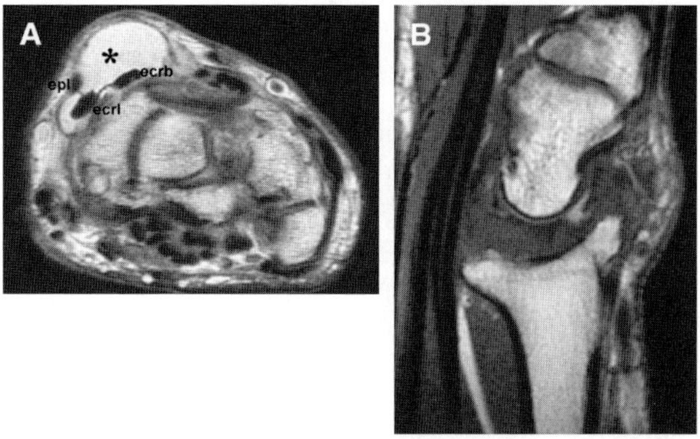

Fig. 10. Tenosynovitis of the extensor pollicis longus, extensor carpi ulnaris brevis, and extensor carpi ulnaris longus tendons associated with postfracture deformity of the distal radius. (*A*) Axial T2-weighted image at the level of the proximal carpal row demonstrates prominent tenosynovial effusion (*asterisk*) involving the extensor carpi radialis longus (ecrl), extensor carpi radialis brevis (ecrb), and extensor pollicis longus (epl) tendons. (*B*) Sagittal T1-weighted image demonstrates a healed fracture of the distal radius with a large dorsal spur.

tendon has decreased vascularity. The rupture usually develops between 3 weeks and 3 months following injury [58,59].

MRI characteristics of EPL tenosynovitis include thickening of the EPL tendon sheath and fluid surrounding the tendon. Stenosing tenosynovitis, noted in chronic cases, is displayed by the presence of low-signal scar tissue about the tendon sheath. Heterogeneity of the tendon consistent with either tendinosis or partial rupture may be seen, but care should be taken not to confuse normal increased signal related to magic-angle effect with tendon disease. In cases of rupture, MRI is useful for locating the retracted tendon margins and for assessing the size of the tendon gap. In acute cases, fluid will help to outline the torn edges. However, chronic tears will often have scar tissue filling the tendon gap, obscuring the torn ends.

Extensor digitorum, extensor indicis, and extensor digiti minimi are susceptible to lacerations because of their superficial position. The ruptures may also be closed injuries, however. MRI can be useful in making the diagnosis of tendon lacerations, because they can be missed clinically when the laceration occurs proximal to the interconnecting junctura. Function of the middle and little fingers' extensor tendons may be preserved through ring finger interconnecting junctura contributing to the distal ends of these tendons when lacerated. Primary surgical repair is mandatory in this type of injury. Digital extensor tendon injuries at the wrist and distal forearm are usually related to deep lacerations and are associated with significant proximal tendon retraction [60,61].

Tenosynovitis of the extensor carpi ulnaris within the sixth compartment is common. Instability of the tendon is frequently associated with the tenosynovitis. Ulnar subluxation of the tendon during supination and volar flexion can occur secondary to disruption of the ulnar aspect of the extensor carpi ulnaris (ECU) tunnel. Causes for dislocation of the ECU tendon include recurrent instability, distal radial fractures with disruption of the extensor retinaculum, and posttraumatic distal radioulnar subluxation.

The MRI characteristics of tenosynovitis of the ECU tendon include thickening of the tendon sheath, tenosynovial effusion, and peritendinous inflammatory changes (Fig. 11). Peritendinous low signal intensity and irregular tendon margins may be seen with chronic stenosing tenosynovitis. Partial tears secondary to chronic attrition of the tendon in patients who have underlying instability or chronic stenosing tenosynovitis [62] demonstrate heterogeneity and splits within the tendon. Closed, nonrheumatoid ruptures of the ECU tendon are rare and have been described in tennis and hockey players [63,64].

Ligaments

Scapholunate instability

Scapholunate instability is the most common carpal instability. It may occur after a traumatic extension injury to the wrist or result from repetitive stress, as in chronic crutch walking [65]. Weakness and pain about the dorsal radial aspect of the wrist are frequent complaints. On clinical examination, a positive scaphoid shift test may be found [66]. This result consists of a click elicited when bringing the wrist from ulnar to radial deviation while the scaphoid tuberosity is stabilized by the examiner's thumb.

The diagnostic work-up of scapholunate instability includes conventional postero-anterior (PA) and lateral radiographs of the wrist. Radiographic signs of scapholunate instability may be seen in advanced stages when the scapholunate and radioscaphoid ligaments are fully torn. These include (1) scapholunate interval widening of more than 3 mm on the PA view; (2) cortical ring sign, in which the scaphoid tuberosity is seen in profile; and (3) disruption of the proximal carpal arc with a step-off in the contour of the scapholunate interval. On the lateral view, a scapholunate angle of more than 70° is consistent

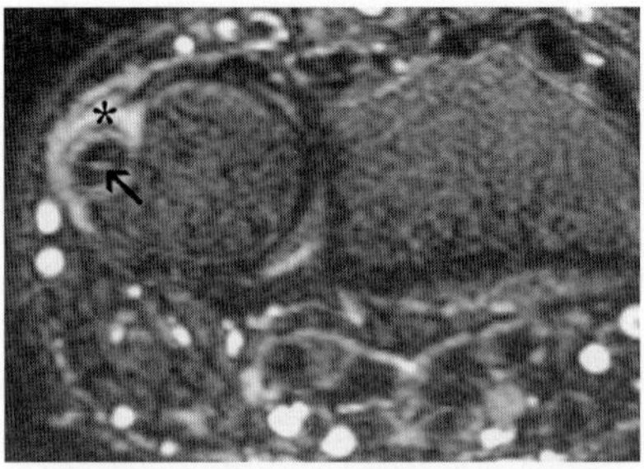

Fig. 11. Partial tear of the extensor carpi ulnaris longus tendon. Axial fat-suppressed T2-weighted image shows intrasubstance longitudinal split of the ECU tendon (*arrow*) associated with peritendinous edema (*asterisk*) at the level of the ulnar styloid.

with scapholunate dissociation. Progressive instability will lead to a dorsal intercalated segment instability pattern of the wrist and, ultimately, to degenerative arthritis [65,67]. The instability is considered static if the abnormalities are noted on static radiographs of the wrist. In some cases, the instability will only become apparent on dynamic radiographic evaluation with clenched-fist PA view or cineradiography.

On MRI, direct visualization of a scapholunate ligament tear may be achieved. Complete tears are characterized by a distinct area of discontinuity within the ligament, outlined by fluid-like T2 hyperintensity, or by complete absence of the ligament (Fig. 12). Fluid signal at the attachment sites of the ligament can also be seen. On MR arthrography, complete tears are outlined by contrast material extravasating through a full-thickness defect. Widening of the scapholunate interval is seen when more than two portions of the ligament are involved. It is believed that injury and tearing of the dorsal portion of the scapholunate ligament must be present for instability to occur [68,69]. Ancillary signs include associated tears of the volar extrinsic radiocarpal ligaments, scaphoid or lunate chondromalacia, bone marrow contusions or fractures (see Fig. 12A), ganglion cysts (usually dorsal), and secondary osteoarthritis. Partial tears are characterized by focal thinning or irregularity in a portion of the ligament (Fig. 13). Partial tears more commonly affect the weaker volar ligamentous attachment [18].

MR arthrography appears to have greater sensitivity in the evaluation of partial tears than routine MRI or conventional arthrography [13,70–72]. MR arthrographic findings include contrast leak or imbibition into a portion of the

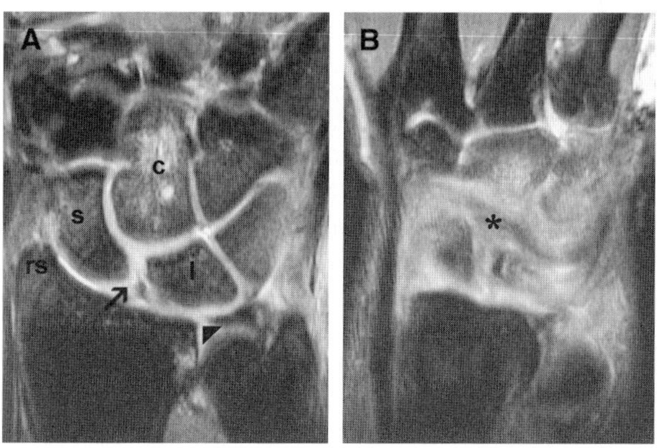

Fig. 12. Scapholunate ligament tear. (*A, B*) Coronal fat-suppressed T2-weighted images demonstrate full-thickness disruption of the scapholunate ligament at its scaphoid insertion (*arrow*), resulting in widening of the scapholunate interval. Associated bone marrow contusions of the lunate, capitate, scaphoid, and radial styloid are present. Also noted are radial avulsion of the triangular fibrocartilage (*arrowhead*) and partial-thickness rupture of the dorsal intercarpal ligament (*asterisk*). c, capitate; l, lunate; rs, radial styloid; s, scaphoid.

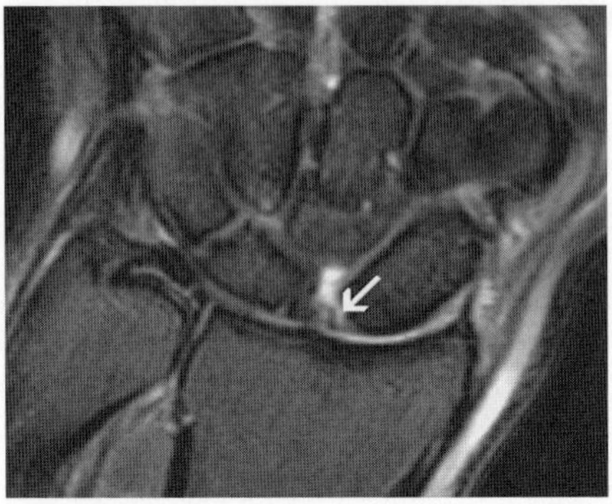

Fig. 13. Scapholunate ligament partial tear. Coronal fat-suppressed T2-weighted image shows a partial tear of the volar portion of the scapholunate ligament outlined by fluid (*arrow*).

injured scapholunate ligament. Ligamentous stretching and elongation without tear can also be seen on MR images.

Lunotriquetral instability

Disruption of the lunotriquetral ligament can be seen as a result of perilunate instability or ulnocarpal abutment. Concurrent static or dynamic patterns of midcarpal instability or volar intercalated segmental instability may also be found. The instability develops secondary to volar tilt of the lunate, along with the scaphoid, secondary to disruption of the lunate attachment to the triquetrum. MR detection of lunotriquetral ligament tears is more difficult, given the smaller size of this structure; therefore, lower sensitivity, specificity, and accuracy have been found as compared with arthroscopy and surgery [13,73].

Triangular fibrocartilage complex

Tears of the TFCC manifest clinically with ulnar-sided wrist pain and tenderness. On physical examination, an audible click or pain may be elicited with rotation of the forearm. Palmer and Werner [15] divided TFCC tears into traumatic and degenerative types. Traumatic tears include central perforation, ulnar avulsion with or without distal ulnar fracture, distal avulsion, and radial avulsion with or without sigmoid notch fracture [15]. Central perforations typically occur 2 to 3 mm medial to the radial insertion site of the TFCC. Unstable ulnar avulsions may be associated with fractures of the ulnar styloid (Fig. 14). Distal avulsion of the TFCC at the insertion into the lunate or triquetrum is indicative of a tear of the ulnolunate or ulnotriquetral ligament or both. Radial avulsion of the TFCC occurs at the distal aspect of the sigmoid notch and may be associated with a radial fracture (Fig. 15). Degenerative tears of the TFCC are part of the spectrum of ulnocarpal abutment syndrome.

On MRI, partial tears of the TFCC can be depicted as fluid-signal intensity on T2-weighted images extending only to one articular surface, more frequently to the proximal articulating surface with the DRUJ [13]. Full-thickness

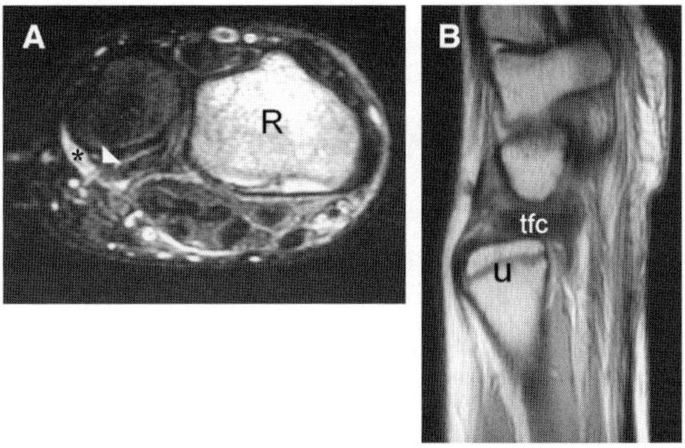

Fig. 14. Ulnar avulsion of the triangular fibrocartilage. (*A*) Axial fat-suppressed T2-weighted image demonstrates complete avulsion of the volar radioulnar ligament (*arrowhead*) outlined by fluid (*asterisk*) in this patient with distal radial fracture. (*B*) Sagittal T1-weighted image shows dorsal subluxation of the distal ulna. R, radius; tfc, triangular fibrocartilage; U, ulna.

defects can be outlined either by joint fluid or intra-articular contrast material. No specific MR signs help to differentiate traumatic from degenerative tears. The age of the patient, location of the tear, and presence of associated lesions such as bruises or fractures may help in this regard. The location of the injury should always be reported. Tears located in the periphery have better blood supply and may be treated with primary repair. By contrast, central lesions are avascular and are treated with debridement.

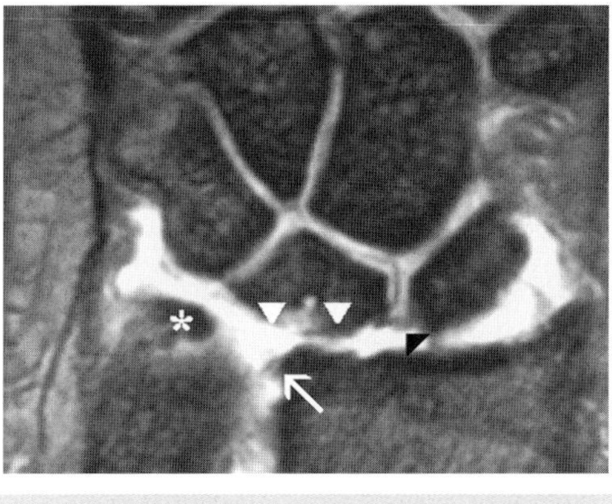

Fig. 15. Radial avulsion of the triangular fibrocartilage. Coronal gradient echo T2*-weighted image shows complete avulsion of the triangular fibrocartilage (*asterisk*) from its attachment to the radius at the distal aspect of the sigmoid notch (*arrow*). Fluid outlines loss of cartilage along the articulating surfaces of the lunate and distal radius (*white arrowheads*) in keeping with secondary osteoarthritis and probable abutment. Scapholunate ligament indicated by black arrowhead.

Nerves

Carpal tunnel syndrome

The most common neuropathy of the upper extremity is the carpal tunnel syndrome, with an estimated incidence of nearly 1% annually, or almost 2.8 million new cases per year, and prevalence of 0.125% to 5.8% [74]. The syndrome is most often found in patients between 30 and 60 years of age, has a male/female ratio of 1:5, and is bilateral in as many as 50% of patients. Clinical complaints include often transient and reversible pain and paresthesia in the median nerve distribution.

In wrist flexion, in asymptomatic individuals, the median nerve moves radially and posteriorly and becomes interposed between the flexor tendons [75]. The median nerve is more likely to remain adjacent to the flexor retinaculum during wrist flexion in patients who have carpal tunnel syndrome. This lack of motion of the median nerve may predispose it to compression and subsequent carpal tunnel syndrome. Other theories proposed to account for carpal tunnel syndrome include repeated compression of the median nerve with subsequent ischemia, subendoneurial edema, synovitis, and eventual fibrosis, as well as reduced gliding and tethering of the nerve due to scar tissue [76].

Increased incidence of carpal tunnel syndrome has been associated with repetitive flexion and extension of the wrist and has been described in swimmers, motocross riders, body-builders, and wheelchair athletes [77–80]. Many other pathologic processes may compress the median nerve within the tunnel, including anomalous muscles, ganglion cysts (Fig. 16), fracture fragments, bony spurs, inflammatory synovial pannus, amyloid deposits, and rice bodies.

Carpal tunnel syndrome is usually an easy clinical and electromyographic diagnosis. Clinical evidence of carpal tunnel syndrome includes a positive Phalen's test (worsened paresthesia following 1 minute of maximal passive wrist flexion) and a positive Tinel's sign (paresthesia in the median territory elicited

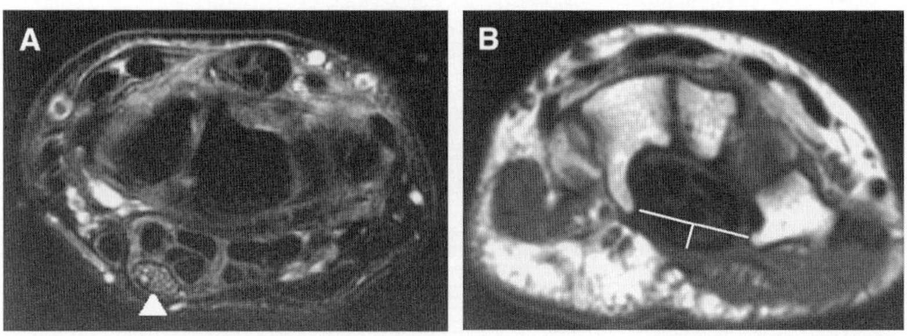

Fig. 16. Carpal tunnel syndrome. (*A*) Axial fat-suppressed T2-weighted image at the proximal carpal tunnel demonstrates high signal intensity and enlargement of the median nerve (*arrowhead*). (*B*) Axial proton-density–weighted image at the level of the transverse carpal ligament shows increased bowing ratio, determined by dividing the palmar displacement of the retinaculum (*short line*) by the distance between the hook of the hamate and the tubercle of the trapezium (*long line*).

by gentle tapping over the carpal tunnel) [81]. These clinical tests, however, are not foolproof, and some symptomatic patients fail to show decreased median nerve conduction velocity [82]. MRI evaluation in this select group of patients can be useful [82,83]. MRI can also depict space-occupying lesions within the carpal tunnel, such as anomalous muscles, persistent median artery, carpal tunnel lipomatosis, ganglion cysts, and synovial hypertrophy.

Disagreement exists in the literature on the most sensitive and most specific MRI findings of carpal tunnel syndrome. Nevertheless, these findings may be divided into four major categories: (1) increased size of the nerve, (2) nerve flattening, (3) bowing of the flexor retinaculum, and (4) increased T2 signal within the median nerve (see Fig. 16A). Significantly increased cross-sectional area of the median nerve is noted in patients who have carpal tunnel syndrome as compared with asymptomatic individuals [84]. Comparison of the cross-sectional area of the nerve at the radiocarpal joint and at the pisiform bone level is best performed on axial MR images. In patients who have carpal tunnel syndrome, the size of the nerve should be about two to three times bigger at the pisiform level compared with the radiocarpal joint level. The ratio between the major and minor axis of the nerve, both at the level of the distal radioulnar joint and at the level of the hook of the hamate, may be used to assess flattening of the nerve. A ratio of three is usually indicative of disease. In normal individuals, the flexor retinaculum at the level of the hook of the hamate should be flat or slightly convex. The degree of bowing is determined by dividing the distance of palmar displacement of the retinaculum by the distance between the hamate's hook and the tubercle of the trapezium (Fig. 16B). In normal patients, the ratio varies from 0 to 0.15 (mean 0.05); in carpal tunnel syndrome, the ratio varies from 0.14 to 0.26 (mean 0.18) [85]. Increased T2 signal within the median nerve may be difficult to assess, because the normal median nerve, like many other nerves in the body, often reveals a slightly increased signal on fat-suppressed T2-weighted fast spin echo images. Intense increased signal, however, is fairly diagnostic of a diseased nerve.

MRI is particularly useful for identifying space-occupying lesions within the carpal tunnel. A variety of median nerve sheath tumors can be identified and often have distinct MR characteristics, including intermediate signal on T1-weighted images and relative homogeneous increased signal on fluid-sensitive sequences. The target sign indicating central low-signal postcontrast enhancement is a fairly specific sign for neurilemmomas.

Another lesion of the median nerve is the fibrolipomatous hamartoma, which has a pathognomic striated increased signal, dubbed "coaxial cable–like," compatible with fat. Other masses within the carpal tunnel, such as ganglions, bursa, fracture fragments, proliferative synovitis, and aberrant muscles, can also be easily displayed on MRI. Aberrant muscles may be identified by their isointense to muscle signal on all pulse sequences.

MRI is useful in identifying persistent median artery or vein within the carpal tunnel. This finding is important to recognize to avoid inadvertent injury to the vessels during surgery. MRI has also been used in the assessment of persistent carpal tunnel syndrome after surgical release. Scar tissue engulfing the nerve, adhesions, persistent tenosynovitis, and incomplete release of the retinaculum may be identified.

Because the diagnostic accuracy of MRI signs of carpal tunnel syndrome is still controversial, particularly when no mass effect is identified, and disagreement exists as to the specificity of nerve swelling and flattening, the presence of MRI indications of carpal tunnel syndrome should not be taken as sole proof of the condition. It should be reviewed in light of the clinical history, physical examination, and electrodiagnostic studies.

Ulnar tunnel syndrome

Compression of the ulnar nerve, although more commonly seen at the elbow, can occasionally occur at the wrist in Guyon's canal. The loss of sensation on the dorsal ulnar hand, present in proximal ulnar compressive neuropathy, can aid in distinguishing elbow and forearm ulnar neuropathy from Guyon's or ulnar tunnel syndrome.

The ulnar nerve can undergo compression at three potential sites within Guyon's canal: (1) zone 1, extending from the proximal edge of the palmar carpal ligament to the bifurcation of the ulnar nerve into the deep motor and superficial sensory branches; (2) zone 2, extending from the bifurcation of the ulnar nerve just distal to the fibrous arch of the hypothenar muscles and containing the deep motor branch of the ulnar nerve; and (3) zone 3, which is parallel to zone 2 and contains the superficial sensory branch of the ulnar nerve.

The clinical presentation can provide clues to the site of ulnar nerve compression: combined motor and sensory deficit is seen in zone 1 lesions, zone 2 lesions display pure motor deficit, and isolated sensory deficits are noted in zone 3 lesions. Most patients undergo ulnar nerve compression at either zone 1 or zone 3; in more than 50% of the cases, the compression occurs in more than one zone [86].

Ulnar nerve compression within Guyon's canal can either be idiopathic (45%) or secondary to trauma (26%) [86]. A displaced hook of the hamate fracture or enlarged hook of the hamate are well-known offending entities (Fig. 17).

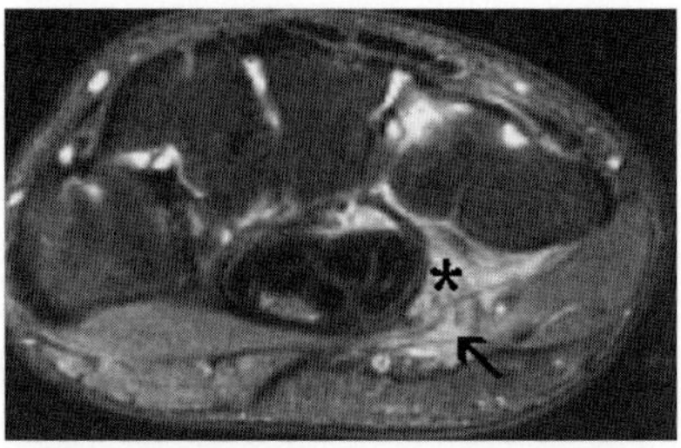

Fig. 17. Hook of the hamate fracture and ulnar neuropathy. Axial fat-suppressed T2-weighted image demonstrates a hook of the hamate fracture (*asterisk*) associated with extensive perineural edema at the level of Guyon's canal (*arrow*).

Isolated compressive neuropathy of the deep terminal motor branch of the ulnar nerve in bikers has been termed handlebar palsy [87] and is related to prolonged riding with the hands pressed against the handlebars. Because no sensory fibers are affected, the patients are not aware of the ongoing nerve compression until a severe nerve lesion develops.

Other causes for ulnar tunnel syndrome include space-occupying lesions, such as tumors, musculotendinous variants, aberrant fibrous bands, and enlarged bursae, and vascular lesions, such as ulnar artery aneurysm and thrombosis [88].

MRI findings of Guyon's canal include increased size and increased signal in the nerve and its branches, best appreciated on axial MR images. The nerve can usually be distinguished from the adjacent bright signal vessels by its closer proximity to the pisiform and hamate bones. Space-occupying lesions such as ganglions, lipomas, and hemangiomas, posttraumatic scarring, and obliteration of the fat around the nerves may be seen. Careful attention should be paid to the presence of aberrant muscles, a common cause of Guyon's canal syndrome. Hook of the hamate fractures are often associated with edema and scarring in the adjacent Guyon's canal. Muscle denervation, edema, and atrophy in the hypothenar and intrinsic muscles should be sought, but this is a less common finding.

References

[1] Strauch B, de Moura W. Digital flexor tendon sheath: an anatomic study. J Hand Surg [Am] 1985;10:785–9.

[2] Bencteux P, Simonet J, el Ayoubi L, et al. Symptomatic palmaris longus muscle variation with MRI and surgical correlation: report of a single case. Surg Radiol Anat 2001;23:273–5.

[3] Schuurman AH, van Gils AP. Reversed palmaris longus muscle on MRI: report of four cases. Eur Radiol 2000;10:1242–4.

[4] Meyer FN, Pflaum BC. Median nerve compression at the wrist caused by a reversed palmaris longus muscle. J Hand Surg [Am] 1987;12(3):369–71.

[5] Zeiss J, Guilliam-Haidet L. MRI demonstration of anomalous muscles about the volar aspect of the wrist and forearm. Clin Imaging 1996;20:219–21.

[6] Mayfield JK. Wrist ligamentous anatomy and pathogenesis of carpal instability. Orthop Clin North Am 1984;15:209–16.

[7] Bozentka DJ. Scapholunate instability. The University of Pennsylvania Orthopaedic Journal 1999;12:27–32.

[8] Berger RA. The anatomy of the ligaments of the wrist and distal radioulnar joints. Clin Orthop 2001;383:32–40.

[9] Taleisnik J. The ligaments of the wrist. J Hand Surg [Am] 1976;1:110–8.

[10] Smith DK. MR imaging of normal and injured wrist ligaments. Magn Reson Imaging Clin N Am 1995;3:229–48.

[11] Theumann NH, Pfirmann CWA, Antonio GE, et al. Extrinsic carpal ligaments: normal MR arthrographic appearance in cadavers. Radiology 2003;226:171–9.

[12] Smith DK. Dorsal carpal ligaments of the wrist: normal appearance on multiplanar reconstructions of three-dimensional Fourier transform MR imaging. AJR Am J Roentgenol 1993;161:119–25.

[13] Brown RR, Fliszar E, Cotton A, et al. Extrinsic and intrinsic ligaments of the wrist: normal and pathologic anatomy at MR arthrography with three-compartment enhancement. Radiographics 1998;18:667–74.

[14] Berger RA. The gross and histologic anatomy of the scapholunate interosseous ligament. J Hand Surg [Am] 1996;21:170–8.

[15] Palmer AK, Werner FW. The triangular fibrocartilage complex of the wrist—anatomy and function. J Hand Surg [Am] 1981;6:153–62.
[16] Sasao S, Beppu M, Kihara H, et al. An anatomical study of the ligaments of the ulnar compartment of the wrist. Hand Surg 2003;3:219–26.
[17] Nishikawa S, Toh S. Anatomical study of the carpal attachment of the triangular fibrocartilage. J Bone Joint Surg Br 2002;84:1062–5.
[18] Zlatkin MB, Rosner J. MR imaging of ligaments and triangular fibrocartilage complex of the wrist. Magn Reson Imaging Clin N Am 2004;12:301–31.
[19] Yoshioka H, Ueno T, Tanaka T, et al. High-resolution MR imaging of the triangular fibrocartilage complex (TFCC): comparison of microscopy coils and a conventional small surface coil. Skeletal Radiol 2003;32:575–81.
[20] Sahin G, Dogan BE, Demirtas M. Virtual MR arthroscopy of the wrist joint: a new intraarticular perspective. Skeletal Radiol 2004;33:9–14.
[21] Saupe N, Prussmann KP, Luechinger R, et al. MR imaging of the wrist: comparison between 1.5- and 3-T MR imaging—preliminary experience. Radiology 2005;234:256–64.
[22] Prendergast N, Rauschning W. Normal anatomy of the hand and wrist. Magn Reson Imaging Clin N Am 1995;3:197–212.
[23] Totterman SM, Miller RJ. MR imaging of the triangular fibrocartilage complex. Magn Reson Imaging Clin N Am 1995;3:213–28.
[24] Cobb TK, Dalley BK, Posteraro RH, et al. Anatomy of the flexor retinaculum. J Hand Surg [Am] 1993;18:91–9.
[25] Zeiss J, Jakab E, Khimji T, et al. The ulnar tunnel at the wrist (Guyon's canal): normal MRI anatomy and variants. AJR Am J Roentgenol 1992;158:1081–5.
[26] Erickson SJ, Cox IH, Hyde JS, et al. Effect of tendon orientation on MRI imaging signal intensity: a manifestation of the "magic angle" phenomenon. Radiology 1991;181: 389–92.
[27] Timins ME, O'Connell SE, Erickson SJ, et al. MR imaging of the wrist: normal findings that may simulate disease. Radiographics 1996;16(5):987–95.
[28] Pfirrmann CW, Theumann NH, Chung CB, et al. What happens to the triangular fibrocartilage complex during pronation and supination of the forearm? Analysis of its morphology and diagnostic assessment with MRI arthrography. Skeletal Radiol 2001;30:677–85.
[29] Smith DK. Scapholunate interosseous ligament of the wrist: ME appearances in asymptomatic volunteers and arthrographically normal wrists. Radiology 1994;192:217–21.
[30] Smith DK, Snearly WN. Lunotriquetral interosseous ligament of the wrist: MR appearances in asymptomatic volunteers and arthrographically normal wrists. Radiology 1994;191: 199–202.
[31] Palmer AK, Glisson RR, Werner FW. Relationship between ulnar variance and triangular fibrocartilage complex thickness. J Hand Surg [Am] 1984;9:681–2.
[32] Kang HS, Kindynis P, Brahme SK, et al. Triangular fibrocartilage and intercarpal ligaments of the wrist: MR imaging. Cadaveric study with gross pathologic and histologic correlation. Radiology 1991;181:401–4.
[33] Mikic Z. Age changes in the triangular fibrocartilage of the wrist joint. J Anat 1978;126: 367–84.
[34] Singer G, Ashworth CR. Anatomic variations and carpal tunnel syndrome: 10 year experience. Clin Orthop 2001;392:330–40.
[35] Lanz U. Anatomical variations of the median nerve in the carpal tunnel. J Hand Surg [Am] 1977;2:44–53.
[36] Siegel DB, Kuzma G, Eakins D. Anatomic investigation of the role of the lumbrical muscles in carpal tunnel syndrome. J Hand Surg [Am] 1995;20:860–3.
[37] Schon R, Kraus E, Boller O, et al. Anomalous muscle belly of the flexor digitorum superficialis associated with carpal tunnel syndrome: case report. Neurosurgery 1992;31:969–97.
[38] Drape JL, Tardif-Chastenet de Gery S, Silbermann-Hoffman O, et al. Closed ruptures of the flexor digitorum tendons: MRI evaluation. Skeletal Radiol 1998;27:617–24.

[39] Saitoh S, Hata Y, Murakami N, et al. Scaphoid nonunion and flexor pollicis longus tendon rupture. J Hand Surg [Am] 1999;24:1211–9.
[40] Kato N, Nemoto K, Arino H, et al. Ruptures of flexor tendons at the wrist as a complication of fracture of the distal radius. Scand J Plast Reconstr Surg Hand Surg 2002;36:245–8.
[41] Concannon MJ, Duffy FJ Jr, Palmer WE, et al. Late rupture of a flexor tendon after electrical injury: localization using magnetic resonance imaging. A case report. Ann Plast Surg 1996;36:84–7.
[42] Boyes JH, Stark HH. Flexor tendon grafts in the fingers and thumb. A study of factors influencing results in cases. J Bone Joint Surg Am 1971;53:1332–42.
[43] Kumar BA, Tolat AR, Threepuraneni G, et al. The role of magnetic resonance imaging in late presentation of rupture of the flexor digitorum profundus tendon in the finger. J Hand Surg [Br] 2000;25:95–7.
[44] Rubin DA, Kneeland JB, Kitay GS, et al. Flexor tendon tears in the hand: use of MRI imaging to diagnose degree of injury in a cadaver model. AJR Am J Roentgenol 1996;166:615–20.
[45] Irwin LR, Outhwaite J, Burge PD. Rupture of the flexor carpi radialis tendon associated with scapho-trapezial osteoarthritis. J Hand Surg [Br] 1992;17:343–5.
[46] Rennie WR, Muller H. Linburg syndrome. Can J Surg 1998;41(4):306–8.
[47] Glajchen N, Schweitzer M. MRI features in de Quervain's tenosynovitis of the wrist. Skeletal Radiol 1996;25:63–5.
[48] Witt J, Pess G, Gelberman TH. Treatment of de Quervain's tenosynovitis. J Bone Joint Surg Am 1991;73:218–21.
[49] Viegas S. Trigger thumb of de Quervain's disease. J Hand Surg [Am] 1986;11:235–6.
[50] Watson F. Nonarthritic inflammatory problems of the hand and wrist. Emerg Med Clin North Am 1985;3:275–82.
[51] Costa CR, Morrison WB, Carrino JA. MRI features of intersection syndrome of the forearm. AJR Am J Roentgenol 2003;181:1241–9.
[52] Hanlon DP, Luellen JR. Intersection syndrome: a case report and review of the literature. J Emerg Med 1999;6:969–71.
[53] de Lima JE, Kim HJ, Albertotti F, et al. Intersection syndrome MR imaging with anatomical comparisons of the distal forearm. Skeletal Rad 2004;33:627–31.
[54] Grundberg AB, Reagan DS. Pathologic anatomy of the forearm. Intersection syndrome. J Hand Surg [Am] 1985;10:299–302.
[55] Beatty JD, Remedios D, McCullough CJ. An accessory extensor tendon of the thumb as a cause of dorsal wrist pain. J Hand Surg [Br] 2000;25:110–1.
[56] Payne AJ, Harris NJ, Kehoe NJ. Bilateral delayed extensor pollicis longus rupture following bilateral undisplaced distal radial fractures. Orthopedics 2000;23:163.
[57] Hirasawa Y, Katsumi Y, Akiyoshi T, et al. Clinical and crioangiographic studies on rupture of the E.P.L. tendon after distal radial fractures. J Hand Surg [Br] 1990;15:51–7.
[58] Bonatz E, Kramer TD, Masear VR. Rupture of the extensor pollicis longus tendon. Am J Orthop 1996;25:118–22.
[59] Skoff HD. Post fracture extensor pollicis longus tenosynovitis and tendon rupture: a scientific study and personal series. Am J Orthop 2003;32:245–7.
[60] Rockwell WB, Butler PN, Byrne BA. Extensor tendon: anatomy, injury and reconstruction. Plast Reconstr Surg 2000;106:1592–603.
[61] Kameyama M, Shiraishi T. Traumatic rupture of the extensor digitorum communis and extensor digiti minimi at the musculotendinous junction associated with volar dislocation of the distal radioulnar joint. A case report. Hand Surg 2000;5:165–8.
[62] Crimmins CA, Jones NF. Stenosing tenosynovitis of the extensor carpi ulnaris. Ann Plast Surg 1995;35:105–7.
[63] Xarchas KC, Leviet D. Non rheumatoid closed rupture of extensor carpi ulnaris tendon. Report of a case in a professional athlete. Acta Orthop Belg 2002;68(4):399–402.
[64] Wang C, Gill TJ 4th, Zarins B, et al. Extensor carpi ulnaris tendon rupture in an ice hockey player: a case report. Am J Sports Med 2003;31(3):459–61.

[65] Taleisnik J. Current concepts review: carpal instability. J Bone Joint Surg Am 1988;70: 1262–7.
[66] Taleisnik J, Linscheid RL. Scapholunate instability. In: Cooney WP, Linsheid RL, Dobyns JH, editors. The wrist: diagnosis and operative treatment. Philadelphia: Mosby; 1998. p. 501–26.
[67] Dagum AB, Hurst LC, Finzel KC. Scapholunate dissociation: an experimental kinematic study of two types of indirect soft tissue repairs. J Hand Surg [Am] 1997;22:714–9.
[68] Linscheid RL, Dobyns JH, Beabout JW, et al. Traumatic instability of the wrist: diagnosis, classification and pathomechanics. J Bone Joint Surg Am 2002;84:142.
[69] Ruby LK, An KN, Linscheid RL, et al. The effect of scapholunate ligament section on scapholunate motion. J Hand Surg [Am] 1987;12:767–71.
[70] Scheck RJ, Kubitzek C, Hierner R, et al. The scapholunate interosseous ligament in MR arthrography of the wrist: correlation with non-enhanced MRI and wrist arthroscopy. Skeletal Radiol 1997;26:263–71.
[71] Scheck RJ, Romagnolo A, Hierner R, et al. The carpal ligaments in MR arthrography of the wrist: correlation with standard MRI and wrist arthroscopy. J Magn Reson Imaging 1999;9: 468–74.
[72] Zanetti M, Bram J, Hodler J. Triangular fibrocartilage and intercarpal ligaments of the wrist: does MR arthrography improve standard MRI? J Magn Reson Imaging 1997;7:590–4
[73] Zlatkin MB, Chao PC, Osterman AL, et al. Chronic wrist pain: evaluation with high-resolution MR imaging. Radiology 1989;173:723–9.
[74] De Krom MC, Knipschild PG, Kester AD, et al. Carpal tunnel syndrome: prevalence in the general population. J Clin Epidemiol 1992;45(4):373–6.
[75] Zeiss J, Skie M, Ebraheim N, et al. Anatomic relations between the median nerve and flexor tendons in the carpal tunnel: MRI evaluation in normal volunteer. AJR Am J Roentgenol 1989;153:533–6.
[76] Rempel D, Dahlin L, Lundborg G. Pathophysiology of nerve compression syndrome: response of peripheral nerves to loading. J Bone Joint Surg Am 1999;81:1600–10.
[77] Mauer UM, Rath SA. Stress-induced carpal tunnel syndrome in athletes. Schweiz Z Sportmed 1992;40:131–5.
[78] Lorei MP, Hershman EB. Peripheral nerve injuries in athletes. Treatment and prevention. Sports Med 1993;16:130–47.
[79] Krivickas LS, Wilbourn AJ. Peripheral nerve injuries in athletes: a case series of over 200 injuries. Semin Neurol 2000;20(2):225–32.
[80] Boninger ML, Robertson RN, Wolff M, et al. Upper limb nerve entrapments in elite wheelchair racers. Am J Phys Med Rehabil 1996;75(3):170–6.
[81] Katz JN, Larson MG, Sabra A, et al. The carpal tunnel syndrome: diagnostic utility of the history and physical examination findings. Ann Intern Med 1990;112:321–7.
[82] Bordalo-Rodriques M, Amin P, Rosenberg ZS. MR imaging of common entrapment neuropathies at the wrist. Magn Reson Imaging Clin N Am 2004;12:265–79.
[83] Horch RE, Allman KH, Laudenberger J, et al. Median nerve compression can be detected by magnetic resonance imaging of the carpal tunnel. Neurosurgery 1997;41:76–82.
[84] Jarvik JG, Yuen E, Haynor DR, et al. MR nerve imaging in a prospective cohort of patients with suspected carpal tunnel syndrome. Neurology 2002;58:1597–602.
[85] Mesgarzadeh M, Triolo J, Schneck CD. Carpal tunnel syndrome. MR imaging diagnosis. Magn Reson Imaging Clin N Am 1995;3:249–64.
[86] Murata K, Shih JT, Tsai TM. Causes of ulnar tunnel syndrome: a retrospective study of 31 subjects. J Hand Surg [Am] 2003;28:647–51.
[87] Capitani D, Beer S. Handlebar palsy—a compression syndrome of the deep terminal (motor) branch of the ulnar nerve in biking. J Neurol 2002;249:1441–5.
[88] Yoshii S, Ikeda K, Murakami H. Ulnar nerve compression secondary to ulnar artery true aneurysm at Guyon's canal. J Neurosurg Sci 1999;43(4):295–7.

Clin Sports Med 25 (2006) 433–443
CLINICS IN SPORTS MEDICINE

Imaging of the Painful Shoulder in Throwing Athletes

Josh B. Moosikasuwan, MD[a], Theodore T. Miller, MD[a,*], David M. Dines, MD[b]

[a]Department of Radiology, North Shore University Hospital, 825 Northern Boulevard, Great Neck, NY 11021, USA
[b]Department of Orthopaedic Surgery, Albert Einstein College of Medicine at Long Island Jewish Medical Center, 270-05 76th Avenue, New Hyde Park, NY 11040, USA

Throwing athletes are prone to shoulder injuries due to the extreme positioning of the shoulder in the various phases of the throw, the adaptive changes that develop over time to allow an advantageous arc of motion, and the chronic, repetitive nature of an activity that places such a high demand on the shoulder joint. The injuries are often particular to a specific phase of the throw and are well demonstrated with MRI. In this article, the authors review the phases of the throw, MRI techniques, and the MR appearances of the injuries associated with particular phases.

PHASES OF THE THROW

Baseball-throwing motion may be divided into six phases: wind-up, early cocking, late cocking, acceleration, deceleration, and follow-through. The position of the humerus during these phases changes in three dimensions: vertically in the coronal plane, horizontally in the anterior–posterior direction, and rotationally. Vertically, the humerus begins in minimal mild abduction during the wind-up phase and proceeds to 90° abduction in the early cocking phase, where it changes minimally and is maintained in 90° to 100° of abduction until it decreases at the end of the throw. In the horizontal plane, the humerus begins in a neutral position, is extended 15° posteriorly in the early cocking phase, starts to move forward in the late cocking phase, and is in approximately 35° and 60° of horizontal adduction in the deceleration and follow-through phases, respectively. Rotationally, the arm begins in internal rotation during the wind-up phase, is maximally externally rotated in the late cocking phase, and is then quickly internally rotated, ranging from 0° to 30° of internal rotation during

*Corresponding author. Department of Radiology, North Shore University Hospital, 825 Northern Boulevard, Great Neck, NY 11021. *E-mail address:* tmiller@nshs.edu (T.T. Miller).

0278-5919/06/$ – see front matter
doi:10.1016/j.csm.2006.02.005

sportsmed.theclinics.com

the deceleration and follow-through phases, respectively [1]. These glenohumeral relationships are peculiar to baseball throwing because the throw is usually performed mildly "side-arm," whereas football throwing is a more overhead activity.

IMAGING TECHNIQUES

Conventional MRI, supplemented with MR arthrography, can accurately diagnose injuries sustained by the throwing athlete, such as rotator cuff tears and tendinosis, as well as labral and capsuloligamentous pathologic conditions [2–4]. MR arthrography requires the intra-articular injection of 12 mL or more of a dilute gadolinium solution (1:250 or 2 mmol/L) to distend the joint capsule and outline the labral and articular surface tears of the rotator cuff [5]. At a concentration of 2 mmol/L, the paramagnetic effect of gadolinium and hence its signal intensity on T1-weighted images in a 1.5 Telsa magnetic field are optimal [6]. Indirect MR arthrography with intravenous administration of gadolinium may also be performed; this is dependent on diffusion of contrast into the joint space from the highly vascular synovium. Though it is less invasive than direct MR arthrography, lack of joint distention makes this technique less useful for labral tears [7].

Imaging of the shoulder may be performed with the arm in a neutral position or may be performed with the arm in the abducted and externally rotated (ABER) position by having the patient place the hand behind the head. The ABER position mimics the late cocking phase of the throw, stretches the anterior capsuloligamentous structures, in particular the anterior band of the inferior glenohumeral ligament, and allows better visualization of the posterosuperior aspect of the labrum and the undersurface of the supraspinatus tendon [8–12]. If the patient is unable to tolerate the ABER position, full external rotation of the conventionally positioned arm will similarly stretch the anterior capsule [12,13], but this position does not simulate the cocking phase.

MECHANISM OF INJURY AND IMAGING FINDINGS—THE LATE COCKING PHASE

The extreme positioning of the humerus in maximum external rotation and 90° of abduction can, over time, stretch the anterior capsule and ligaments, leading to anterior capsular laxity and resultant microinstability or even frank anterior humeral translation. Microinstability may be assessed clinically by a positive "apprehension test" in which the patient has a sense of apprehension as his or her arm approaches the ABER position. Posterosuperior or "internal" impingement, in which the posterior aspect of the supraspinatus tendon and the anterior aspect of the infraspinatus tendon are compressed against the posterosuperior aspect of the labrum and the glenoid, may ensue as a result of microinstability and anterior translation of the humeral head. Although this compression can be a normal finding with overhead movements [14–16], it may also produce posterior shoulder pain [17,18]. Internal impingement may be assessed clinically with the "relocation test of Jobe," in which, with the arm in the ABER position, the examiner holds the humeral head and pushes it anteriorly to produce pain and then posteriorly to relieve the pain. This test reproduces the impingement of the supraspinatus and infraspinatus tendons on the posterosuperior glenoid rim that occurs from anterior humeral subluxation in a shoulder with lax anterior restraints [19–21]. Decreased range of motion may also be present and may be seen on clinical examination as loss of internal rotation ("glenohumeral internal rotation deficiency," defined relative to the contralateral nonthrowing arm), weakness of scapular retraction, and weakness of upward rotation of the humerus. These can all contribute to loss of control and velocity during the throw, referred to as the "dead arm" syndrome [22,23]. Microinstability may also allow superior translation of the humeral head, which may then impinge the supraspinatus and infraspinatus tendons against the acromion or clavicle; this is referred to as secondary impingement [14].

Internal impingement may lead to "kissing" lesions on the glenoid and humeral sides of the joint due to repetitive impaction. On the humeral side, the supraspinatus and infraspinatus tendons and greater tuberosity are affected, whereas on the glenoid side, the posterosuperior aspect of the labrum and subchondral bone are affected. Kaplan and colleagues [23], Giaroli and colleagues [24], and Giombini and colleagues [25] all found similar constellations of abnormalities on MR imaging. In the study of Giaroli and colleagues, all six of their patients with clinically and arthroscopically diagnosed internal impingement had undersurface tears of the supraspinatus or infraspinatus tendons (Fig. 1) and had posterosuperior labral pathologic conditions, such as abnormal signal, fraying, or frank tears [24]. In a retrospective study of nine throwing athletes who had severe internal impingement, Kaplan and colleagues [23] found that all nine had posterosuperior labral lesions, eight with labral fraying and one with a tear, found on both MRI and arthroscopy. All had infraspinatus tendinopathy, and three had supraspinatus tendinopathy. Similarly, in the prospective study by Giombini and colleagues [25] of 11 water polo players complaining of shoulder pain, posterosuperior labral injury and partial tears of the undersurface of the rotator cuff were detected in all 11 athletes on both MRI and arthroscopy. Rotator cuff tendinopathy and tears involve the posterior aspect of the supraspinatus tendon or the anterior aspect of the infraspinatus tendon [17,18].

The bony changes that can occur in the posterior aspect of the greater tuberosity include subcortical cysts subjacent to the attachment of the supraspinatus and infraspinatus tendons (Fig. 2), flattening or focal indentation of the humeral head mimicking a Hill-Sachs defect (Figs. 3 and 4), and bone marrow edema, whereas subchondral sclerosis may occur in the posterosuperior aspect of the glenoid (Fig. 5) [23–25]. In Kaplan's [23] nine cases, eight had sclerosis in the posterosuperior aspect of the glenoid, whereas in Giombini's study [25], four had erosions of the posterosuperior glenoid, and five had osteochondral defects in the posterior aspect of the humeral head on radiographs.

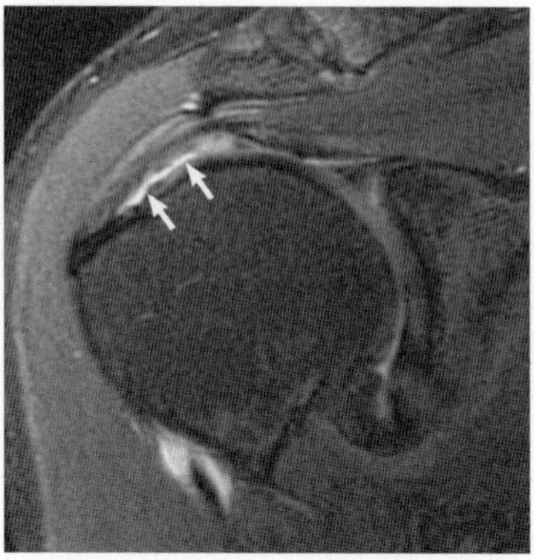

Fig. 1. Extensive articular surface tear of the supraspinatus tendon. Coronal fat-suppressed T2-weighted image shows extensive but shallow tearing of the articular surface of the supraspinatus tendon (*arrows*).

In addition, in the abducted and externally rotated position in the late cocking phase, the long head of the biceps tendon has a more vertical and posterior course and is twisted at its base. This causes a posteriorly directed torsional force on the labrum and can lead to shearing and peeling back of the labrum from the glenoid, producing superior labral anterior posterior (SLAP) tears [26].

Superior labral lesions were originally described in 1985 by Andrews and colleagues [27]. SLAP tears were initially classified into four types in 1990 by Snyder and colleagues [28], but there are now at least 10 types [3]. Type I lesions involve fraying of the superior aspect of the labrum and are usually not

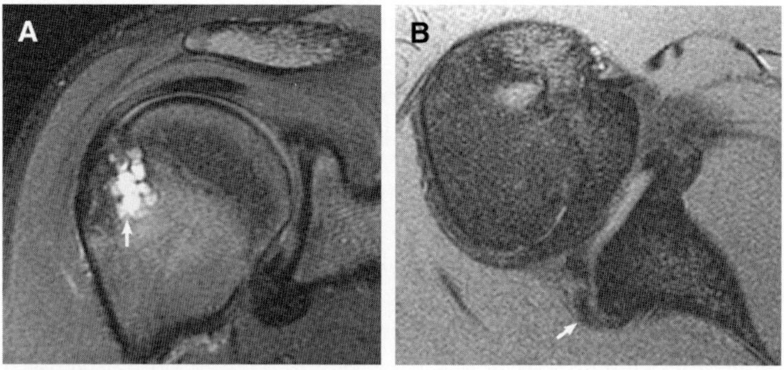

Fig. 2. Subcortical cysts and posterior capsular stripping in a 16-year-old male who had right shoulder pain when throwing for 3 months. (*A*) Subcortical cysts (*arrow*) in the greater tuberosity at the insertion of the supraspinatus tendon are seen as high signal intensity on a fat-suppressed T2-weighted image. (*B*) Axial gradient echo T2-weighted image shows a nondisplaced tear of the posterior labrum and capsular stripping (*arrow*).

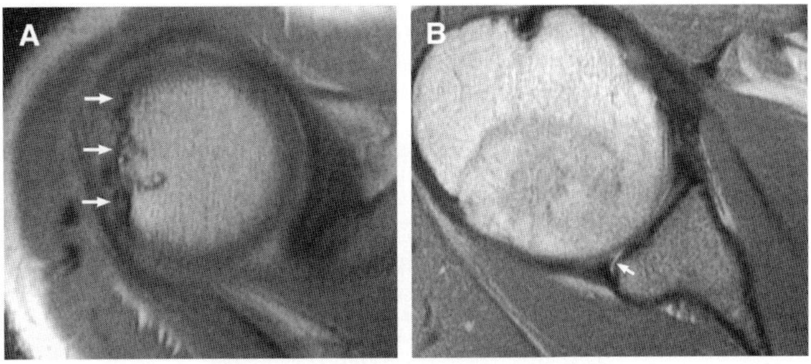

Fig. 3. Posterosuperior labral tear and impaction of the greater tuberosity in a 17-year-old female pitcher who had right shoulder pain and impingement for 5 years. (*A*) Axial proton-density image through the superior humeral head, which should normally be round, shows flattening of the posterosuperior aspect (*arrows*). (*B*) Axial proton-density weighted image demonstrates curvilinear high signal intensity extending from the articular surface into the posterior aspect of the labral (*arrow*), indicating a nondetached tear.

clinically significant and not repaired. In a Type II lesion, there is frank stripping of the superior part of the labrum along with the attached long head of the biceps tendon from the glenoid labrum (Fig. 6). Types III and IV are buckle-handle tears of the labrum that do not or do extend into the long head of the biceps tendon, respectively. Type I and II tears are associated with throwing, whereas Type III and IV tears are associated with a fall on an outstretched arm [29]. Type II lesions are the most common; these have been divided into A, B, and C subtypes, which involve the anterosuperior, posterosuperior (resulting from internal impingement), or entire superior half of the labrum, respectively [30]. MRI findings may be linear abnormal signal intensity within the labrum that extends to the labral surface or frank cleavage of the labrum.

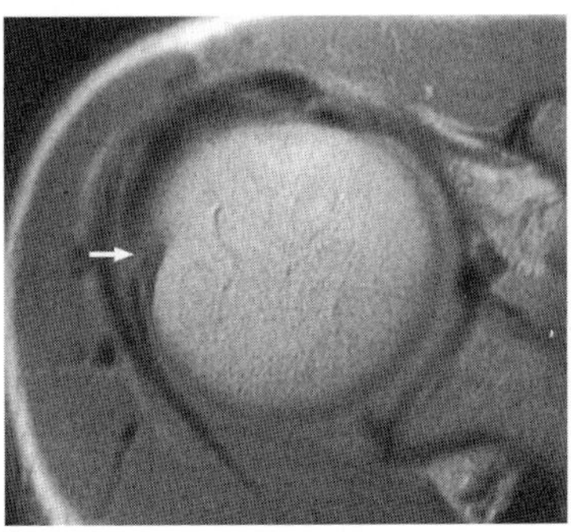

Fig. 4. Axial proton-density image shows a small focal divot in the posterosuperior aspect of the humeral head (*arrow*), mimicking a Hill-Sachs defect, in a 16-year-old male who had pain when throwing for 2 to 3 years.

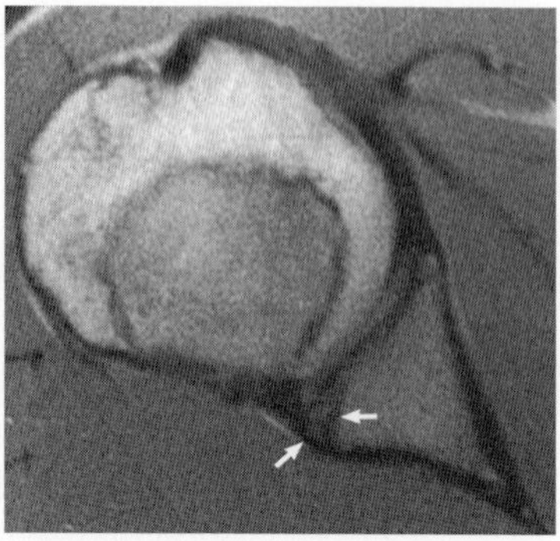

Fig. 5. Posterosuperior glenoid sclerosis in a 15-year-old male who had pain when throwing a baseball. Axial proton-density weighted image at the level of the proximal humeral physis demonstrates decreased signal intensity within the posterosuperior aspect of the glenoid (*arrows*) due to sclerosis.

On MR arthrography, contrast material insinuates into the tears [3]. The sensitivity for detection of SLAP lesions on conventional MRI ranges widely, but it is generally 75% to 86%, with sensitivities reported as low as 41% and as high as 98% in four separate studies [31–34]. The sensitivity for MR arthrography ranges from 82% to 89% [29,35,36]. Arm traction may also be applied to the wrist using 1- to 3-kg weights during MR arthrography with the arm in external rotation to improve accuracy in detecting and characterizing SLAP tears. Using this technique in a cadaver model, two observers detected six of seven and five of seven SLAP tears without traction; these figures increased to seven and six, respectively, with arm traction. In addition, both observers categorized only three of seven SLAP tears correctly without traction but characterized six

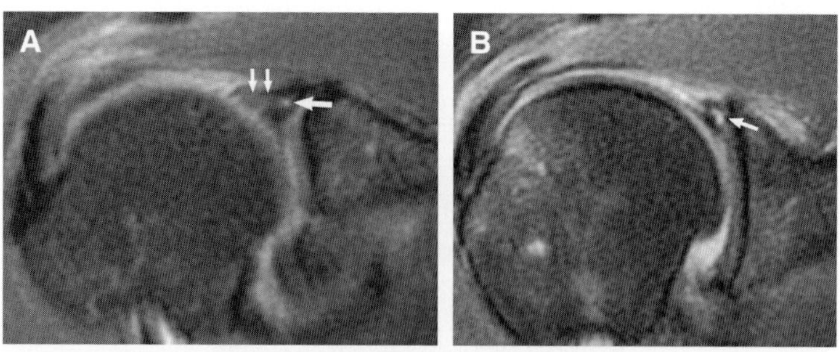

Fig. 6. Type II SLAP tear. (*A*) Oblique coronal fat-suppressed T2-weighted image at the biceps–labral junction demonstrates irregularity of the undersurface of the biceps (*small arrows*), due to fraying and shallow tears, and linear high signal intensity tear (*large arrow*) in the superior aspect of the labrum. (*B*) Oblique coronal fat-suppressed T2-weighted image posterior to the biceps–labral junction shows the high signal intensity tear (*arrow*) in the superior labrum.

correctly with arm traction [13]. In clinical series, undercalling and overcalling of Type I lesions, as well as confusion of Type II lesions with the sublabral recesses and foramen, which are normal anatomic variants, have been cited as potential sources of decreased accuracy [3,29].

Bennett [37] described mineralization of the posterior inferior glenoid in overhead throwing athletes and believed it was due to traction from the long head of the triceps muscle. However, it actually occurs in the area of the attachment of the posterior band of the inferior glenohumeral ligament [38] and represents a sign of chronic capsular traction from the repetitive throwing motion [39]. Although the Bennett's lesion has been associated with posterior shoulder pain during the late cocking, acceleration, and follow-through phases of the throw [40], it is also found in asymptomatic pitchers [39]. Radiographically, the lesion may be best detected with the patient supine, the beam angled 5° cephalad, and the arm abducted 90° and externally rotated 90° [37]. Alternatively, CT can demonstrate the small traction osteophyte as a crescent-shaped focus of calcification in the posteroinferior aspect of the labrum extending toward the humeral head [41,42]. The lesion may also be seen on axial MR images as a focus of signal void when it is calcified, or as having the same signal as the bony glenoid when it is ossified (Fig. 7). Patients who have larger Bennett's lesions (>100 mm^2) tend to have poorer outcomes, with failure to return to their preinjury levels of activity [39].

MECHANISM OF INJURY AND IMAGING FINDINGS—THE DECELERATION PHASE

During the deceleration phase, after ball release, there is strong eccentric contraction of all muscle groups to maintain the humerus within the glenoid fossa. Joint loads and compressive forces can be large enough to cause rotator cuff tears [43]. These compressive forces, combined with internal rotation and anterior displacement of the humerus, can also cause grinding of the humeral head on the biceps tendon and anterosuperior aspect of the labrum and lead

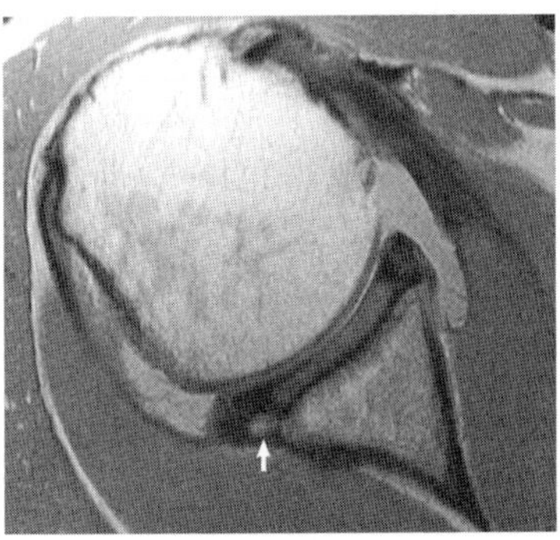

Fig. 7. Bennett's lesion. Axial proton-density weighted image shows an ossified spur (*arrow*) arising from the posterior inferior aspect of the glenoid.

to SLAP tears [27]. Repetitive traction on the superior aspect of the labrum from contraction of the long head of the biceps tendon during the deceleration phase further predisposes to SLAP tears [44].

Coracoid or subcoracoid impingement is another cause of shoulder pain that may occur during the deceleration phase. The pain is anteromedial, is accentuated by cross-arm adduction, internal rotation, and forward flexion (the "coracoid impingement test"), and is due to impingement of the subscapularis between the lesser tuberosity and coracoid [45,46]. Patients who have this type of impingement have a narrow distance between the lesser tuberosity of the humeral head and the lateral aspect of the coracoid. The narrowing may be congenital due to a long or lateral coracoid, posttraumatic resulting from fracture deformity of either the coracoid or humeral head (especially the lesser tuberosity), or iatrogenic resulting from glenoid osteotomy or coracoplasty [45,46].

The coracohumeral distance may be evaluated radiographically on an axillary view or an anteroposterior view that is perpendicular to the scapular plane [47]. Using axial CT images, Gerber and colleagues [48] evaluated 47 normal shoulders with the arm at the side in external, neutral, and internal rotation. They found that the narrowest coracohumeral distance occurred in internal rotation, with an average distance of 8.7 mm. Twenty of these shoulders were then scanned in forward flexion/internal rotation, and the coracohumeral distance decreased to 6.8 mm. Such a decreased coracohumeral distance does not necessarily predict subcoracoid impingement, however. Giaroli and colleagues [49], in a retrospective analysis of axial MR images with the shoulders in neutral or external rotation, found an average coracohumeral distance of 6.2 mm (range 2 to 9 mm) in seven patients who had clinically suspected subcoracoid impingement. However, they found an even narrower average distance of 5.1 mm (range 3 to 10 mm) in nine patients who had shoulder pain but who did not have a specific clinical suspicion of subcoracoid impingement or surgical evidence of such impingement. None of the seven patients who had clinical impingement had secondary signs on MRI, such as edema in the intervening soft tissues or in the marrow of the humerus or coracoid. Giaroli and colleagues concluded that the standard positioning of the shoulder for routine MRI, which is neutral or external rotation, may be inaccurate for evaluating subcoracoid impingement. They caution that, although a narrow coracohumeral distance on MRI may suggest impingement or corroborate the clinical suspicion, the diagnosis of subcoracoid impingement itself remains clinical.

OTHER IMAGING FINDINGS

In contrast to secondary impingement, which is due to superior instability of the humeral head, intrinsic narrowing of the supraspinatus outlet with compression of the subacromial bursa and supraspinatus tendon can also cause pain. This condition is referred to as primary impingement and is not specific to any phase of the throw. It may be caused by acquired structural changes, such as a hooked acromion morphology [50] and acromioclavicular arthrosis

[51], or by congenital changes, such as an accessory acromial ossicle [52] or a thick coracoacromial ligament [53]. Primary impingement is commonly seen in football quarterbacks, because of the direct overhead motion of the throw, and in other overhead athletes, such as tennis players during the serve and freestyle swimmers.

SUMMARY

A wide spectrum of abnormalities can affect the throwing shoulder. Knowledge of the athletic activity or particular phase in which pain occurs can guide the radiologist to the most likely site of involvement on the MRI examinations.

References

[1] Beltran J, Kim DH. MR imaging of shoulder instability injuries in the athlete. Magn Reson Imaging Clin N Am 2003;11:221–38.
[2] Roger B, Skaf A, Hooper AW, et al. Imaging findings in the dominant shoulder of throwing athletes: comparison of radiography, arthrography, CT arthrography, and MR arthrography with arthroscopic correlation. AJR Am J Roentgenol 1999;172:1371–80.
[3] Mohana-Borges AVR, Chung CB, Resnick D. Superior labral anteroposterior tear: classification and diagnosis on MRI and MR arthrography. AJR Am J Roentgenol 2003;181:1449–62.
[4] Tirman PF, Bost FW, Garvin GJ, et al. Posterosuperior glenoid impingement of the shoulder: findings at MR imaging and MR arthrography with arthroscopic correlation. Radiology 1994;193(2):431–6.
[5] Steinbach LS, Palmer WE, Schweitzer MEMR. Arthrography. Radiographics 2002;22:1223–46.
[6] Hajek PC, Sartoris DJ, Neumann CH, et al. Potential contrast agents for MR arthrography: in vitro evaluation and practical observations. AJR Am J Roentgenol 1987;149:97–104.
[7] Bergin D, Schweitzer ME. Indirect magnetic resonance arthrography. Skeletal Radiol 2003;32:551–8.
[8] Tirman PF, Bost FW, Steinbach LS, et al. MR arthrographic depiction of tears of the rotator cuff: benefit of abduction and external rotation of the arm. Radiology 1994;192(3):851–5.
[9] Shankman S, Bencardino J, Beltran J. Glenohumeral instability: evaluation using MR arthrography of the shoulder. Skeletal Radiol 1999;7:365–82.
[10] Cvitanic O, Tirman PFJ, Feller JF, et al. Using abduction and external rotation of the shoulder to increase the sensitivity of MR arthrography in revealing tears of the anterior glenoid labrum. AJR Am J Roentgenol 1997;169:837–44.
[11] Lee SY, Lee JK. Horizontal component of partial thickness tears of rotator cuff: imaging characteristics and comparison of ABER view with oblique coronal view at MR arthrography—initial results. Radiology 2002;224:470–6.
[12] Kwak SM, Brown RR, Trudell D, et al. Glenohumeral joint: comparison of shoulder positions at MR arthrography. Radiology 1998;208:375–80.
[13] Chan KK, Muldoon KA, Yeh L, et al. Superior labral anteroposterior lesions: MR arthrography with arm traction. AJR Am J Roentgenol 1999;173:1117–22.
[14] Miniaci A, Fowler PJ. Impingement in the athlete. Clin Sports Med 1993;12(1):91–110.
[15] Halbrecht JL, Tirman P, Atkin D. Internal impingement of the shoulder: comparison of findings between the throwing and nonthrowing shoulders of college baseball players. Arthroscopy 1999;15:253–8.
[16] McFarland EG, Hsu CY, Neira C, et al. Internal impingement of the shoulder: a clinical and arthroscopic analysis. J Shoulder Elbow Surg 1999;8:458–60.
[17] Jobe CM. Posterior superior glenoid impingement: expanded spectrum. Arthroscopy 1995;11(5):530–6.

[18] Walch G, Boileau P, Noel E, et al. Impingement of the deep surface of the supraspinatus tendon on the posterosuperior glenoid rim: an arthroscopic study. J Shoulder Elbow Surg 1992;1:238–45.
[19] Hamner DL, Pink MM, Jobe FW. A modification of the relocation test: arthroscopic findings associated with a positive test. J Shoulder Elbow Surg 2000;9:263–7.
[20] Meister K, Buckley B, Batts J. The posterior impingement sign: diagnosis of rotator cuff and posterior labral tears secondary to internal impingement in overhand athletes. Am J Orthop 2004;33:412–5.
[21] Kvitne RS, Jobe FW. The diagnosis and treatment of anterior instability in the throwing athlete. Clin Orthop Relat Res 1993;291:107–23.
[22] Burkhart SS, Morgan CD, Ben Kibler W. The disabled throwing shoulder: spectrum of pathology. Part I: pathoanatomy and biomechanics. Arthroscopy 2003;19:404–20.
[23] Kaplan LD, McMahon PJ, Towers J, et al. Internal impingement: findings on magnetic resonance imaging and arthroscopic evaluation. Arthroscopy 2004;20:701–4.
[24] Giaroli EL, Major NM, Higgins LD. MRI of internal impingement of the shoulder. AJR Am J Roentgenol 2005;185:925–9.
[25] Giombini A, Rossi F, Pettrone FA, et al. Posterosuperior glenoid rim impingement as a cause of shoulder pain in top level water polo players. J Sports Med Phys Fitness 1997;37:273–8.
[26] Burkhart SS, Morgan CD. The peel-back mechanism: its role in producing and extending posterior type II SLAP lesions and its effect on SLAP repair rehabilitation. Arthroscopy 1998;14:637–40.
[27] Andrews JR, Carson WG, Mcleod WD. Glenoid labrum tears related to the long head of the biceps. Am J Sports Med 1985;13:337–40.
[28] Snyder SJ, Karzel RP, Del Pizzo W, et al. SLAP lesions of the shoulder. Arthroscopy 1990;6:274–9.
[29] Waldt S, Burkaart A, Lange P, et al. Diagnostic performance of MR arthrography in the assessment of superior labral anteroposterior lesions of the shoulder. AJR Am J Roentgenol 2004;182:1271–8.
[30] Morgan CD, Burkhart SS, Palmeri M, et al. Type II SLAP lesions: three subtypes and their relationships to superior instability and rotator cuff tears. Arthroscopy 1998;14:553–65.
[31] Legan JM, Burkhart TK, Goff WB II, et al. Tears of the glenoid labrum: MR imaging of 88 arthroscopically confirmed cases. Radiology 1991;179:241–6.
[32] Gusmer PB, Potter HG, Schatz JA, et al. Labral injuries: accuracy of detection with unenhanced MR imaging of the shoulder. Radiology 1996;200:519–24.
[33] Yoneda M, Izawa K, Hirooka A, et al. Indicators of superior glenoid labral detachment on magnetic resonance imaging and computed tomography arthrography. J Shoulder Elbow Surg 1998;7:2–12.
[34] Connell DA, Potter HG, Wickiewicz TL, et al. Noncontrast magnetic resonance imaging of superior labral lesions: 102 cases confirmed at arthroscopic surgery. Am J Sports Med 1999;27:208–13.
[35] Bencardino JT, Beltran J, Rosenberg ZS, et al. Superior labrum anterior–posterior lesions: diagnosis with MR arthrography of the shoulder. Radiology 2000;214:267–71.
[36] Jee WH, McCauley TR, Katz LD, et al. Superior labral anterior posterior (SLAP) lesions of the glenoid labrum: reliability and accuracy of MR arthrography for diagnosis. Radiology 2001;218:127–32.
[37] Bennett GE. Shoulder and elbow lesions of the professional baseball pitcher. JAMA 1941;117:510–4.
[38] O'Brien SJ, Neves MC, Arnoczky SP, et al. The anatomy of the inferior glenohumeral ligament complex of the shoulder. Am J Sports Med 1990;18(5):449–56.
[39] Wright RW, Paletta GA Jr. Prevalence of the Bennett lesion of the shoulder in major league pitchers. Am J Sports Med 2004;32(1):121–4.
[40] Meister K, Andrews JR, Batts J, et al. Symptomatic thrower's exostosis. Am J Sports Med 1999;27(2):133–6.

[41] De Maeseneer M, Joavisidha S, Jacobson JA, et al. The Bennett lesion of the shoulder. J Comput Assist Tomogr 1998;22:31–4.
[42] Ferrari JD, Ferrari DA, Coumas J, et al. Posterior ossification of the shoulder: the Bennett lesion. Etiology, diagnosis and treatment. Am J Sports Med 1994;22:171–5.
[43] Blevins FT. Rotator cuff pathology in athletes. Sports Med 1997;24:205–20.
[44] Yeh M, Lintner D, Luo Z. Stress distribution in the superior labrum during throwing motion. Am J Sports Med 2005;33:395–401.
[45] Dines DM, Warren RF, Inglis AE, et al. The coracoid impingement syndrome. J Bone Joint Surg [Br] 1990;72:314–6.
[46] Paulson MM, Watnik NF, Dines DM. Coracoid impingement syndrome, rotator interval reconstruction, and biceps tenodesis in the overhead athlete. Orthop Clin North Am 2001;32:485–93.
[47] Ferrick MR. Coracoid impingement: a case report and review of the literature. Am J Sports Med 2000;28:117–9.
[48] Gerber C, Terrier F, Zehnder R. The subcoracoid space: an anatomic study. Clin Orthop 1997;215:132–8.
[49] Giaroli EL, Major NM, Lemley DE, et al. Coracohumeral interval imaging in subcoracoid impingement syndrome on MRI. AJR Am J Roentgenol 2006;186:242–6.
[50] Bigliani LU, Ticker JB, Flatlow EL, et al. The relationship of acromial architecture to rotator cuff disease. Clin Sports Med 1991;10:823–38.
[51] Cone RO 3rd, Resnick D, Danzig L. Shoulder impingement syndrome: radiographic evaluation. Radiology 1984;150:29–33.
[52] Park JG, Lee JK, Phelps CT. Os acromiale associated with rotator cuff impingement: MR imaging of the shoulder. Radiology 1994;193:255–7.
[53] Farley TE, Neumann CH, Steinbach LS, et al. The coracoacromial arch: MR evaluation and correlation with rotator cuff pathology. Skeletal Radiol 1994;23:641–5.

Clin Sports Med 25 (2006) 445–464
CLINICS IN SPORTS MEDICINE

MRI of the Postoperative Shoulder

Jim Wu, MD[a], Aaron Covey, MD[b], Lee D. Katz, MD[c,*]

[a]Department of Diagnostic Radiology, Beth Israel Deaconess Medical Center, 330 Brookline Avenue, Shapiro 4th Floor, Boston, MA 02215, USA
[b]Department of Orthopaedic Surgery and Rehabilitative Medicine, Yale University School of Medicine, 800 Howard Avenue, New Haven, CT 06510, USA
[c]Department of Diagnostic Radiology and Orthopaedic Surgery and Rehabilitative Medicine, Yale University School of Medicine, 333 Cedar Street, New Haven, CT 06510, USA

Pain in the postoperative shoulder is difficult for all individuals involved. The patient has already undergone a surgical procedure and is presenting now with pain possibly relating to a complication of the procedure or re-injury. In addition, the patient typically has undergone a series of maneuvers, from physical therapy to cortisone injection, without relief of the symptoms. For the orthopaedic surgeon the possibility of a complication of the procedure is disheartening. Finally, for the radiologist the postoperative shoulder usually is more difficult to interpret because of a change in the normal anatomy, not knowing exactly what was accomplished at surgery or what techniques or types of equipment were used, and, more typically, the presence of artifact.

Evaluation of the postoperative shoulder at our institution usually is accomplished with MR arthrography. Occasionally the study can be performed as a noncontrast study or possibly as a CT arthrogram of the shoulder in cases of claustrophobia or contraindications, such as a cardiac pacemaker or metal located somewhere in the body.

IMAGING TECHNIQUE

When imaging the postoperative shoulder, as in the nonoperated shoulder, a dedicated phase array shoulder coil should be used [1]. The imaging parameters often do not differ from standard nonoperated shoulder protocols; however, attention should be given to sequences that can reduce metallic susceptibility artifact. At our institution we use 3- to 4-mm slice thickness for most planes, a 13- to 16-cm field of view, and a 256 to 192 matrix. The patient is imaged with the arm adducted and in external rotation. Some studies have advocated additional sequences in the abducted external rotation position (ABER) to provide tension and better demonstrate the anteroinferior capsulolabral structures, especially following Bankart repair [2,3]. This additional

*Corresponding author. *E-mail address*: Lee.Katz@yale.edu (L.D. Katz).

0278-5919/06/$ – see front matter
doi:10.1016/j.csm.2006.03.003

sportsmed.theclinics.com

sequence requires relocalization and can lengthen image time; however, it is useful when evaluating failed Bankart repairs. Unfortunately, the position can be uncomfortable and occasionally, in the surgically unstable shoulder, anterior dislocation can be provoked.

Susceptibility Artifact Considerations

A major problem with postoperative imaging is susceptibility artifact from the screws, sutures, tacks, suture anchors, and shavings. The foreign material causes intravoxel dephasing, which leads to loss of signal intensity. Most evident on gradient echo images, the artifact can be reduced by using fast spin-echo techniques, which use multiple 180 degree refocusing pulses [1,3–6]. Frequency-selective fat saturation technique is highly dependent on uniform field homogeneity, which becomes distorted by surgical hardware leading to poor fat saturation. Short tau inversion recovery (STIR) can be substituted for frequency-selective fat saturation; however, the drawback is reduced signal-to-noise [1,3,4,6,7]. Other parameters that can improve image quality include increasing the receiver bandwidth and decreasing voxel size [1,4,5,7,8].

MR Arthrography

Many initial studies on postoperative shoulder imaging were performed without MR arthrography [1,9–14]. Subsequent studies have advocated the use of direct MR arthrography in the postoperative shoulder, and direct MR arthrography is used in all postoperative patients at our institution [1–3,5,7]. MR arthrography improves the identification of rotator and labral retears. Several studies have shown that partial tears of the rotator cuff cannot be distinguished adequately from granulation tissue in the tendon from the healing response [3,6,7,9]. In these cases MR arthrography can be particularly useful, because contrast can be seen extending into the partial tear and can help define the margins of the tendon for preoperative planning [6]. One pitfall is that in the operated shoulder the presence of contrast in the subacromial-subdeltoid space does not indicate a full-thickness rotator cuff tear as it would in the nonoperated shoulder. The joint is no longer watertight following surgery [3,5,6,11]. Conversely, the absence of contrast in the subacromial-subdeltoid space does not exclude a full-thickness tear, because scar tissue may prevent contrast from extending through the entire defect [5,6,11]. Arthrography also distends the capsule, allowing for evaluation of the capsular anatomy and the anterior band of the inferior glenohumeral ligament (AIGHL) [2,3,6,15].

The arthrogram portion of the procedure is performed under fluoroscopy. Once the needle tip is documented to be intra-articular with several milliliters of iodinated contrast, or air if allergy is present, a volume of a mixture of gadolinium in normal saline is injected. For a 1.5 T magnet the usual concentration is 1 mL in 250 mL of normal saline. For lower field strength magnets, the concentration can be doubled to 2 mL in 250 mL of normal saline. The effect of shortening the relaxation time of the water produces a bright signal on a T1-weighted fat-suppressed image. The movement of the gadolinium–water complex into an adjacent space is consistent with a rotator cuff tear.

Over the last 15 years, the Yale group has performed more than 6000 MR arthrograms. There have been four major complications, including three cases of suspected infection requiring washout. Only two of the three cases grew a pathogen. The other case appeared to be reflex sympathetic dystrophy that slowly resolved with time.

ROTATOR CUFF TEAR

Overview

The most common concern in the patient who has postoperative pain is retear of the rotator cuff repair. The patient usually presents with a known incident and details a history of acute pain associated with loss of motion. The diagnostic criteria are similar to the preoperative evaluation with the presence of fluid signal on a T2-weighted image that extends through the entire tendon substance. In the case of MR arthrography, simply seeing the contrast extend into the subacromial-subdeltoid space is not enough to diagnose a retear. The normal postoperative shoulder does not need to be watertight, so a small amount of leakage can be expected (Fig. 1). The presence of a definite gap in the tendon makes the diagnosis more substantial (Fig. 2).

The location of the retear usually occurs at the tendon–bone interface. In addition, some tears occur at a second site approximately 1.5 cm medial to the reattachment site (Fig. 3). This tear may result from increasing tension following reattachment in a tendon that already contains abnormal architecture. Slight irregularities of the undersurface of the tendon should not be called partial surface tears.

The time course following surgery is another important point in evaluating the patient who has postoperative pain. The concern for pain following surgery would be infection. As with any septic joint, the MRI appearance is one in which there is an effusion, and with the introduction of IV contrast there is

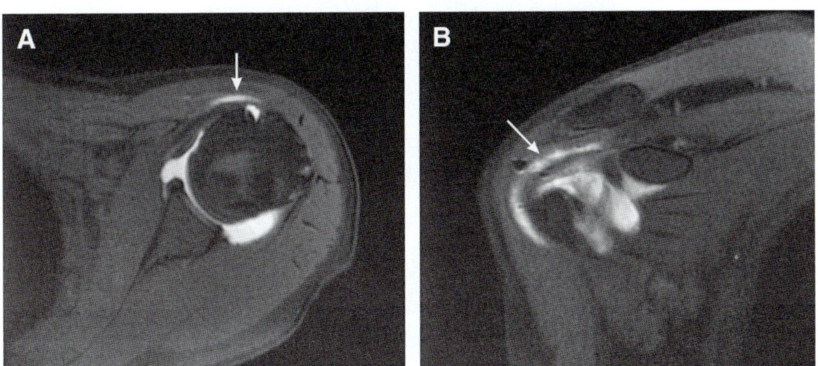

Fig. 1. Intact rotator cuff repair with small amount of leakage. (*A*) T1 fat-suppressed axial with contrast seen in the subdeltoid space (*arrow*). (*B*) T1 fat-suppressed coronal oblique with contrast seen in the subdeltoid space. The rotator cuff repair is maintained.

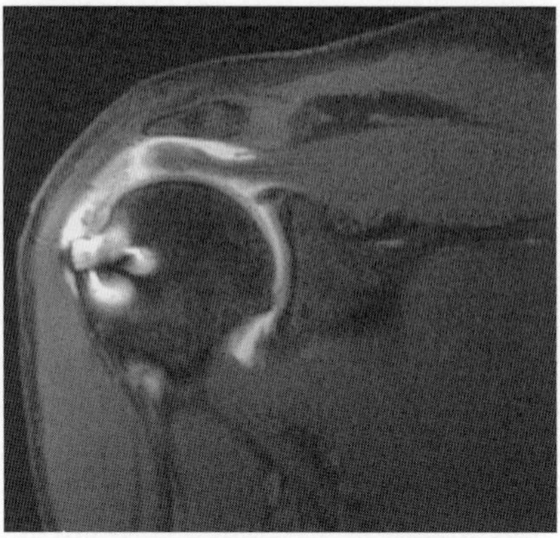

Fig. 2. Retear of the rotator cuff repair at the greater tuberosity. T1 fat-suppressed coronal oblique demonstrating a retear with retraction of the supraspinatus tendon and contrast extending up into the subacromial/subdeltoid space.

prompt enhancement not only to the joint but also to the surrounding musculature (Fig. 4). These patients often are tapped, cultured, and sent to surgery for a washout and possible removal of hardware.

Shortly following surgery and usually in the perioperative period two different types of problems arise. The first is adhesive capsulitis, in which there is a general inflammatory response with loss of motion and pain. The patient, if sent for arthrography, generally is uncomfortable and demonstrates pain as the needle approaches the shoulder capsule. The volume of contrast that is administered is reduced, usually to a total of less than 8 mL. The MRI

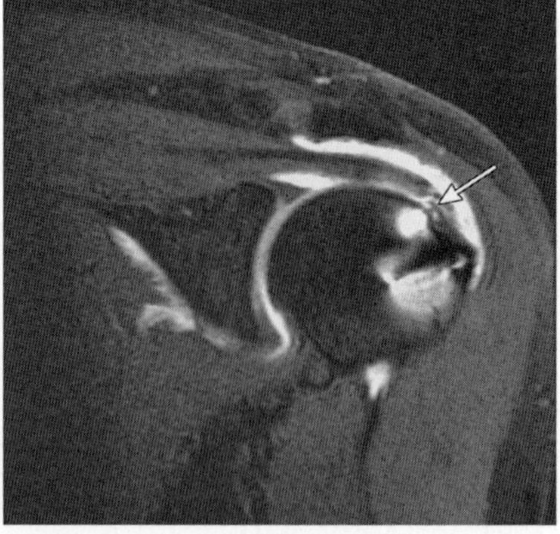

Fig. 3. Retear of the rotator cuff repair away from the greater tuberosity. T1 fat-suppressed coronal oblique demonstrating tear medial to the reattachment site. Contrast seen leaking into the subacromial-subdeltoid space (*arrow*).

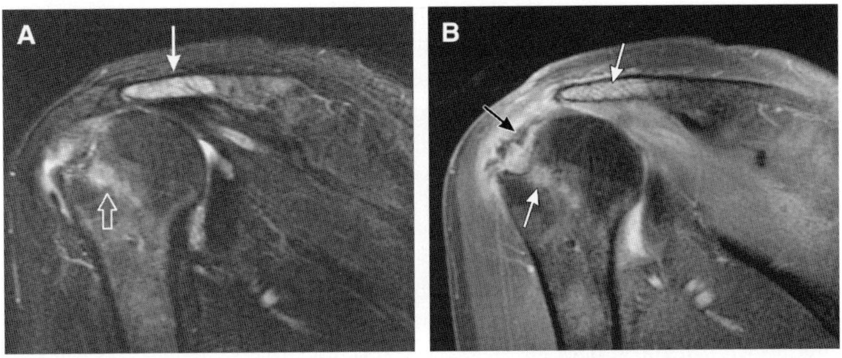

Fig. 4. Osteomyelitis of the humerus and acromion. (*A*) T2 fat-suppressed coronal oblique with edema of the acromion (*arrow*), no evidence of rotator cuff, and an additional area of edema just medial to the site of attachment (*open arrow*). (*B*) Post IV Contrast fast spoiled gradient echo demonstrating enhancement of the soft tissues, acromion, and humerus consistent with infection (*white arrows*). In addition, serpiginous low signal structure (*black arrow*) represents necrotic supraspinatus tendon.

findings do not show a clear cause for the pain, but the patient's history and the lack of volume that can be injected point toward the diagnosis (Fig. 5). There were some nonspecific MRI findings, such as thickening of the axillary pouch and a lack of contrast flowing into the subcoracoid portion of the subscapularis bursa. These patients usually are treated with physical therapy, anti-inflammatory medications, and if necessary, surgical manipulation under anesthesia.

We have encountered several cases of subacromial bursitis; one case appeared to be a hypersensitivity reaction possibly attributable to the suture

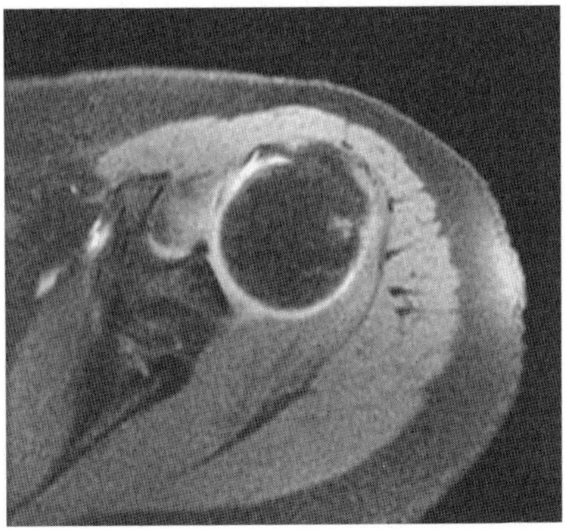

Fig. 5. Adhesive capsulitis. T1 fat suppressed axial image demonstrates a paucity of contrast surrounding the humeral head consistent with lack of distention secondary to small injected volume. There is also contrast seen extending into the subcoracoid region of the subscapularis bursa.

material. MR arthrography is extremely useful in making this diagnosis. The MR arthrogram essentially is normal, with no contrast extending into the subacromial-subdeltoid bursae. Correspondingly, on the conventional T2-weighted image there is a large effusion with surrounding inflammation (Fig. 6). In our experience, a patient went back to surgery and the deltoid sutures were removed, with resolution of the pain syndrome. This diagnosis also can be considered if a subacromial injection of anesthetic relieves the pain syndrome.

Surgical Considerations

There is no treatment algorithm available for the management of partial-thickness rotator cuff tears. Partial tears are a common finding in the asymptomatic aging athlete. In those patients who have shoulder pain, partial tears often are found in conjunction with other lesions. When such tears are found on imaging they are not necessarily the source of the patient's symptoms.

Most partial-thickness rotator cuff tears can be managed nonoperatively. Failure of improvement after 3 to 6 months of conservative treatment has been recommended before the consideration of surgery for symptomatic partial-thickness rotator cuff tears. Several factors, however, such as coexisting shoulder pathology, patient lifestyle, and activity level, also are important factors.

The operative treatment of partial-thickness tears includes two controversial considerations: debridement only versus rotator cuff repair, and whether to perform an acromioplasty or not. Although some surgeons perform the surgery entirely arthroscopically, others use arthroscopically assisted or open technique. In addition to assessment and repair of the cuff, arthroscopic technique allows for direct visualization of rotator cuff and other shoulder pathology in the glenohumeral and subacromial spaces.

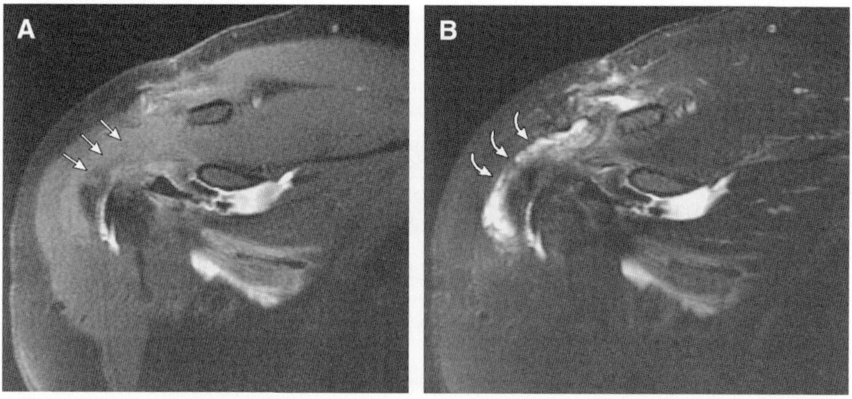

Fig. 6. Subacromial bursitis. (*A*) T1 fat-suppressed image demonstrating no contrast extending into the subacromial bursa (*small arrows*). The rotator cuff repair is intact. (*B*) T2 fat-suppressed coronal oblique demonstrating edema and fluid consistent with inflammation of the bursa (*small curved arrows*).

Neer [16] proposed that partial-thickness tears represent an intermediate stage in the spectrum of impingement syndrome that ranges from edema in the tendons to full-thickness tear. The coracoacromial arch and osteophytes that form in this region have been implicated as the structures that impinge onto the rotator cuff tendon with repetitive shoulder elevation. This impingement is the basis for subacromial decompression surgery in which the anterior undersurface portion of the acromion is removed and the coracoacromial ligament is released [17]. Some surgeons debride the rotator cuff tear, remove of the impinging structures, and perform a subacromial bursectomy for definitive treatment. Others debride the cuff without performing an acromioplasty.

Coinciding with improvements in arthroscopic technique, repairing the partially torn rotator cuff has gained more popularity recently. Though there is no consensus regarding the degree of tear depth that warrants repair, there is evidence that the depth of the tear is an important prognostic indicator [18]. Many surgeons recommend repair for tears of greater than 50% depth [19]. Operative treatment is most beneficial in active patients, traumatic tears, and in those with bursal-sided tears [20].

Repair of the partial tendon tear may involve an in situ repair of the tear or a completion of the tear followed by a repair [21,22]. In the arthroscopic repair technique, bioabsorbable or metallic anchors are placed lateral to the articular margin of the humeral head in the area of the rotator cuff footprint. Typically, one or two sutures are loaded onto the anchors. They are passed through the tendon and tied so as to attach the tendon to the bone. In the open technique, either anchors or transosseous tunnels are used for the same purpose.

Similar to partial tears, the mere presence of a full-thickness tear does not warrant operative treatment. For those tears that fail adequate nonoperative management, however, surgery has shown reliable pain relief and, to a lesser extent, improvement in strength and function. The surgeon may choose to perform a subacromial decompression with the repair. In addition, other findings, such as type II superior labrum anterior to posterior (SLAP) lesions, biceps tendinopathy, acromioclavicular (AC) joint arthrosis, or labral lesions, often are addressed at the time of the repair.

Repair can be performed arthroscopically, with arthroscopic assistance, or open. The advantages of using the arthroscope for diagnosis are the visualization of the cuff from the subacromial and glenohumeral joint spaces, the ability to use arthroscopic technique for cuff mobilization, and the assessment of other shoulder pathology.

When the tendon's distal attachment is intact the cuff defect is amenable to a side-to-side suture or marginal convergence repair. More commonly, however, the tendinous insertion has avulsed and a tendon-to-bone repair is necessary. For larger tears, a combination of side-to-side and end-to-side is used. In the setting of a chronic tear with significant retraction, stump immobility creates a challenge because repair of the tendon medial to the footprint, so-called "partial repair," has led to poor clinical results. It is imperative that the cuff repair is not performed with excess tension. As such, for larger tears careful mobilization techniques are used.

The edges of the tendon are trimmed if they appear nonviable, and the attachment to bone begins. Some make a formal bony trough between the articular surface and the greater tuberosity; others rasp the bone to create a decorticated surface for the repair. Attachment of the tendon to bone is performed by way of bone tunnels, suture anchors, or a combination of the two.

Bone tunnels can be placed only by way of the open technique. As many tunnels as are necessary are placed at the greater tuberosity, approximately 0.5 in from each other. Nonabsorbable suture that is passed through the tendon is shuttled through the bone tunnels, reapproximating the tendon to the footprint.

For arthroscopic repair, suture anchors currently are the standard and tacks have fallen out of favor. Suture anchors may be used exclusively or in combination with bone tunnels in open repair. There are metallic and bioabsorbable anchors commercially available. Placement most often is in the sulcus that lies just medial to the greater tuberosity and lateral to the articular surface. Anchors can be single or double loaded with suture. The suture is placed through the tendon and tied, thus securing the tendon to bone. A double-row technique, unique in that it incorporates two coronal plane rows, is starting to gain favor because it increases the surface area of the tendon insertion to bone.

Although most rotator cuff tears are amenable to surgical repair, some are considered irreparable. Factors that may prevent successful repair include large size of the tear, immobility, and a high degree of fatty infiltration into the muscle. Historically, the management of these massive tears has included open or arthroscopic debridement, local tendon transposition (upper subscapularis, teres minor, teres major), extrinsic tendon transfer (trapezius), tendon autografts and allografts, synthetic grafts, and deltoid flap reconstruction.

Currently, the most common surgical treatment of massive rotator cuff tears is arthroscopic debridement. Muscle transfers do have a role in treatment, however. The indication for a latissimus dorsi tendon transfer is irreparable massive posterosuperior rotator cuff tear in a patient who has intolerable shoulder pain and subjectively unacceptable dysfunction [23]. The functional goal of this surgery is to achieve active external rotation. The latissimus dorsi tendon is sharply dissected from its humeral insertion and pulled though the interval between the deltoid and teres minor where it is sutured over the humeral head to the upper subscapularis tendon.

Successful open surgical repair of the subscapularis has been reported when there is no advanced degeneration of the tendon [24,25]. When fatty degeneration is present in chronic tears, however, direct repair is less likely to yield success [26]. For irreparable tears of the anterior portion of the rotator cuff that have failed conservative measures, pectoralis major transfer represents an option.

Either the superior portion or the entire pectoralis major tendon can be used for transfer [27,28]. The tendon can be passed over or under the conjoined tendon and is affixed to the medial aspect of the greater tuberosity by way of anchors or transosseous sutures. Using the entire pectoralis major muscle in the transfer, Gerber and associates [29] showed improvement in pain, abduction strength, and ability to perform activities of daily living in a group of 28 patients. Those patients who also had an irreparable supraspinatus tear had worse outcomes compared with those who had intact or reparable supraspinatus lesions.

MRI Findings

The appearance of the shoulder following surgery for impingement depends on several factors, including the operative technique (open, mini-open, arthroscopic), type of fixation devices used (transosseous sutures, suture anchors, tendon-to-tendon repairs), and whether or not subacromial decompression has been performed [1,5]. Open procedures are considered the gold standard and technically are easier to perform. No special equipment is necessary and there are good long-term results [3,30,31]. Open procedures are associated with higher morbidity, more blood loss, and longer initial recovery time, however [30]. Moreover, in an open procedure the deltoid tendon is detached from its acromial attachment to expose the repair site and reattached at the conclusion of the surgery. Deltoid dehiscence thus can occur as a major complication (Fig. 7). Arthroscopic procedures cause less postoperative pain, enable faster rehabilitation, have fewer complications, and do not require takedown of the deltoid tendon; however, arthroscopy is more demanding technically and has slightly lower success rates than open repair [3,6,30,31].The mini-open procedure is a combination of the two techniques and involves a longitudinal split of the anterolateral deltoid muscle without takedown of the deltoid insertion [6,30]. The surgical technique depends on the presence and severity of impingement, degree and type of tendon tear, presence of other intra-articular pathology, and surgeon expertise and preference [3].

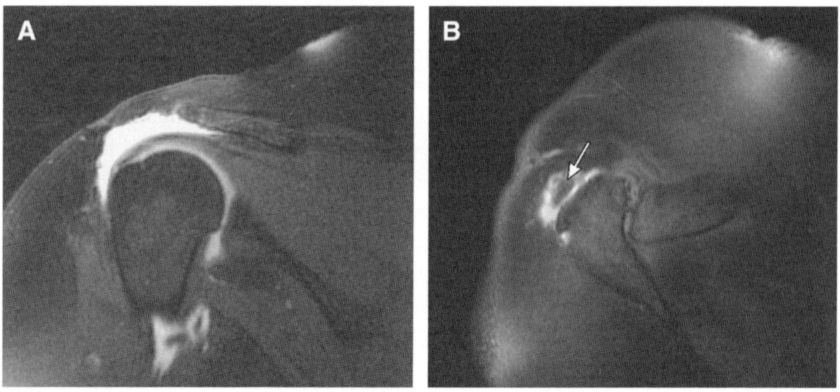

Fig. 7. Deltoid dehiscence. (*A*) T2 fat-suppressed coronal oblique demonstrating fluid within a space created by breakdown of the deltoid repair. (*B*) T1 fat-suppressed axial demonstrating the end of the retracted deltoid tendon floating in the fluid (*arrow*).

Partial rotator cuff tears involve debriding the frayed tissue, a procedure that typically is performed arthroscopically [1,6,32]. Large partial tears may be converted into full-thickness tears at surgery and repaired as full-thickness tears. Small proximal full-thickness tears can be debrided of frayed tissue and side-to-side tendon sutures can be applied [1]. Larger tears greater than 3 cm and retracted tears require mobilization of the free end of the rotator cuff and reattachment of the tendon back to the tuberosity if possible [1,6]. The greater tuberosity often is freshened to expose bleeding bone to facilitate healing and attachment of the rotator cuff tendon [6,30]. The tendon is reattached with sutures or suture anchors. The suture anchors can be metallic, titanium, plastic, or bioabsorbable polymers, each creating various artifacts on MRI [6]. At our institution, similar to other centers, repairs of partial tears are considered when the tear involves greater than 50% of the tendon thickness [6]. Smaller tears often are managed by conservative measures [32].

MRI findings following rotator cuff surgery can be divided into intratendinous and extratendinous findings. For intratendinous findings, the repaired cuff tendons often demonstrate some signal abnormality following repair and many patients have occult partial- and small full-thickness tears [1,13,14]. Intermediate to high signal in the cuff tendon on T1-, proton density-, and T2-weighted sequences is common and expected [3,6]. Spielmann and colleagues [13] evaluated 15 asymptomatic patients following rotator cuff repair and found that only 10% had normal tendons on MRI imaging. In the remainder, tendinosis was seen in 53%, partial tears in 17%, and full-thickness tears in 20%. Zanetti and coworkers [14] evaluated full-thickness tears in asymptomatic and symptomatic patients following rotator cuff surgery and found similar numbers; however, asymptomatic full-thickness cuff tears averaged 0.8 cm in length and the symptomatic tears averaged 3.2 cm. Healing granulation tissue within the tendon can produce high T2 and STIR signal (fluid signal) within the tendon, mimicking a partial tear [1,8,14,15]. This signal may change from high (same as fluid) to intermediate signal with increasing time following surgery [8]. In these cases, several authors advocate MR arthrography [1,3,14,15]. With MR arthrography, the tendon contour and contrast tracking into the defects can aid in the diagnosis of partial tears and better define the margins of torn tendons for surgical planning. Bursal or articular surface tendon irregularity is expected and should not be called a partial tear [1].

As for extratendinous findings, virtually all patients have loss of the subacromial and peribursal fat following rotator cuff surgery [1,6,8,13,15]. Joint effusion and fluid in the subacromial-subdeltoid space is expected even in asymptomatic patients [1,3,6,13,15]. Following repair, the joint is no longer watertight and observing contrast in the subacromial-subdeltoid space does not correlate with full-thickness rotator cuff tears [3,6]. Moreover, mild marrow edema in the humeral head can last for several years [1,6]. Susceptibility artifact is seen commonly at the site of repair from the various tendon attachment devices. In tendon-to-bone repair, a surgical trough with adjacent metallic susceptibility artifact is seen at the superolateral humeral head [6,8,15]. Mild superior subluxation of the humeral head can occur also because of capsular tightening, scarring, cuff atrophy, or bursectomy [3,8,15]. Scarring in the subacromial area, around tendons, the joint capsule, and adjacent soft tissues can occur and may influence repeat surgery or change surgical approach from open to arthroscopic [8]. Artifact in the deltoid and at its proximal attachment can be seen following open or mini-open procedures [8].

SUBACROMIAL DECOMPRESSION

Surgical Considerations

Acromioplasty refers to surgical removal of the anterior inferior hook of the acromion, which is implicated in the pathogenesis of impingement syndrome. The result is a flat acromial undersurface. Subacromial decompression involves an acromioplasty with removal of the coracoacromial ligament, bursectomy, subacromial osteophyte removal, and adhesion removal. This procedure is performed most commonly in isolation in cases of impingement syndrome, less than 50% partial thickness tears, and massive, irreparable tears. (See previous discussion for details of impingement syndrome, partial-, and full-thickness tear surgery). It also can be used in combination with repair in greater than 50% partial-thickness tears and full-thickness tears. This procedure can be performed open or arthroscopically.

Pathology of the acromioclavicular joint is seen frequently in the active and athletic populations primarily from trauma, and in the elderly from a degenerative process. Initial treatment is with nonsteroidal anti-inflammatory drugs and corticosteroid injections; however, surgery can be used for those who fail conservative treatment. It is important to distinguish those patients who have AC joint pain from joint instability (in which a stabilization procedure may be warranted) or isolated meniscal pathology (in which an isolated meniscal procedure may be indicated) from most patients who have focal AC osteoarthritis. In this latter group, in which degenerative changes have occurred in the articulation, isolated excision of the AC joint is the treatment of choice.

The traditional open approach involves an incision over the AC joint and division and detachment of the deltoid and trapezius muscular fascia followed by excision of 2 cm of distal clavicle [33]. If necessary, a subacromial decompression may be performed by way of the same incision. Arthroscopic technique spares the deltoid and trapezial fibers and can be done through portals just over the AC joint (superior approach) or by way of those portals used for traditional shoulder arthroscopy (subacromial approach). Snyder and colleagues [34] report 94% good or excellent outcome at an average of 2 years following arthroscopic distal clavicle resection by way of the subacromial approach. There is no consensus as to the appropriate amount of distal clavicle or medial acromion that should be resected. Although Snyder and colleagues [34] removed an average of 14.8 mm of distal clavicle, Levine [35], who reports 88% excellent or good outcomes, resected an average of 5.4 mm. Care is taken to keep the superior capsule of the AC joint intact to avoid postoperative instability.

Subacromial decompression for impingement can be performed alone or more commonly in conjunction with rotator cuff repair. This procedure also can be performed as an open, arthroscopic, or mini-open procedure [1,3,6]. A burr or shaver is used to remove the anterior third and inferior aspect of the acromion, with care not to remove too much cortical bone [1,3,6,8]. Aggressive decompression can predispose to deltoid detachment or acromion fracture. The subdeltoid bursa often is inflamed and resected [1,6]. Complete or partial removal of the coracoacromial ligament usually is performed also [8]. If there are clinical or imaging signs of acromioclavicular osteoarthritis, the inferior osteophytes with or without the lateral aspect of the clavicle (Mumford procedure) can be resected [1,6,8].

MR findings

The typical MRI appearance following subacromial decompression includes a flattened acromial surface, type 1 shape, and nonvisualization of the anterior third of the acromion [1,3,6]. There is shortening of the anterior acromion and decreased signal on T1- and T2-weighted images in the distal acromion from marrow fibrosis [1,3]. Artifact is common from the shavings created by the burr. The coracoacromial ligament typically is absent and scar tissue may fill in at the postoperative site [1,3,6]. There can be widening of the AC joint if the distal clavicle is resected [3]. These findings are seen best on the sagittal images [2,3].

LABRAL ABNORMALITIES

Patients who have undergone labral repair generally fall into two categories: those who have had SLAP repairs for an athletic-type injury or trauma of some sort, and those who have undergone Bankart repairs for shoulder dislocation.

Surgical Considerations

Snyder and associates [36] coined the term SLAP lesion in 1990. Snyder and others attempted to classify SLAP lesions [37,38]. In assessing a SLAP lesion, the surgeon must have a thorough understanding of the normal anatomy and the normal variants commonly seen in the superior labrum and biceps insertion region. Without such an understanding, aberrant but nonpathologic anatomy may be mistake for a SLAP lesion [39,40].

After the diagnostic portion of the arthroscopy is performed, any degenerative labral tissue is debrided. The bony surface of the superior glenoid is abraded in preparation for the repair. The biceps anchor is repaired with either bioabsorbable tacks or bioabsorbable or metallic suture anchors. Of 102 patients who have type II SLAP lesions treated with suture anchor techniques, Burkhart and colleagues [41] report 97% excellent or good results. This group included 44 baseball pitchers, 37 of whom were able to return to preinjury level of activity.

Reported complications of SLAP repair include penetration of titanium screws used for biceps anchor fixation device into the glenoid articular cartilage, loosening of a screw used for fixation, loose bioabsorbable tack material in the joint necessitating arthroscopic removal, adhesive capsulitis, and failed repair [42–44].

During a diagnostic arthroscopy in a patient who has anterior instability, the extent of the lesion is defined. Many types of lesions have been described with variable involvement of the following structures: labrum, glenoid rim, capsule, inferior glenohumeral ligament (IGHL), or middle glenohumeral ligament. The IGHL may be avulsed from the humerus, a so-called "HAGL" lesion. Chondral defects may be present (glenoid labrum articular disruption). In chronic cases, the labrum tends to scar ectopically beneath the glenoid rim to the scapular neck.

Surgery most commonly is performed arthroscopically. The ectopically scarred tissue of the anterior labral ligament complex (LLC) is released and mobilized. This mobilization stops once the release reaches the 6:00 position (relative to the glenoid), but should be extended in the case of atraumatic instability. Next, the anterior portion of the scapular neck is decorticated to prepare the attachment site for the repaired LLC.

Bioabsorbable anchors are gaining favor over metal anchors because of the danger of implant dislocation or misplacement with resultant arthritis. The first anchor is placed into the 5:00 to 5:30 position of the glenoid. Anchors that are too superficial create chondral injury to the humeral head, whereas those pushed in too deep may suffer suture abrasions. Anchors placed too shallow with reference to the glenoid rim may penetrate the glenoid's subchondral bone and cause anchor arthritis.

An anchor suture is passed through the IGHL and labrum at the most inferior position, about 1 cm lateral to the glenoid rim. Depending on the size of the lesion, three to four suture anchors are used. The ligament shift occurs in an inferosuperior and lateromedial direction. The magnitude of the shift depends on the anterior laxity and tissue redundancy. If warranted, a concomitant posterior capsular plication, SLAP repair, or rotator interval closure may be performed.

Most patients who have multidirectional instability are well managed with a rigorous physician-directed home exercise program [45]. There are many soft tissue and bony procedures available, however, that are designed to stabilize the glenohumeral joint for cases that have failed at least 6 months of conservative treatment. To be a candidate for soft tissue surgery, glenoid hypoplasia or aplasia must be ruled out as a cause of the clinical shoulder instability.

Many capsular plication surgeries have been described. The Putti-Platt procedure involves dissection of the subscapularis tendon 2.5 cm from its insertion. The scapular neck is roughened to create a bed onto which the lateral stump will adhere. The lateral stump of the tendon is then tensioned and attached to the anterior capsular and labral complex. The medial stump is then lapped over the lateral stump, shortening the capsule and subscapularis muscle. Recurrent instability and loss of motion are common after this procedure. In a review of 101 patients, Fredriksson and colleagues [46] report a 20% recurrent instability rate, and all patients had a decrease in range of motion.

In 1980, Neer and Foster [47] described the classic inferior capsular shift, which they performed on 32 patients who had multidirectional instability. These authors emphasized capsular detachment from the humeral neck by using a T-shaped incision with the stem of the T aimed at the glenoid and in between the middle and inferior glenohumeral ligaments. The top of the T is parallel to the humeral anatomic neck 1 cm from the capsule's lateral insertion. The inferomedial flap is mobilized first, tensioned, and attached by suture to the remnant lateral capsule or adjacent subscapularis stump. The superomedial flap is advanced distally and sutured to the superior and anterior lateral capsule remnant and subscapular stump. This procedure reduces capsular redundancy and obliterates the axillary pouch. This procedure has been modified many times. Currently, it is more common to make the shift on the glenoid side.

The Eden-Hybbinette procedure uses a bone block, typically an iliac graft, to extend the anterior glenoid and theoretically impart stability. There are many variations regarding the graft shape, placement technique, and type of fixation for this procedure. In 41 cases, Paavolainen [48] reported 3 with recurrent instability, an average loss of 10% of external rotation, and 10% development of degenerative joint disease.

The use of arthroscopy for multidirectional instability is evolving. Thermal or radiofrequency capsular shrinkage has been used. High failure rates, worrisome case reports of articular cartilage and nerve damage, and concerns about the effect of these modalities on the tissue have limited the attractiveness of these procedures to many surgeons [49]. Arthroscopic suture capsule plication has been reported with promising results, but remains a technically difficult procedure.

Anterior instability with injury to the anterior inferior labrum, adjacent capsule, and anterior band of the inferior glenohumeral ligament accounts for 95% of glenohumeral instability and typically is because of trauma [1,6]. Atraumatic instability has a higher likelihood of being multidirectional and can be because of inherent laxity of the joint capsule [1]. There are more than 100 procedures reported for treatment of instability and they can be divided into anatomic or nonanatomic repair [1,3,6].

Anatomic repairs involve direct reattachment of the labrum and adjacent capsular structures to the anterior inferior glenoid as in the classic Bankart repair [1,2]. The Bankart repair involves removal and stabilization of the anterior capsulolabral structures by way of the deltopectoral interval [2,6,15]. Osseous drill holes are placed in the anterior inferior glenoid at the junction of the labrum and articular cartilage in the 3:00, 4:00, and 5:00 positions. The sutures are then attached to the labrum and anterior band of the inferior glenohumeral ligament that make up the capsulolabral complex [2,6]. The use of suture anchors has helped make arthroscopic Bankart repairs more widespread [2]. Suture anchors are placed along the articular margin of the anterior inferior glenoid rim through the subscapularis and the sutures on the anchors are tied to the capsulolabral complex [2,15]. These suture anchors can be made of titanium or bioabsorbable material, such as polylactic acid [5,6,50]. Bioabsorbable tacks or staples also can be used [6]. Glenoid fractures associated with instability and involving more than 25% of the glenoid surface are repaired by an open procedure with screw fixation. Occasionally bone graft is necessary if there is significant bone loss [1,6].

Nonanatomic procedures can involve manipulation of either soft tissue or bone block structures. Putti-Platt and Magnusson-Stack procedures involve indirect tightening of the anterior capsule by way of shortening and manipulation of the subscapularis [3,12]. Bone block procedures include the Bristow-Helfet and Eden-Hybinette procedures, in which the coracoid is resected and reattached to the anterior inferior glenoid [1,3,12]. A bone block acts as a mechanical stabilizer of the shoulder and prevents recurrent anterior subluxation. Nonanatomic repairs have lost favor amongst surgeons because of persistent pain and other complications; however, knowledge of these procedures and variations of them are important because these patients can present for MR imaging and the anatomy can be distorted [3].

Procedures for shoulder instability can be performed in combination with a capsulorraphy, which can be performed by way of direct suture technique or laser or thermal capsular shrinkage [1,3,6]. In the inferior capsular shift procedure, a horizontal T-shaped incision is made in the anterior capsule [3]. The inferior portion is shifted superiorly and the superior portion is advanced anteroinferiorly with the overlapping tissues sutured over each other. This overlap thickens the anterior inferior capsule and creates greater tension on the humeral side [3]. Laser and thermal-assisted capsular shift also can be performed; however, results are controversial [3,51,52].

MR Findings

Following repair of the anterior capsulolabral complex, there should be anatomic position and morphology of the labrum and capsule without fluid or

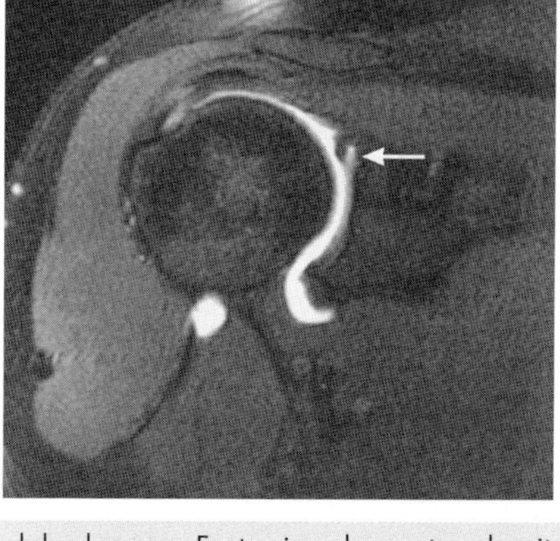

Fig. 8. Normal superior labral recess. Fast spin echo proton density coronal oblique demonstrating prominent fluid within the superior labral recess (*arrow*) but not extending into the labrum. This finding can be a normal variant.

contrast tracking into the labrum [1,2,7]. Fluid or contrast within or dissecting into the labrum indicates a tear; however, this criterion is less accurate when compared with that for nonoperated labra [7]. Following labral surgery, the superior labral recess may become accentuated (Fig. 8). Susceptibility artifact at the repair site is common and can limit interpretation severely. Nonabsorbable or ferromagnetic devices can cause extensive artifact. These devices also may become detached and be responsible for postoperative pain (Fig. 9). Conversely, absorbable polylactic acid suture anchors can be difficult to see and present as subtle drill tracks, which can disappear with time [1,2]. Metallic anchors causing susceptibility artifact also can mimic retears [1,7]. MR arthrography is useful particularly when evaluating continued pain following instability repair [7]. Contrast can aid in the diagnosis of labral retears and distend the capsule for evaluation of the capsulolabral structures (Fig. 10). Imaging in the ABER position has been described to improve visualization of the repaired

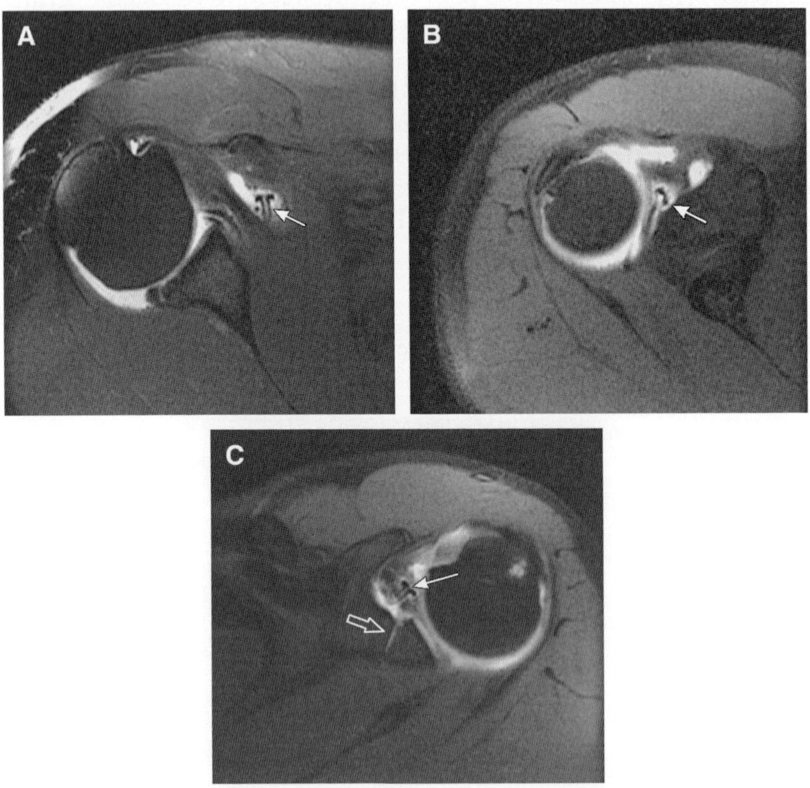

Fig. 9. Loose hardware. (*A,B,C*) Three images from several patients demonstrating various surgical tacks that have become dislodged and may reflect the cause of the painful shoulder from recurrence of the labral abnormality or the loose body itself. The hardware track in the glenoid is identified (*open arrow*).

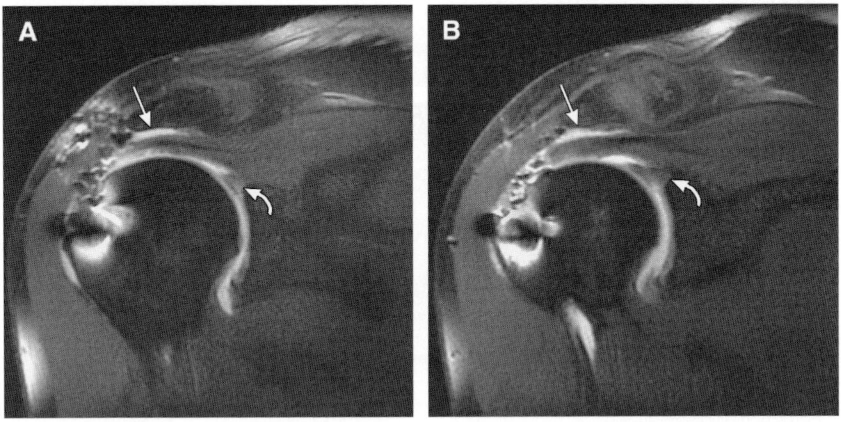

Fig. 10. SLAP tear in a patient who had a prior rotator cuff repair. (*A*) T2 fat-suppressed coronal oblique demonstrating rotator cuff repair intact and leakage of contrast into the subacromial space (*arrow*). (*B*) T1 fat-suppressed coronal oblique demonstrating contrast extending into labrum (*curved arrow*) consistent with a tear.

structures [2]. Moreover, the capsule and glenohumeral ligaments can become thickened following repair, which is best seen with MR arthrography [2,6]. The normal AIGHL should abut the humeral head covering its entire margin and the transition from the AIGHL to the labrum should be seamless [2].

Following capsular shift surgery, the anterior capsule, especially at the anteroinferior aspect, should be smaller than before surgery. Tirmin and coworkers [53] described measurement of the anterior and posterior capsular distances. The anterior capsular distance (A) is measured between the base of the labrum and the anterior capsule. The posterior capsule distance (P) is the distance between the posterior-most aspect of the humeral head and the posterior capsule, measured 1 cm lateral to the most medial aspect of the humeral head. A P/A ratio of greater than 1 is a predictor of good outcome [6,15]. Rand and colleagues [15] showed a change of the P/A ratio from 0.64 preoperatively to 2.36 postoperatively in their series. A nodular thickened capsule is a common appearance [15]. Furthermore, the anterior capsular insertion is typically type 1 or 2 following repair [2]. Joint distention with MR arthrography is necessary to visualize these capsular and joint findings [7].

Thickening and abnormal contour of the subscapularis muscle and tendon can occur. The subscapularis can be traverse during Bankart repair or directly manipulated as in the Putti-Platt procedure [1,3]. Alterations of the coracoid process and anterior margin of the glenoid are seen in bone block procedures. A bony mass with extensive scar tissue can be seen at the anterior inferior glenoid from the Bristow-Helfet or Eden-Hybinette procedures [3,12]. In these procedures, the labral and capsular abnormalities are not repaired and are persistent on repeat imaging [3].

SUMMARY

The postoperative shoulder is a complicated area depending on the patient, the patient's age, the type of technique and equipment that was used, and imaging of the shoulder using MRI. This article has discussed the surgical and radiologic considerations faced in trying to assess patients who have had surgery to explain the rationale of the operation and then try to understand if there is an abnormality that can explain the post-operative pain. MR arthrography has been shown to be a safe and effective technique for evaluating the postoperative shoulder.

References

[1] Zanetti M, Hodler J. MR imaging of the shoulder after surgery. Magn Reson Imaging Clin N Am 2004;12:169–83.

[2] Sugimoto H, Suzuki K, Mihara K, et al. MR arthrography of shoulders after suture-anchor bankart repair. Radiology 2002;224:105–11.

[3] Mohana-Borges AV, Chung CB, Resnick D. MR imaging and MR arthrography of the postoperative shoulder: spectrum of normal and abnormal findings. Radiographics 2004;24: 69–85.

[4] White LM, Buckwalter KA. Technical considerations: CT and MR imaging in the postoperative orthopedic patient. Semin Musculoskelet Radiol 2002;6(1):5–17.

[5] Rand T, Trattnig S, Breitenseher M, et al. The postoperative shoulder. Top Mag Res Imag 1999;10(4):203–13.

[6] Zlatkin MB. MRI of the postoperative shoulder. Skel Radiol 2002;31:63–80.

[7] Wagner SC, Schweitzer ME, Morrison WB, et al. Shoulder instability: accuracy of MR imaging performed after surgery in depicting recurrent injury—initial findings. Radiology 2002;222:196–203.

[8] Gusmer PB, Potter HG, Donovan WD, et al. MR imaging of the shoulder after rotator cuff repair. AJR 1997;168:559–63.

[9] Owen RS, Iannotti JP, Kneeland JB, et al. Shoulder after surgery: MR imaging with surgical validation. Radiology 1993;186:443–7.

[10] Gaenslen ES, Satterlee CC, Hinson GW. Magnetic resonance imaging for evaluation of failed repairs of the rotator cuff. J Bone Joint Surg Am 1996;78:1391–6.

[11] Magee TH, Gaenslen ES, Seitz R, et al. MR imaging of the shoulder after surgery. AJR 1997;168:925–8.

[12] Vahlensieck M, Lang P, Wagner U, et al. Shoulder MRI after surgical treatment of instability. Eur J Radiol 1999;30:2–4.

[13] Spielmann AL, Forster BB, Kokan P, et al. Shoulder after rotator cuff repair: MR imaging findings in asymptomatic individuals—initial experience. Radiology 1999;213:705–8.

[14] Zanetti M, Jost B, Hodler J, et al. MR imaging after rotator cuff repair: full thickness defects and bursitis-like subacromial abnormalities in asymptomatic subjects. Skel Radiol 2000;29: 314–9.

[15] Rand T, Freilinger W, Breitenseher M, et al. Magnetic resonance arthrography (MRA) in the postoperative shoulder. Mag Res Imag 1999;17(6):843–50.

[16] Neer CS 2nd. Impingement lesions. Clin Orthop Relat Res 1983;173:70–7.

[17] Neer CS 2nd. Anterior acromioplasty for the chronic impingement syndrome in the shoulder: a preliminary report. J Bone Joint Surg Am 1972;54(1):41–50.

[18] Burkhart SS. Reconciling the paradox of rotator cuff repair versus debridement: a unified biomechanical rationale for the treatment of rotator cuff tears. Arthroscopy 1994;10(1):4–19.

[19] Weber SC. Arthroscopic debridement and acromioplasty versus mini-open repair in the treatment of significant partial-thickness rotator cuff tears. Arthroscopy 1999;15(2): 126–31.

[20] Cordasco FA, Backer M, Craig EV, et al. The partial-thickness rotator cuff tear: is acromioplasty without repair sufficient? Am J Sports Med 2002;30(2):257–60.
[21] Lo IK, Burkhart SS. Transtendon arthroscopic repair of partial-thickness, articular surface tears of the rotator cuff. Arthroscopy 2004;20(2):214–20.
[22] Gartsman GM, editor. Shoulder arthroscopy. 1st edition. Philadelphia: Saunders; 2003.
[23] Craig EV, editor. Master technique in orthopaedic surgery: the shoulder. 2nd edition. Philadelphia: Lippincott Williams & Wilkins; 2004.
[24] Deutsch A, Altchek DW, Veltri DM, et al. Traumatic tears of the subscapularis tendon. Clinical diagnosis, magnetic resonance imaging findings, and operative treatment. Am J Sports Med 1997;25(1):13–22.
[25] Gerber C, Hersche O, Farron A. Isolated rupture of the subscapularis tendon. J Bone Joint Surg Am 1996;78(7):1015–23.
[26] Goutallier D, Postel JM, Bernageau J, et al. Fatty muscle degeneration in cuff ruptures: pre- and postoperative evaluation by CT scan. Clin Orthop Relat Res 1994;304:78–83.
[27] Wirth MA, Rockwood CA Jr. Operative treatment of irreparable rupture of the subscapularis. J Bone Joint Surg Am 1997;79(5):722–31.
[28] Resch H, Povacz P, Ritter E, et al. Transfer of the pectoralis major muscle for the treatment of irreparable rupture of the subscapularis tendon. J Bone Joint Surg Am 2000;82(3):372–82.
[29] Jost B, Puskas GJ, Lustenberger A, et al. Outcome of pectoralis major transfer for the treatment of irreparable subscapularis tears. J Bone Joint Surg Am 2003;85-A(10):1944–51.
[30] Neault MA, Guanche CA. Arthroscopic rotator cuff repair. Oper Tech Sports Med 2002;10(2):93–8.
[31] Brislin K, Rubenstein D, Wetzler M, et al. Operative repair of anterior instability and rotator cuff tears in athletes. Oper Tech Sports Med 2002;10(2):64–8.
[32] Conway JE. The management of partial thickness rotator cuff tears in throwers. Oper Tech Sports Med 2002;10(2):75–85.
[33] Grimes DW, Garner RW. The degeneration of the acromioclavicular joint. Treatment by resection of the distal clavicle. Orthop Rev 1980;9(9):41–4.
[34] Snyder SJ, Banas MP, Karzel RP. The arthroscopic Mumford procedure: an analysis of results. Arthroscopy 1995;11(2):157–64.
[35] Levine WN, Barron OA, Yamaguchi K, et al. Arthroscopic distal clavicle resection from a bursal approach. Arthroscopy 1998;14(1):52–6.
[36] Snyder SJ, Karzel RP, Del Pizzo W, et al. SLAP lesions of the shoulder. Arthroscopy 1990;6(4):274–9.
[37] Maffet MW, Gartsman GM, Moseley B. Superior labrum-biceps tendon complex lesions of the shoulder. Am J Sports Med 1995;23(1):93–8.
[38] Morgan CD, Burkhart SS, Palmeri M, et al. Type II SLAP lesions: three subtypes and their relationships to superior instability and rotator cuff tears. Arthroscopy 1998;14(6):553–65.
[39] Williams MM, Snyder SJ, Buford D Jr. The Buford complex—the "cord-like" middle glenohumeral ligament and absent anterosuperior labrum complex: a normal anatomic capsulolabral variant. Arthroscopy 1994;10(3):241.
[40] Williams MM, Snyder SJ. A sublabral foramen must not be confused with a Bankart lesion. Arthroscopy 1994;10(5):586.
[41] Burkhart SS, Morgan CD, Kibler WB. Shoulder injuries in overhead athletes. The "dead arm" revisited. Clin Sports Med 2000;19(1):125–58.
[42] Resch H, Gosler K, Thoeni H, et al. Arthroscopic repair of superior glenoid labral detachment (the SLAP lesion). J Shoulder Elbow Surg 1993;1993(2):147–55.
[43] Snyder SJ, Banas MP, Karzel RP. An analysis of 140 injuries to the superior glenoid labrum. J Shoulder Elbow Surg 1995;4(4):243–8.
[44] Field LD, Savoie FH 3rd. Arthroscopic suture repair of superior labral detachment lesions of the shoulder. Am J Sports Med 1993;21(6):783–90.
[45] Burkhead WZ Jr, Rockwood CA Jr. Treatment of instability of the shoulder with an exercise program. J Bone Joint Surg Am 1992;74(6):890–6.

[46] Fredriksson AS, Tegner Y. Results of the Putti-Platt operation for recurrent anterior dislocation of the shoulder. Int Orthop 1991;15(3):185–8.

[47] Neer CS 2nd, Foster CR. Inferior capsular shift for involuntary inferior and multidirectional instability of the shoulder: a preliminary report. J Bone Joint Surg Am 1980;62(6): 897–908.

[48] Paavolainen P, Bjorkenheim JM, Ahovuo J, et al. Recurrent anterior dislocation of the shoulder. Results of Eden-Hybbinette and Putti-Platt operations. Acta Orthop Scand 1984;55(5): 556–60.

[49] Karas SG, Noonan TJ, Horan M. Outcomes of shoulder instability treated with radiofrequency thermal capsulorraphy. Presented at the 19th Annual Meeting of the Arthroscopy Association of North America. Miami Beach, FL, April 16, 2001.

[50] Major NM, Banks MC. MR imaging of complications of loose surgical tacks in the shoulder. AJR 2003;180:377–80.

[51] Favorito PJ, Langenderfer MA, Colosimo AJ, et al. Arthroscopic laser-assisted capsular shift in the treatment of patients with multidirectional shoulder instability. Am J Sports Med 2002;30(3):322–8.

[52] Savoie FH 3rd, Field LD. Thermal versus suture treatment of symptomatic capsular laxity. Clin Sports Med 2000;19(1):63–75.

[53] Tirmin PF, Stauffer AE, Crues JV. Saline magnetic resonance arthrography in the evaluation of glenohumeral instability. Arthroscopy 1993;9:550–9.

Clin Sports Med 25 (2006) 465–487

CLINICS IN SPORTS MEDICINE

ELSEVIER SAUNDERS

Entrapment Neuropathies of the Shoulder and Elbow in the Athlete

Jenny T. Bencardino, MD[a,*], Zehava Sadka Rosenberg, MD[b]

[a]Department of Radiology, Huntington Hospital, North Shore Long Island Jewish Health System, 5 Twelvepence Court, Melville, NY 11747, USA

[b]Department of Radiology, Hospital for Joint Diseases, New York University Medical Center, 305 East 17th Street, New York, NY 10003, USA

Entrapment neuropathy secondary to nerve compression by mechanical or dynamic forces may be a cause of upper extremity pain and weakness in the athlete. Anatomically narrow passages predispose individual nerves to entrapment neuropathies. Dynamic changes within these narrow tunnels during repetitive athletic activity can produce further compression of a nerve with only minimal anatomic variation [1]. Nerve compression may also be produced by space-occupying lesions such as tumors, cysts, inflammatory processes; or by post-traumatic conditions such as hematoma, myositis ossificans, and scar formation. Other causes for nerve compression are associated with hormonal alterations and systemic diseases, such as pregnancy, oral contraceptive ingestion, diabetes mellitus, and hypothyroidism.

Muscle weakness, with or without associated sensory loss, sharp burning pain, and paresthesias over a localized skin area, may be associated with entrapment neuropathies. In chronic instances, muscle atrophy and vegetative disturbances can occur. Although electromyographic and nerve conduction studies remain the preferred diagnostic method for entrapment neuropathies, MRI may play a role when the deep course of some nerves, such as the posterior interosseous nerve, may result in unreliable electromyographic analysis.

The treatment of entrapment neuropathies includes conservative measures such as immobilization, local heat, and anti-inflammatory medications. In refractory cases, percutaneous steroid injections and surgical release of the nerve may be required.

Other than MRI, most imaging techniques are insensitive for detecting entrapment neuropathies. Exostosis, osteophytes, fracture callus, and anatomic osseous variants, which may contribute to nerve compression, can occasionally be depicted using conventional radiography and CT. Direct visualization of the nerve, however, is best achieved with MRI.

*Corresponding author. *E-mail address*: jennybencardino@yahoo.com (J.T. Bencardino).

0278-5919/06/$ – see front matter
doi:10.1016/j.csm.2006.03.005

sportsmed.theclinics.com

In the setting of entrapment neuropathies, MRI can confirm the presence of nerve compression or entrapment, assess for space-occupying lesions, and exclude other lesions that can present in a similar clinical fashion to entrapment neuropathy (eg, rotator cuff tear). Normal peripheral nerves are depicted on MR images as low-to-intermediate signal intensity structures highlighted by fat. MRI neurography and high resolution studies often depict the honeycomb, fascicular pattern of the nerves. Spurious mild increased signal of the nerve is often seen on water-sensitive sequences.

MRI features of peripheral entrapment neuropathy can be subdivided into direct signs involving the nerve, and indirect signs related to muscle denervation. Direct evidence of peripheral entrapment include changes in signal intensity, size, and position of the affected nerve. Focal changes in the nerve are particularly useful in distinguishing the mild increased nerve signal normally seen on fluid-sensitive images from true neuropathy. Nerve edema can result in focal effacement of the fascicular pattern of the larger nerves.

Denervation muscle injury follows a pattern of signal alteration characterized by normal T1 signal and interstitial T2 hyperintensity in the acute setting, and increased T1 signal with normal T2 signal consistent with muscle atrophy and fatty infiltration in chronic cases [2,3]. Often, increased signal on both T1 and fluid-sensitive images is noted, indicating an ongoing denervation process. The distribution pattern of denervated muscles can isolate the exact site of entrapment as well as depict variations in muscle innervation.

MRI is also useful in identifying the cause for entrapment. Osseous abnormalities such as bony spurs, fracture fragments, and callous can easily be identified. Mass occupying lesions such as tumors, aberrant muscles, ganglia, bursa, and scar tissue are also well-depicted with MRI.

PATHOPHYSIOLOGY OF NERVE DISORDERS

The classification of nerve disorders is based on the severity of the injury and its potential for reversibility. The least severe nerve injury is neuropraxia, or first-degree nerve injury. Distortion of the myelin about the nodes of Ranvier caused by ischemia, mechanical compression, or electrolyte imbalance produces temporary loss of nerve conduction. Neuropraxia has the greatest potential for complete recovery, usually within 2 or 3 months. A more extensive injury caused by interruption of the axon with secondary Wallerian degeneration distal to the site of injury is defined as axonotmesis, or second-degree nerve injury. The supporting connective tissue surrounding the axon and Schwann cells, however, is preserved, and the recovery period, ranging from weeks to months, depends on the distance between the site of injury and the end organs. Complete disruption of the nerve and its supporting structures is seen in neurotmesis, or third-degree nerve injury. This is the most severe degree of injury, with no potential for regeneration.

Neurotmesis has been further divided by Sunderland [4] into three subtypes: (1) third-degree nerve injury, in which the endoneurium is disrupted with intact perineurium and epineurium; (2) fourth-degree nerve injury, in which all neural elements, sparing the epineurium, are disrupted; (3) and fifth-degree nerve injury, in which there is complete transection and discontinuity of the nerve. Surgical end-to-end anastomosis or nerve grafting depends heavily on the chronicity of the process.

MRI TECHNIQUE

MRI study of the upper extremity is routinely performed using dedicated phase-array coils, with the patient in a supine position and the arm by the side. The nerves of the upper extremity are in general best visualized on axial images. T1-weighted sequences provide superb anatomical resolution. Water-sensitive sequences such as fat-suppressed T2-weighted and Short-tau inversion recovery (STIR) sequences are useful in identifying signs of neuritis/neuropathy and acute denervation muscle injury. Acute axonal nerve lesions are manifested by T2 hyperintensity and increased girth of the nerve at and distal to the site of injury. Proximal increased girth may also be encountered. Increased T2 signal and post-gadolinium enhancement of denervated muscle fibers is most likely related to fluid shift from intracellular to extracellular compartment, and changes in the intramuscular vascular bed leading to capillary engorgement and increased muscular blood volume [5,6]. These changes were noted as early as 24 hours after complete transection of the sciatic nerve in rats [7]. MRI has also been successfully used experimentally as an indicator of nerve degeneration, healing, and reinnervation [8]. New contrast media, such as superparamagnetic iron oxide, may be useful in detecting macrophage invasion into the degenerating nerve distal to an axonal lesion [9]. Other agents such as gadofluorine M-enhanced MRI may aid in the assessment of nerve regrowth and regeneration [10].

In the following pages, the authors review the normal anatomy, the MRI anatomy, and the MRI manifestations of sports-induced entrapment/compressive neuropathies of the upper extremity.

SUPRASCAPULAR NERVE

Normal Anatomy

The suprascapular nerve originates from the upper trunk of the brachial plexus, receiving fibers from C5 and C6 nerve roots. The nerve innervates the supraspinatus and infraspinatus muscles and provides sensation to the glenohumeral and acromioclavicular joints. After traversing the supraclavicular fossa, the suprascapular nerve, with its accompanying vein and artery, enters the suprascapular notch, making a sharp turn around the scapular spine. There the nerve travels within scapular notch or scapular incisura–a fibro-osseous tunnel bridged superiorly by the scapular ligament. The suprascapular vessels travel above the notch. At the scapular notch, the suprascapular nerve divides into the supraspinatus and infraspinatus nerves. In about 50% of the population, the infraspinatus nerve travels within a second more inferior and posterior tunnel roofed by the spinoglenoid ligament [1,11].

MRI Anatomy

The suprascapular nerve and its accompanying vessels, well-outlined by fat, are initially best identified on oblique coronal T1-weighted images within the suprascapular notch, at the junction of the glenoid with the scapular neck, just medial to the superior glenoid rim (Fig. 1A). As the suprascapular neurovascular bundle enters the spinoglenoid notch, it is better seen on axial MR images (Fig. 1B). A prominent suprascapular vein, which in some instances is responsible for compressive neuropathy, is not infrequently noted in the vicinity of the nerve.

Pathology: Suprascapular Nerve Syndrome

The clinical and imaging manifestations of entrapment neuropathies of the suprascapular nerve and its branches vary depending on the location of compression. Entrapment of the suprascapular nerve at the scapular incisura results in supraspinatus and infraspinatus muscle denervation, whereas distal entrapment at the spinoglenoid notch may depict isolated involvement of the infraspinatus muscle [12].

Overhead activities with repetitive scapular motion, performed during sports such as volleyball and tennis, may produce stretching and compression of the suprascapular nerve and its branches under the suprascapular ligament. Repetitive adduction and internal rotation of the shoulder can stretch the nerve underneath the spinoglenoid ligament [11]. Direct trauma, scapular fractures, or post-traumatic calcification of the suprascapular ligament may also produce compression of the nerve. Peripheral nerve injury, including suprascapular neuropathy, was noted in 28% of patients who had full-thickness tears of the rotator cuff [13]. Iatrogenic injury to the suprascapular nerve can also occur during rotator cuff repair.

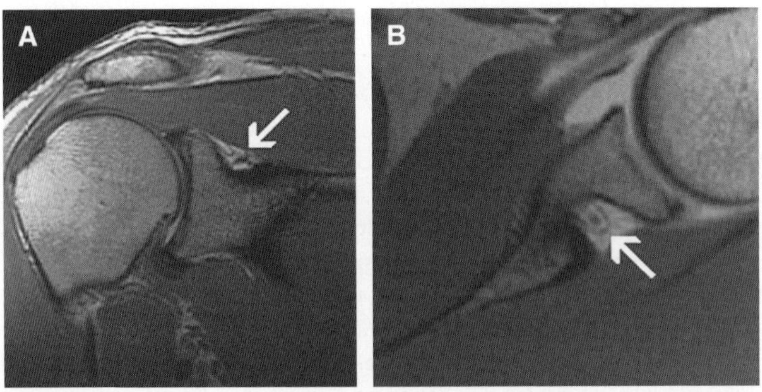

Fig. 1. Normal MR anatomy of the suprascapular nerve. (*A*) Oblique coronal T1-weighted image shows the suprascapular neurovascular bundle (*arrow*) within the suprascapular notch. (*B*) Axial proton density image at the level of the spinoglenoid notch demonstrates the suprascapular nerve (*arrow*) highlighted by fat.

Ganglion cysts at the scapular incisura, typically associated with superior and posterior labral tears, are other causes for suprascapular nerve entrapment [14,15]. Soft tissue masses, osseous tumors, and vascular malformations can also compress the nerve along its course.

MRI is a useful diagnostic modality in patients who have suprascapular nerve entrapment. Acute entrapment is depicted on water-sensitive sequences as hyperintensity involving the affected supraspinatus or infraspinatus muscles (Fig. 2), whereas chronic compression is noted as decreased bulk and fatty infiltration of the involved muscles. The extent of denervation muscle injury [16] can imply the exact site for the entrapment. Involvement of both the supraspinatus and infraspinatus muscles reflects compression at the suprascapular notch, whereas isolated denervation of the infraspinatus muscle is compatible with compression at the spinoglenoid notch.

AXILLARY NERVE

Normal Anatomy

The axillary nerve, as the terminal branch of the posterior cord of the brachial plexus, receives contributions from C5 and C6 nerve roots. The nerve courses along the anterior surface of the subscapularis muscle dorsal to the axillary artery. It then makes a sharp turn posteriorly to travel along the inferior glenohumeral joint surface. Slightly more distally, the nerve, along with the posterior circumflex artery, enters the quadrilateral space. The borders of the quadrilateral space are formed by the long head of the triceps brachii muscle medially, the teres minor muscle superiorly, the teres major muscle inferiorly, and the medial aspect of the proximal humerus laterally. The axillary nerve gives off four branches in the quadrilateral space: two motor branches to the anterior and posterior portions of the deltoid muscle, a sensory branch (the superior lateral brachial cutaneous nerve), and a motor branch to the teres minor muscle [17].

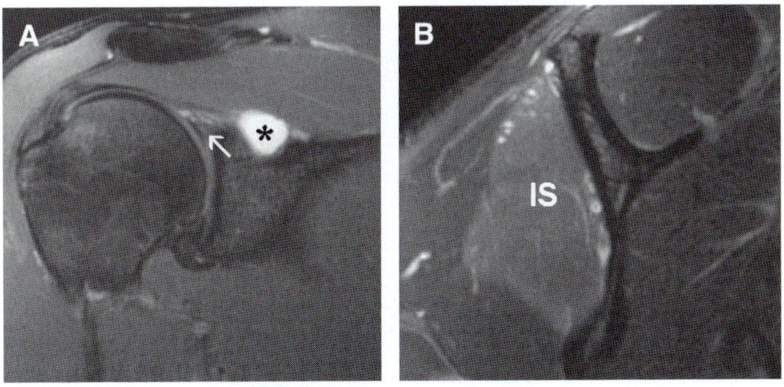

Fig. 2. Suprascapular nerve syndrome. Oblique coronal (*A*) and oblique sagittal (*B*) fat-suppressed, T2-weighted images depict a ganglion cyst (*asterisk*) within the suprascapular notch associated with a tear of the superior labrum (*arrow*). Denervation edema of the infraspinatus muscle (IS) is noted.

The branches to the teres minor and the lateral cutaneous innervation lie closest to the glenoid rim, and thus are most susceptible to injury at that site. Also, the axillary nerve was shown to travel at a fixed distance of approximately 2.5 mm from the inferior glenohumeral ligament throughout its course [18]. An articular branch of the axillary nerve supplies the shoulder joint capsule.

MRI Anatomy

The axillary neurovascular bundle, best visualized on oblique sagittal T1-weighted images of the shoulder, is well highlighted by fat and is seen below the inferior glenoid rim traversing the space between the teres minor muscle superiorly and the teres major muscle inferiorly (Fig. 3). The quadrilateral space is best visualized adjacent to the medial humeral cortex and lateral to the long head of the triceps muscle on oblique coronal images oriented perpendicular to the proximal humeral shaft.

Pathology

Quadrilateral space syndrome

The quadrilateral space syndrome is defined as compression of the axillary nerve within the quadrilateral space. Fractures of the proximal humerus and scapula can produce direct nerve injury [19]. Entrapment of the nerve can be produced by extreme abduction of the arm during athletic endeavors, or even during sleep. Mass effect secondary to tumors, hypertrophy of teres minor muscle in paraplegic patients, or by a fibrous band within the quadrilateral space [19] are other causes of entrapment of the nerve. Symptoms related to this syndrome include shoulder pain and paresthesia. Advanced cases may result in atrophy of the deltoid and teres minor muscles.

Conventional radiography and CT may depict osseous lesions such as fracture callus or bone tumors that could impinge upon the axillary nerve. MRI,

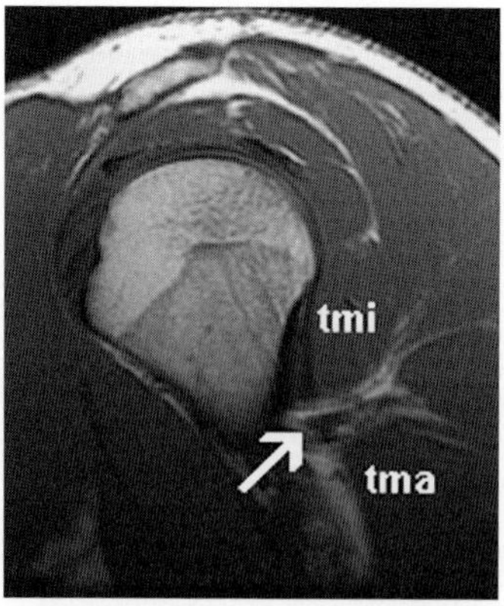

Fig. 3. Normal MR anatomy of the axillary nerve. Oblique sagittal T1-weighted image shows the axillary neurovascular bundle (*arrow*) traveling in between the teres minor muscle (tmi) and teres major muscle (tma).

electromyographic pattern with fibrillation potentials and positive waves is characteristically encountered in Parsonage-Turner syndrome [32].

The clinical symptoms and signs of Parsonage-Turner syndrome can mimic a wide range of disease entities, such as rotator cuff disease, cervical radiculopathy, spinal cord tumor, and peripheral nerve compression. Differentiation of the entity from compressive neuropathy of the suprascapular nerve can be particularly confusing. Useful features in distinguishing Parsonage-Turner syndrome from suprascapular nerve entrapment include the more insidious onset of pain and lack of spontaneous resolution of symptoms noted in the latter entity. MRI detection of paralabral ganglions or other impinging mass lesions within the suprascapular notch is also supportive of suprascapular nerve entrapment [34]. MRI can also be useful in excluding other disease entities such as rotator cuff tear, which can clinically mimic Parsonage-Turner syndrome.

Diffuse increased signal intensity on fluid-sensitive sequences consistent with interstitial muscle denervation edema can be seen on MR imaging during the acute stage of Parsonage-Turner syndrome [34]. The supraspinatus and infraspinatus muscles are the most commonly affected muscles, but the deltoid can also be involved (Fig. 6A). Muscle atrophy manifested by decreased muscle bulk may be visualized later on (Fig. 6B).

ULNAR NERVE

Normal Anatomy

The ulnar nerve continues directly from the medial cord of the brachial plexus, and contains motor and sensory fibers arising from the C8 and T1 roots. The ulnar nerve crosses from the anterior to the posterior compartment at mid-arm level, piercing the intermuscular septum. The ulnar nerve may pass under the arcade of Struthers, present in 70% of individuals, approximately 8 cm proximal to the medial epicondyle [35] . The arcade of Struthers, made of fibers from

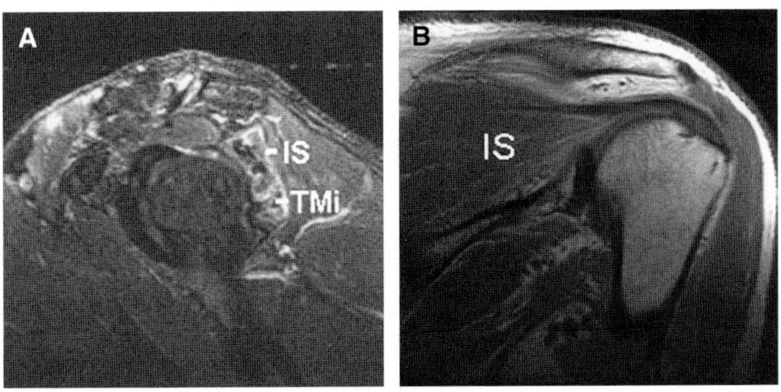

Fig. 6. Parsonage-Turner syndrome. Oblique sagittal fat-suppressed, T2-weighted (*A*) and oblique coronal proton density (*B*) images demonstrate denervation edema and fatty infiltration of the infraspinatus (IS) and teres minor (TMi) muscles.

the deep fascia of the distal arm, connects the medial intermuscular septum to the medial head of the triceps muscle.

The ulnar nerve is quite superficial at the elbow, where it descends posterior to the medial epicondyle within the cubital tunnel. The floor of the cubital tunnel is formed by the elbow capsule and portions of the ulnar collateral ligament, and the roof of the tunnel is formed by the arcuate ligament (Osborne ligament) or cubital tunnel retinaculum, extending from the medial epicondyle to the medial olecranon process (Fig. 7). It has been postulated that the cubital tunnel retinaculum is a remnant of the anconeus epitrochlearis muscle [36].

The ulnar nerve enters the anterior compartment of the forearm between the humeral and ulnar heads of the flexor carpi ulnaris muscle. It then continues in the forearm between the flexor carpi ulnaris and the flexor digitorum profundus muscles, and splits into superficial and deep ulnar branches in the region of Guyon's canal at the wrist.

In the elbow and forearm, the ulnar nerve supplies the elbow joint, the flexor carpi ulnaris muscle, and the ulnar half of the flexor digitorum profundus to the fourth and fifth fingers. The superficial motor branch of the ulnar nerve innervates the palmaris brevis, whereas the deep motor branch supplies the hypothenar muscles, third and fourth lumbricals, all interossei, adductor pollicis, flexor pollicis brevis-deep head, flexor digiti minimi, abductor digiti minimi, and opponens digiti minimi muscles. The ulnar nerve and its branches also provide sensation to the medial palm, and to the palmar and distal dorsal skin of the fifth finger and medial one half of the fourth finger.

MRI Anatomy

The ulnar nerve is clearly highlighted by fat throughout its course in the elbow and proximal forearm. The nerve is easily visualized on axial images as it traverses the cubital tunnel behind the medial epicondyle, roofed by the arcuate ligament (see Fig. 7) [37–39]. Lateral to the nerve, the accompanying recurrent ulnar vessels can often be identified. When imaging the elbow at 90° of flexion,

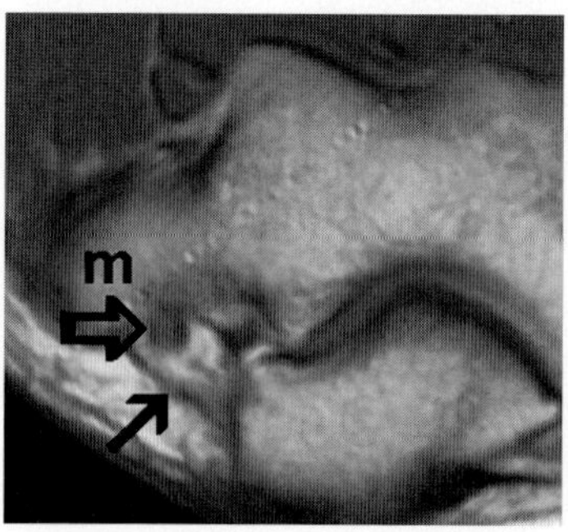

Fig. 7. Normal MRI anatomy of the ulnar nerve at the cubital tunnel. Axial proton density image depicts the ulnar nerve (*open arrow*) behind the medial epicondyle (m). The arcuate ligament (*arrow*) is seen.

reduction in the size of the cubital tunnel may render identification of the ulnar nerve difficult. Distal to the elbow joint, the ulnar nerve is commonly highlighted by fat as it travels in between the ulnar and humeral heads of the flexor carpi ulnaris muscle (Fig. 8). More distally, the nerve is found anterior to the flexor digitorum profundus muscle. The normal nerve is low in signal on T1-weighted images, but can demonstrate mild hyperintensity on fluid-sensitive images.

Pathology

Compressive neuropathy of the ulnar nerve at the elbow is the second most common neuropathy in the upper extremity, exceeded only by carpal tunnel syndrome. There are several potential sites of compression of the ulnar nerve at the distal arm and elbow. Entrapment at the cubital tunnel is the most common, likely related to the superficial course of the nerve rendering it more susceptible to direct trauma. The cubital tunnel experiences dynamic changes during flexion and extension of the elbow. Reduction in the size of the cubital tunnel during flexion is in part secondary to progressive tightening of the overlying arcuate ligament [40]. At 90° of elbow flexion, the greatest tightness of the arcuate ligament is achieved. Further decrease in the volume of the cubital tunnel and medial displacement of the ulnar nerve during elbow flexion are secondary to medial bulging of both the ulnar collateral ligament and the medial head of the triceps.

The arcade of Struthers, the edge of the medial intermuscular septum, thickened arcuate ligament, and the deep flexor pronator aponeurosis (4 cm distal to the medial epicondyle) are other potential sites of compressive ulnar neuropathy.

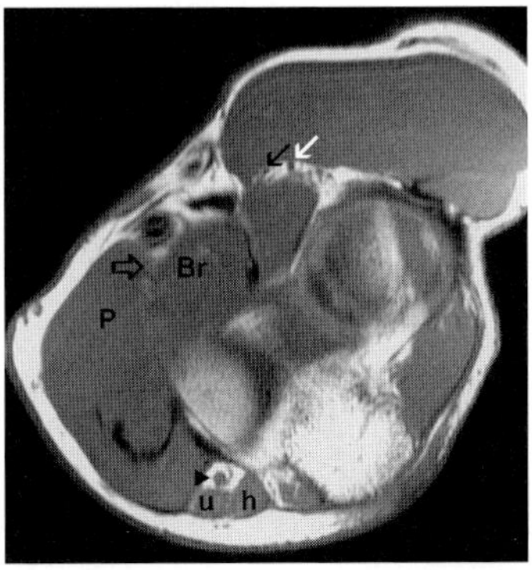

Fig. 8. Normal MRI anatomy of the nerves at the elbow joint. Axial proton density image shows the ulnar nerve (*arrowhead*) traveling in between the ulnar (u) and humeral (h) heads of the flexor carpi ulnaris muscle. The median nerve (*open arrow*) is identified in the interfascial plane between the brachialis (Br) and pronator-flexor (P) muscle groups. The superficial, sensory branch of the radial nerve (*black arrow*) and the posterior interosseous nerve (*white arrow*) are visualized.

CUBITAL TUNNEL SYNDROME

Physiologic and compressive cubital tunnel syndromes have been described. Compressive cubital syndrome may have acute, subacute, or chronic presentation. Normal loss in volume and increased pressure within the tunnel during elbow flexion result in physiologic cubital tunnel syndrome. This can be seen in "sleep palsy," as the arm is held in flexion for prolonged periods of time.

Blunt trauma to the cubital tunnel is a typical cause of acute external compression syndrome of the ulnar nerve. External compressive forces typically cause injury to the more superficial sensory fibers. Subacute compression syndrome has been described in hospitalized, bedridden, or wheelchair-bound patients, and following surgery.

The anconeous epitrochlearis muscle, an accessory muscle that traverses the cubital tunnel, has also been implicated as a cause of chronic external compressive ulnar neuropathy (Fig. 9) [41]. Other causes include callus formation from distal humeral and supracondylar fractures, elbow dislocation, and avulsed medial epicondylar apophysis. In athletes, a frequent cause of chronic cubital tunnel syndrome is lateral shift of the ulna, commonly associated with chronic laxity of the ulnar collateral ligament (Fig. 10). Tardy ulnar palsy refers to a delayed neuropathy presenting 15 to 20 years after a childhood capitellar epiphyseal injury and secondary cubitus valgus [42]. Congenital hypoplasia of the capitellum may also cause lateral shift of the ulna with traction on the ulnar nerve. Lastly, masses such as tumors, distended bursae, ganglions, hematoma, inflammatory pannus, gouty tophi, loose bodies, and osteophytes can result in chronic cubital tunnel syndrome.

Friction neuritis and compressive ulnar neuropathy have also been associated with subluxation or dislocation of the ulnar nerve at the level of the cubital

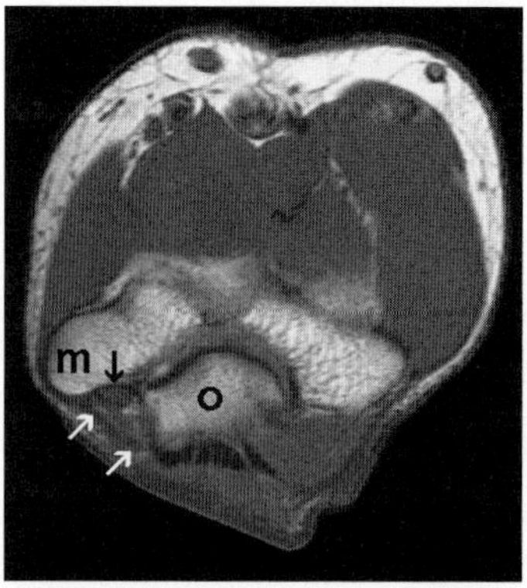

Fig. 9. Anconeus epitrochlearis. Axial T1-weighted image depicts an accessory muscle (*white arrows*) spanning from the medial epicondyle (m) to the olecranon process (o). The ulnar nerve is somewhat enlarged (*black arrow*).

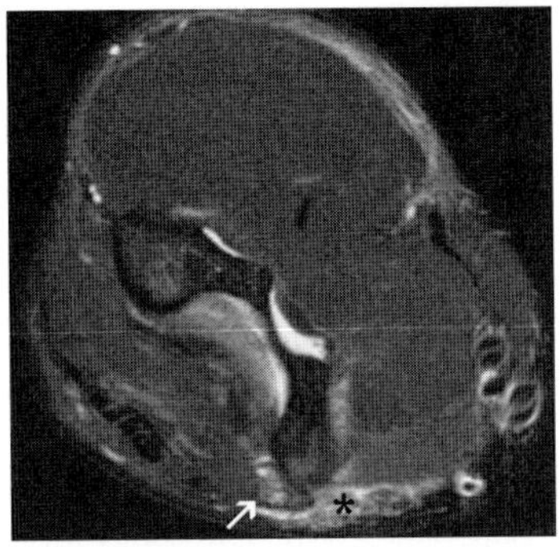

Fig. 10. Ulnar neuritis. Axial fat-suppressed, T2-weighted image at the level of the medial epicondyle shows enlargement and thickening of the ulnar nerve (*arrow*) associated with tears of the ulnar collateral ligament and common flexor tendon (*asterisk*).

tunnel (Fig. 11). Asymptomatic subluxation of the ulnar nerve can be seen in up to 16% of individuals. During elbow flexion, medial excursion of the ulnar nerve may be accentuated. Ulnar nerve instability has been described in association with congenital absence (see Fig. 11), laxity or tear of the arcuate ligament, trochlear hypoplasia, and post-traumatic cubitus valgus deformity. Dislocation of the medial head of the triceps muscle over the medial epicondyle, the snapping triceps syndrome, has been implicated as one more cause of ulnar nerve dislocation [43].

Clinical symptoms of cubital tunnel syndrome include nocturnal paresthesias involving the fourth and fifth fingers, elbow pain radiating to the hand, and sensory symptoms related to prolonged flexion of the elbow. If weakness occurs, it may affect finger abduction, thumb abduction, pinching of the thumb and forefinger, and eventually power grip. In the differential diagnosis of cubital tunnel syndrome, compressive ulnar neuropathy at the wrist, lower cervical

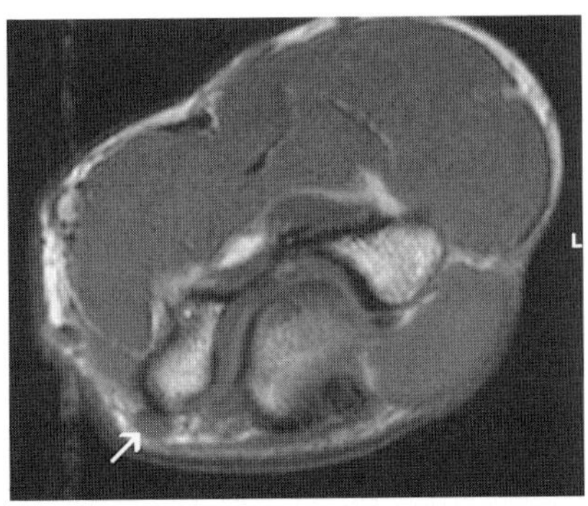

Fig. 11. Ulnar nerve subluxation. Axial proton density image shows an anteriorly subluxed and swollen ulnar nerve (*arrow*). The arcuate ligament is absent.

radiculopathy, thoracic outlet syndrome, amyotrophic lateral sclerosis, and other cord lesions should be considered.

Ulnar nerve thickening and intraneural edema are MRI findings indicative of cubital tunnel syndrome. The arcuate ligament should always be assessed for thickening, tearing, or congenital absence. Medial subluxation or dislocation of the nerve may be seen on standard axial MR images. When ulnar nerve subluxation is clinically suspected and abnormal shift of the nerve is not apparent on conventional MRI examination, repeat imaging in elbow flexion may be of help. Ganglia, soft tissue tumors, osseous spurs, and anomalous muscles such as the anconeus epitrochlearis responsible for compressive ulnar neuropathy can be easily diagnosed using MRI. Signal abnormality or atrophy of the flexor carpi ulnaris and flexor digitorum profundus at the level of the proximal forearm are valuable complementary features in the MRI diagnosis of ulnar neuropathy.

The initial management of acute and subacute ulnar neuropathy at the elbow is conservative. Rest and avoidance of pressure on the nerve may suffice. If symptoms persist, splint immobilization is warranted. For refractory cases, which may be associated with muscle weakness, surgical management, including medial epicondylectomy and anterior ulnar transposition, is often indicated. Fluid-sensitive MR images may reveal ulnar nerve hyperintensity long after the surgery. Intense intraneural edema, however, is more likely to reflect persistent neuritis. Tethering of the nerve and engulfing scar can also be identified (Fig. 12).

MEDIAN NERVE

Normal Anatomy

The median nerve supplies the radial side of the flexor portion of the forearm and hand, and is formed by the blending of the lateral and medial cords of the brachial plexus. It contains both motor and sensory fibers from the C5, C6, C7, C8 and T1 nerve roots. The median nerve descends in the arm in close relationship to the brachial artery. It has no branches at the level of the arm. At

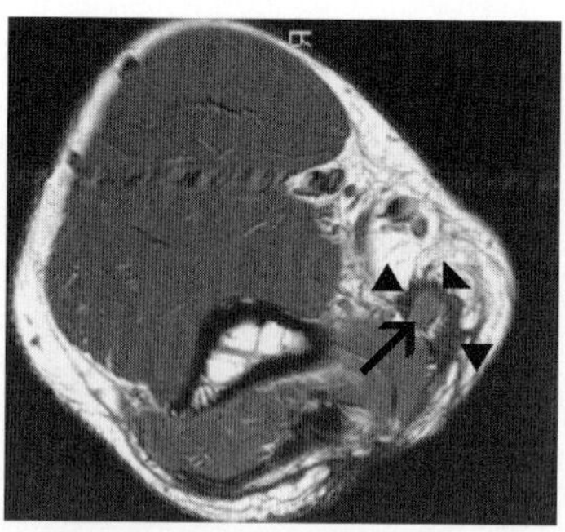

Fig. 12. Subcutaneous anterior transposition of the ulnar nerve. Axial T1-weighted image shows a mildly swollen ulnar nerve (*arrow*) surrounded by a thickened fascial sling and scar tissue (*arrowheads*).

the elbow, the median nerve is found medial and parallel to the brachial artery as it travels in between the bicipital aponeurosis (lacertus fibrosus) and parochialism muscle. The median nerve then courses into the forearm deep to the pronator teres muscle [35]. The median nerve supplies all superficial ventral muscles of the forearm, except for the flexor carpi ulnaris muscle, including the pronator teres, flexor carpi radialis, palmaris longus, and flexor digitorum superficialis.

Approximately 2 to 5 cm below the level of the medial epicondyle, in close proximity to the bifurcation of the brachial artery into the radial and ulnar arteries, the median nerve gives off the anterior interosseous nerve. This courses over the flexor digitorum profundus and along the interosseous membrane toward the wrist joint. All the ventral deep muscles of the forearm, including the radial half of the flexor digitorum profundus, the flexor pollicis longus, and the pronator quadratus muscles, are innervated by the anterior interosseous nerve, except for the ulnar half of the flexor digitorum profundus, which is supplied by the ulnar nerve.

MRI Anatomy

Prominence of the pronator teres and parochialism muscles often obliterates the perifascial fat planes, making it difficult to visualize the median nerve on MR images at the level of the elbow (see Fig. 8). In the proximal forearm, easier identification can be achieved as the nerve travels in the fat plane between the superficial humeral and deep ulnar heads of the pronator teres muscle and underneath the lacertus fibrosus.

Pathology: Pronator Syndrome

The pronator syndrome is the most common cause of median nerve entrapment at the elbow. Elbow fractures and dislocations [44], accessory muscles such as Gantzer's muscle (the accessory head of the flexor pollicis longus muscle), soft tissue masses, and dynamic forces at the elbow have also been implicated. Honeymooner's paralysis is related to median nerve compression secondary to prolonged pressure of a lover's head against a partner's forearm.

Clinical signs of median neuropathy include weak pronation of the forearm, weak flexion, and radial deviation of the wrist associated with thenar atrophy and inability to oppose or flex the thumb.

Numbness in the median nerve distribution with repetitive pronation/supination of the forearm, but not with flexion and extension of the elbow, is a frequent presenting symptom of pronator teres syndrome. On physical examination, forearm pain elicited by resistance to pronation or resistance to isolated flexion of the third and fourth proximal interphalangeal joints can be observed. Electromyographic studies may show only mildly reduced conduction velocities.

There are four potential compression sites within the spectrum of pronator teres syndrome: (1) the supracondylar process/ligament of Struthers, (2) the lacertus fibrosus, (3) the pronator teres muscle, and (4) the proximal arch of the flexor digitorum superficialis muscle [45].

The supracondylar process syndrome is the least common compression neuropathy of the median nerve. The supracondylar process or avian spur arises from the distal humerus about 5 to 7 cm above the elbow joint (Fig. 13) [46]. The lack of radiographic identification of the supracondylar process does not exclude the presence of compressive median neuropathy caused by the ligament of Struthers. This structure, which spans from the supracondylar process to the medial epicondyle, may cause median nerve, and to a lesser extent ulnar nerve entrapment [46]. The compression is worsened with extension and supination.

The median nerve travels deep to the lacertus fibrosus at the level of the elbow. This latter structure emanates from the distal bicipital tendon coursing obliquely over the pronator-flexor group of muscles to insert on the antebrachial fascia. Compression of the pronator muscle and median nerve may be secondary to a thickened lacertus fibrosus.

The most frequent etiology for pronator syndrome is dynamic compression of the median nerve between the superficial humeral and deep ulnar heads of the pronator teres muscle [47]. In up to 50% of anatomic specimens, fibrous bands can be found dorsal to the humeral head or to the nerve itself. Median nerve compression by these bands is more pronounced in pronation and elbow extension, when the distance between the two heads of the pronator teres muscle is narrowed. The fibrous arch of origin of the flexor digitorum superficialis muscle is the most distal as well as the second-most common site of median nerve compression at the elbow.

When there is clinical suspicion of pronator syndrome, MRI examination of the upper extremity should cover all potential compression sites from the distal one third of the arm to the proximal two thirds of the forearm [48]. Denervation edema or atrophy in the flexor-pronator group of muscles, including the

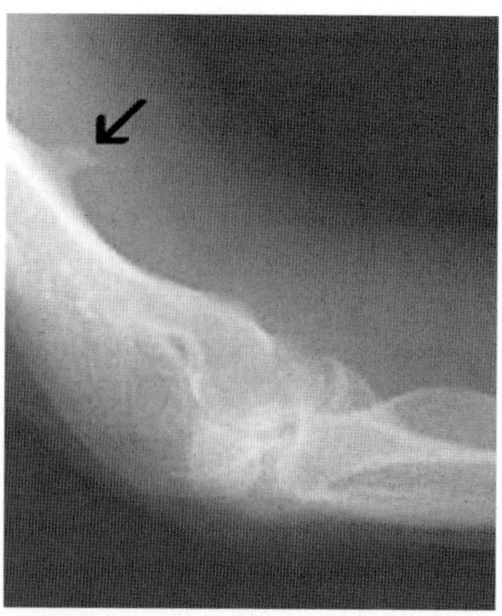

Fig. 13. Supracondylar process. Lateral radiograph of the elbow depicts an osseous spur emanating from the distal humerus approximately 5–7 cm above the elbow joint.

pronator teres, the flexor carpi radialis, the palmaris longus, and the flexor digitorum superficialis muscles, can be seen in patients who have pronator syndrome (Fig. 14). Space-occupying lesions such as nerve sheath tumors (Fig. 15), ganglions, and bursae can also be depicted.

RADIAL NERVE

Normal Anatomy

The radial nerve, a terminal branch of the posterior cord of the brachial plexus, supplies the extensor musculature of the arm and forearm as well as the overlying skin. The radial nerve carries motor and sensory fibers from the C5, C6, C7, C8, and T1 nerve roots. The nerve descends between the medial and long heads of the triceps muscle in the proximal arm. At the proximal humeral shaft, the radial nerve traverses within the humeral spiral groove. In the distal arm, the nerve perforates the lateral intermuscular septum, traveling in between the brachioradialis and parochialism muscles. Motor branches of the radial nerve near the elbow innervate the lateral head of the triceps.

The radial nerve enters the radial tunnel at the radiocapitellar joint. This tunnel begins and is bounded posteriorly by the capitellum, and terminates at the level of the supinator muscle [35]. The brachioradialis, the extensor carpi radialis longus, and extensor carpi radialis brevis muscles form the anterolateral margin of the tunnel, whereas the parochialism muscle outlines the medial margin. Near the radial head, the radial nerve divides into the motor, posterior interosseous nerve, and the sensory, superficial branch. The superficial sensory branch passes into the forearm deep to the brachioradialis. The posterior interosseous nerve crosses into the posterior compartment between the superficial and deep heads of the supinator muscle to supply nine muscles on the extensor aspect of the forearm. As it enters the supinator muscle, the posterior interosseous nerve dives under the arcade of Frohse, a fibrous arch formed by the proximal thickened edge of the superficial head of the supinator muscle.

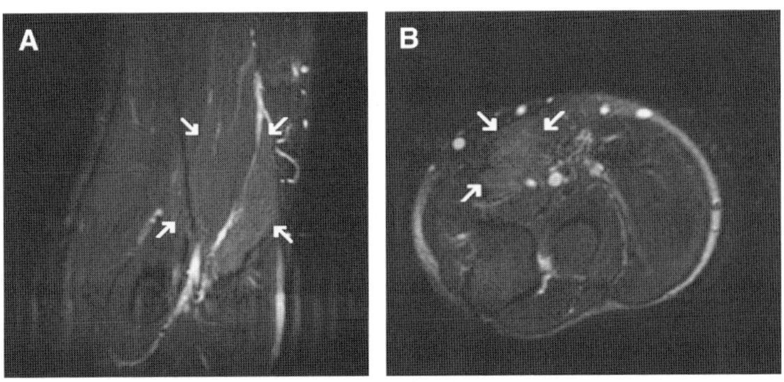

Fig. 14. Pronator syndrome. Oblique coronal and axial fat-suppressed, T2-weighted images show diffuse T2 hyperintensity of the pronator teres muscle consistent with acute denervation edema (*arrows*).

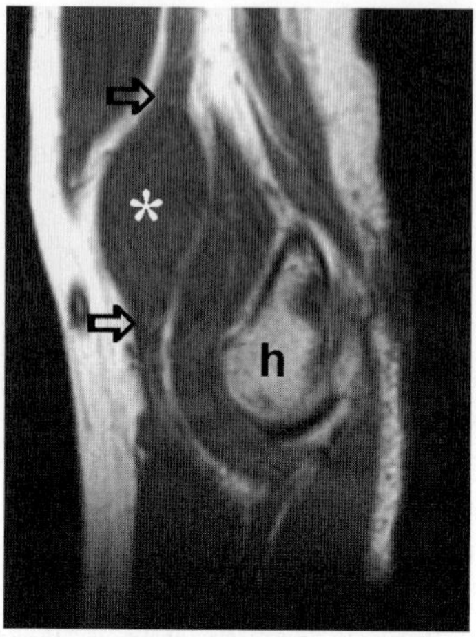

Fig. 15. Median nerve neurofibroma. Sagittal T1-weighted image shows a fusiform mass (*asterisk*) arising from the median nerve. Comet tail sign is noted proximally and distally (*open arrows*). h, distal humerus.

The posterior interosseous nerve innervates the supinator, extensor carpi ulnaris, extensor digitorum communis, extensor digiti quinti, abductor pollicis longus, extensor indicis proprius, and extensor pollicis longus and brevis muscles.

MRI Anatomy

At the level of the elbow, the radial nerve is best visualized on axial images as it courses between the parochialism, brachioradialis, and extensor carpi radialis longus and brevis muscles (see Fig. 8) [37–39]. The division of the radial nerve into the superficial radial branch and the deep posterior interosseous nerve is usually identified proximal or at the radiocapitellar joint (see Fig. 8). The branches of the radial nerve may be difficult to differentiate from the adjacent accompanying vessels. A hypointense band at the proximal edge of the superficial head of the supinator muscle is consistent with the arcade of Frohse. A similar, low-signal, linear band is noted along the medial edge of the extensor carpi radialis brevis. In the proximal forearm, the posterior interosseous nerve is frequently observed as it runs in between the superficial and deep heads of the supinator muscle.

Pathology

At the level of the arm, radial nerve injury is frequently post-traumatic secondary to displaced humeral shaft fracture, inappropriate use of axillary crutches, proximal prolonged tourniquet application,, and lateral or posterior arm intramuscular injection. In weight lifters, compressive radial neuropathy has been described beneath the lateral head of the triceps muscle during extension against resistance. Soft tissue masses such as ganglia, and tumors can also cause entrapment of the nerve (Fig. 16).

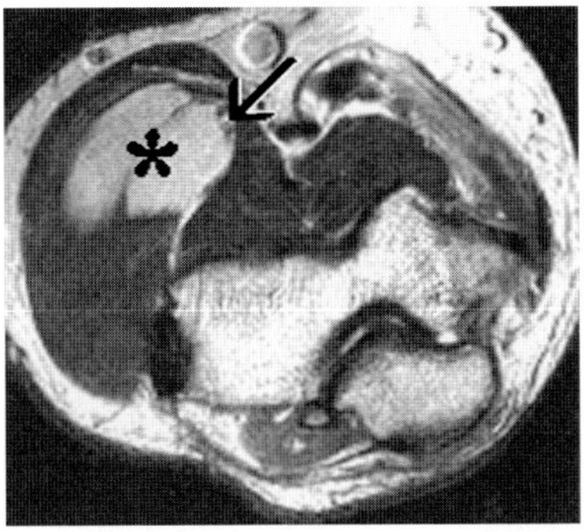

Fig. 16. Radial nerve entrapment by lipoma. Axial T2-weighted image at the level of the distal arm demonstrates a large intramuscular lipoma (*asterisk*) displacing the radial nerve branches (*arrow*).

Radial nerve entrapment at the elbow mainly affects the posterior interosseous nerve, and can be subdivided into two major categories: (1) the radial tunnel syndrome, which is a painful condition without motor deficits; and (2) the posterior interosseous nerve syndrome, which is a motor neuropathy [49]. Deep forearm pain, pain radiating to the neck and shoulder, and a "heavy" sensation of the affected arm are common presenting symptoms [49]. On physical examination, tenderness over the radial nerve along the radial tunnel, pain on resisted supination, and the presence of a Tinel's sign over the radial forearm can be found. In up to 90% of patients, the electromyographic studies reveal no significant abnormalities. Of 79 surgical decompressions, 77% had excellent recovery and 20% were judged to have good outcome [49].

Radial tunnel syndrome

Compressive neuropathy of the posterior interosseous nerve at the radial tunnel without motor deficit is the hallmark of radial tunnel syndrome [50]. There is controversy about the neurogenic etiology of the entity, because its main manifestation is pain at the radial tunnel without muscle weakness [51]. The clinical diagnosis is often confounding, because radial tunnel syndrome can masquerade as or coexist with lateral epicondylitis. Recalcitrant lateral epicondylitis, which is refractory to conservative treatment, should raise the suspicion of radial tunnel syndrome.

Dynamic compression within the radial tunnel may be secondary to repeated pronation and supination or forceful extension of the forearm. Tennis players [35], swimmers, housewives, welders, conductors, and violinists are frequently affected. The condition most commonly involves patients in the fourth to sixth decade of life without significant gender predilection.

The posterior interosseous nerve can be compressed within the radial tunnel at several sites, which include, from proximal to distal: (1) at the radiocapitellar joint by fibrous bands; (2) at the tendinous edge of the extensor carpi radialis brevis muscle; (3) at the radial recurrent artery and branches (leash of Henry); (4) at the arcade of Frohse, the proximal edge of the supinator muscle [52]; and (5) at the distal end of the supinator muscle by a fibrous band [34].

The utility of electromyographic studies in diagnosing radial tunnel syndrome is somewhat limited because of the deep location of the posterior interosseous nerve. Surgical release of the arcade of Frohse often relieves the symptoms.

Posterior interosseous nerve syndrome

The posterior interosseous nerve syndrome is defined as a motor neuropathy. Potential causative factors include trauma, space-occupying lesions, and inflammatory processes. Compression sites for posterior interosseous nerve syndrome are the same as those for the radial tunnel syndrome (see above). Clinically, deep forearm pain and muscle weakness with loss of extension of all the digits and decrease of wrist dorsiflexion can be noted. Complete sparing of the extensor carpi radialis longus and frequent sparing of the extensor carpi radialis brevis are often observed as the branches to these muscles often originate proximal to the takeoff of the posterior interosseous nerve. On the contrary, the extensor carpi ulnaris longus is always affected. The initial management of posterior interosseous nerve syndrome is conservative, except in the presence of masses, fractures, or dislocation, which may require surgical intervention. When there is lack of improvement following 6 to 8 weeks of conservative treatment, surgical decompression may be warranted.

Radial tunnel syndrome and posterior interosseous nerve syndrome have similar MR imaging manifestations of acute denervation, manifested as increased T2 signal; and chronic denervation, manifested as increased T1 signal in the muscles supplied by the posterior interosseous nerve [53–56]. Isolated or concomitant involvement of the supinator (Fig. 17) and extensor muscles is seen (Fig. 18). Muscle signal alterations in more proximal muscles, such as the extensor carpi radialis longus, the anconeus, and the triceps muscles, are indicative of radial nerve entrapment above the radial tunnel. Mass effect

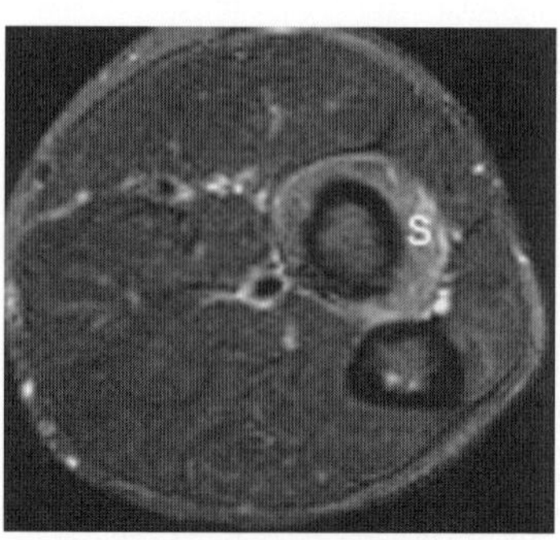

Fig. 17. Radial tunnel syndrome. Axial fat-suppressed, T2-weighted image at the level of the radial tuberosity demonstrates selective denervation edema of the supinator muscle (S).

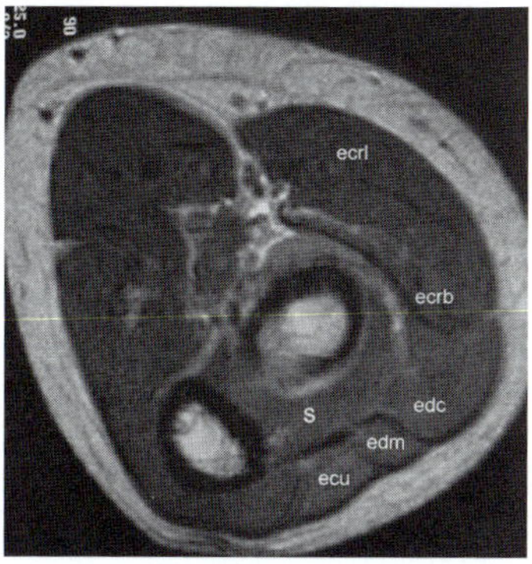

Fig. 18. Posterior interosseous nerve syndrome. Axial T2-weighted image at the level of the radial tuberosity shows mild atrophy and diffuse interstitial hyperintensity of the supinator and extensor muscles with sparing of the extensor carpi radialis longus. ecu, extensor carpi ulnaris muscle; edc, extensor digitorum communis muscle; edm, extensor digiti minimi muscle; ecrb, extensor carpi radialis brevis muscle; ecrl, extensor carpi radialis longus muscle.

exerted by a thickened arcade of Frohse, thickened medial edge of the extensor carpi radialis brevis muscle, prominent recurrent radial vessels, neurogenic tumors, and distended bursae can be easily depicted by MRI.

SUMMARY

In conclusion, MRI is a useful diagnostic method for evaluating nerve disease at the shoulder and elbow. MRI can depict the normal anatomy of the nerves, confirm and identify the cause of the neuropathy, identify the site of entrapment based on muscle denervation patterns, and detect unsuspected space-occupying lesions. MRI can also narrow down the differential diagnosis of nerve disease, such as in the case of suprascapular nerve syndrome versus Parsonage-Turner syndrome, or radial tunnel syndrome versus lateral epicondylitis. Large prospective studies with surgical correlation, however, are still necessary to better elucidate MRI's exact role in the assessment of entrapment neuropathies of the upper extremity.

References

[1] Pecina MM, Krmpotic-Nemanic J, Petkiewicz AD. Tunnel syndromes in the upper extremities. In: Pecina MM, Krmpotic-Nemanic J, Markiewitz AD, editors. Tunnel syndromes. New York: CRC Press; 1991. p. 29–53.

[2] Uetani M, Kuniaki H, Matsunaga N, et al. Denervated skeletal muscle: MR imaging. Radiology 1983;189:511–5.

[3] Fleckenstein JL, Watumull D, Conner KE, et al. Denervated human skeletal muscle: MR imaging evaluation. Radiology 1993;187:213–8.

[4] Sunderland S. The anatomy and physiology of nerve injury. Muscle Nerve 1990;13:771–84.

[5] Koltzenburg M, Bendszus M. Imaging of peripheral nerve lesions. Curr Opin Neurol 2004;17:621–6.

[6] Bendszus M, Koltzenburg M. Visualization of denervated muscle by gadolinium-enhanced MRI. Neurology 2001;57:1709–11.
[7] Bendszus M, Koltzenburg M, Wessig C, et al. Sequential MR imaging of denervated muscle: experimental study. AJNR Am J Neuroradiol 2002;23:1427–31.
[8] Kikuchi Y, Nakamura T, Takayama S, et al. MRI imaging in the diagnosis of denervated and reinnervated skeletal muscles: experimental study in rats. Radiology 2003;229:861–7.
[9] Bendszus M, Stoll G. Caught in the act: in vivo mapping of macrophage infiltration in nerve injury by magnetic resonance imaging. J Neurosci 2003;23:10892–6.
[10] Bendszus M, Wessig C, Schutz A, et al. Assessment of nerve degeneration by gadofluorine M-enhanced magnetic resonance imaging. Ann Neurol 2005;57:388–95.
[11] Demirhan M, Imhoff AB, Debski RE, et al. The spinoglenoid ligament and its relationship to the suprascapular nerve. J Shoulder Elbow Surg 1998;7:238–43.
[12] Fritz RC, Helms CA, Steinbach LS, et al. Suprascapular nerve entrapment: evaluation with MR imaging. Radiology 1992;182:437–44.
[13] Vad VB, Southern D, Warren RF, et al. Prevalence of peripheral neurological injuries in rotator cuff tears with atrophy. J Shoulder Elbow Surg 2003;12:333–6.
[14] Tirman PF, Feller JF, Janzen DL, et al. Association of glenoid labral cysts with labral tears and glenohumeral instability: radiologic findings and clinical significance. Radiology 1994;190:653–8.
[15] Mittal S, Turcinovic M, Gould ES, et al. Acute isolated suprascapular nerve palsy limited to the infraspinatus muscle: a case report. Arch Phys Med Rehabil 2002;83:565–7.
[16] Elsayes KM, Shariff A, Staveteig PT, et al. Value of magnetic resonance imaging for muscle denervation syndromes of the shoulder girdle. J Comput Assist Tomogr 2005;29:326–9.
[17] Zhao X, Hung LK, Zhang GM, et al. Applied anatomy of the anatomy of the axillary nerve for selective neurotization of the deltoid muscle. Clin Orthop 2001;390:244–51.
[18] Price MR, Tillet ED, Acland RD, et al. Determining the relationship of the axillary nerve to the shoulder joint capsule from an arthroscopic perspective. J Bone Joint Surg Am 2004;86:2135–42.
[19] Sanders TG, Tirman PF. Paralabral cyst: an unusual cause of quadrilateral space syndrome. Arthroscopy 1999;15:631–7.
[20] Visser CP, Coene LN, Brand R, et al. The incidence of nerve injury in anterior dislocation of the shoulder and its influence on functional recovery. A prospective clinical and EMG study. J Bone Joint Surg Br 1999;81:679–85.
[21] Tuckman GA, Devlin TC. Axillary nerve injury after anterior glenohumeral dislocation: MR findings in three patients. AJR Am J Roentgenol 1996;167:695–7.
[22] Bencardino JT, Petchprapa CN, Rybak LK, et al. Teres minor atrophy: a sign of axillary denervation injury following shoulder trauma. Radiology 2002;225:371.
[23] Sofka CM, Lin J, Feinberg J, et al. Teres minor denervation on routine magnetic resonance imaging of the shoulder. Skeletal Radiol 2004;33:514–8.
[24] Visser CP, Coene LN, Brand R, et al. Nerve lesions in proximal humeral fractures. J Shoulder Elbow Surg 2001;10:421–7.
[25] Wong KL, Williams GR. Complications of thermal capsulorrhaphy of the shoulder. J Bone Joint Surg Am 2001;(Suppl 2):51–5.
[26] Bredella MA, Tirman PF, Fritz RC, et al. Denervation syndromes of the shoulder girdle: MR imaging with electrophysiologic correlation. Skeletal Radiol 1999;28:567–72.
[27] Fleckenstein JL, Watumull D, Conner KE, et al. Denervated human skeletal muscle: MR imaging evaluation. Radiology 1993;187:213–8.
[28] Steinmann SP, Moran EA. Axillary nerve injury: diagnosis and treatment. J Am Acad Orthop Surg 2001;9:328–35.
[29] Pellas F, Bolivares JP, Zandotti C, et al. Neuralgic amyotrophy after parvovirus B19 infection. Lancet 1993;342:503–4.
[30] Tsairis P, Dyck P, Mulder DW. Natural history of brachial plexus neuropathy. Report on 99 patients. Arch Neurol 1972;27:109–17.

[31] Lahrmann H, Grisold W, Authier FJ, et al. Neuralgic amyotrophy with phrenic nerve involvement. Muscle Nerve 1999;22:437–42.
[32] Misamore GW, Lehman DE. Parsonage-Turner syndrome (acute brachial neuritis). J Bone Joint Surg Am 1996;78A:1405–8.
[33] Parsonage MJ, Aldren, Turner JW. Neuralgic amyotrophy. The shoulder girdle syndrome. Lancet 1948;1:973–8.
[34] Helms CA, Martinez S, Speer KP. Acute brachial neuritis (Parsonage-Turner syndrome): MR imaging appearance-report of three cases. Radiology 1999;207:255–9.
[35] Morrey BF. Anatomy of the elbow joint. In: Morrey BF, editor. The elbow and its disorders. Philadelphia: W.B. Saunders; 1993. p. 7–42.
[36] O'Driscoll SW, Horii E, Carmichael SW, et al. The cubital tunnel and ulnar neuropathy. J Bone Joint Surg Br 1991;73:613–7.
[37] Rosenberg ZS, Bencardino J, Beltran J. MR features of nerve disorders at the elbow. Magn Reson Imaging Clin N Am 1997;5:545–65.
[38] Rosenberg ZS, Beltran J, Cheung YY, et al. The elbow: MR features of nerve disorders at the elbow. Radiology 1993;188:235–40.
[39] Beltran J, Rosenberg ZS. Diagnoses of compressive and entrapment neuropathies of the upper extremity: value of MR imaging. AJR Am J Roentgenol 1994;163:525–31.
[40] Patel VV, Heidenreich FP Jr, Bindra RR, et al. Morphologic changes in the ulnar nerve at the elbow with flexion and extension: a magnetic resonance imaging study with three-dimensional reconstruction. J Shoulder Elbow Surg 1998;7:368–74.
[41] Dahners LE, Wood FM. Anconeus epitrochlearis, a rare cause of cubital tunnel syndrome: a case report. J Hand Surg [Am] 1984;9:579–80.
[42] Abe M, Ishizu T, Shirai H, et al. Tardy ulnar nerve palsy caused by cubitus varus deformity. J Hand Surg [Am] 1995;20:5–9.
[43] Jacobson JA, Jebson PJ, Jeffers AW, et al. Ulnar nerve dislocation and snapping triceps syndrome: diagnosis with dynamic sonography—report of three cases. Radiology 2001; 220:601–5.
[44] Akansel G, Dalbayrak S, Yilmaz M, et al. MRI demonstration of intra-articular median nerve entrapment after elbow dislocation. Skeletal Radiol 2003;32:537–41.
[45] Spinner M, Linscheid RL. Nerve entrapment syndromes. In: Morrey BF, editor. The elbow and its disorders. Philadelphia: W.B. Saunders; 1993. p. 813–32.
[46] Al-Naib I. Humeral supracondylar spur and Struther's ligament. A rare cause of neurovascular entrapment in the upper limb. Int Orthop 1994;18:393–4.
[47] Hartz CR, Linscheid RL, Gramse RR, et al. The pronator teres syndrome: compressive neuropathy of the median nerve. J Bone Joint Surg Am 1981;63:885–90.
[48] Pecina M, Boric I, Anticevic D. Intraoperatively proven anomalous Struthers' ligament diagnosed by MRI. Skeletal Radiol 2002;31:532–5.
[49] Rinker B, Effron CR, Beasley RW. Proximal radial nerve compression. Ann Plast Surg 2004;52:174–80.
[50] Barnum M, Mastey RD, Weiss AC, et al. Radial tunnel syndrome. Hand Clin 1996;12(4): 679–89.
[51] Rosenbaum R. Disputed radial tunnel syndrome. Muscle Nerve 1999;22:960–7.
[52] Spinner M. The arcade of Frohse and its relationship to posterior interosseous nerve paralysis. J Bone Joint Surg Br 1968;50:809–12.
[53] Ferdinand B, Rosenberg ZS, Schweitzer ME, et al. MRI features of the radial tunnel syndrome. Radiology, in press.
[54] Shah JJ, Bhatti NA. Radial nerve paralysis associated with fractures of the humerus. A review of 62 cases. Clin Orthop 1993;172:171–6.
[55] Konjengbam M, Elangbam J. Radial nerve in the radial tunnel: anatomic sites of entrapment neuropathy. Clin Anat 2004;17:21–5.
[56] Lorei MP, Hershman EB. Peripheral nerve injuries in athletes. Treatment and prevention. Sports Med 1993;16:130–47.

ELSEVIER
SAUNDERS

Clin Sports Med 25 (2006) 489–504

CLINICS IN SPORTS MEDICINE

Imaging of Upper Extremity Stress Fractures in the Athlete

Mark W. Anderson, MD

Department of Radiology, Box 170, University of Virginia Health Sciences Center, 100 Lee Street, Charlottesville, VA 22908, USA

The incidence of stress fractures has been rising over the last several years in our increasingly active society. Although most of these injuries occur in the lower extremities, because of their weight-bearing function [1], they have also been reported to involve multiple sites in the upper extremities. Because of their relative infrequency, clinical diagnosis may be difficult, and diagnostic imaging studies can be exceedingly helpful in arriving at an accurate and timely diagnosis. The purpose of this article is to describe the most common sites of stress injuries in the upper extremity, their underlying pathophysiology, and their spectrum of imaging findings.

STRESS INJURIES TO BONE

The skeleton is a dynamic organ that undergoes constant remodeling in response to applied stresses according to Wolfe's law (bone is formed and retained along the lines of stress within a bone). Cortical and trabecular microdamage occurs as a result of daily activities, and normally osteoclastic resorption of the damaged bone is followed by osteoblastic bone production, resulting in an equilibrium [2].

However, with new or increased physical activity, the degree of remodeling increases, and bone resorption outpaces bone production because there is usually a lag of several weeks before new, lamellar bone is laid down [3]. During this "window of vulnerability," the imbalance between resorption and formation results in a localized weakening of the bone, and if the offending activity is not curtailed, the microdamage will begin to accumulate [3]. At this stage in the stress reaction, periosteal and endosteal new bone is produced in an attempt to buttress the temporarily weakened cortex [4]. Ultimately, if the activity is continued, further weakening of the bone will lead to mechanical failure and the development of a true, macroscopic fracture (stress fracture).

Stress fractures are classically divided into *fatigue fractures* (in which increased physical activity results in damage to normal bone) and *insufficiency fractures* (in

E-mail address: mwa3a@virginia.edu

0278-5919/06/$ – see front matter
doi:10.1016/j.csm.2006.02.006

sportsmed.theclinics.com

which normal activities result in damage to abnormal bone, such as bone weakened by osteoporosis). In this article, the term "stress fracture" is used synonymously with "fatigue fracture."

MECHANISMS OF INJURY

General

Osseous structures are subjected to several different types of stress during physical activities, including tensile, compressive, bending, and shear/torsional forces [5]. One or more of these may result in a stress injury to bone if applied in a repetitive manner. A number of mechanisms have been suggested as possible causes for the development of stress fractures.

Weight bearing

The compressive forces that result from weight-bearing activities are undoubtedly the source of many stress injuries in the lower extremities [6]. In certain sports, such as gymnastics, the upper extremities are also used for weight bearing; this can lead to stress fractures, most typically in the forearm and wrist [5].

Muscle action

Even without weight bearing, muscular actions on bone can generate significant forces that may be torsional, tensile, bending, or even compressive in nature [5]. It has also been suggested that, during training, muscle tends to hypertrophy faster than bone, resulting in an imbalance that may lead to stress injuries, especially early in a training regimen [7,8].

Muscle fatigue

Muscle fatigue is also thought to play a role in the production of stress injuries [9]. Normally, muscles act to "shield" the bones from excessive forces by dynamically dissipating stresses away from the underlying osseous structures so that the force is not concentrated on a focal portion of the bone. As muscles begin to fatigue, this "shock absorbing" effect is lost, and more stress is applied directly to the bone. If a particular muscle group fatigues, this may also result in unopposed pull from an antagonistic muscle group, leading to excessive bending or torsional forces on the bone.

Throwing Injuries

During throwing, tremendous forces are imposed on the shoulder, humeral shaft and elbow, and even the first rib, creating the potential for stress injuries at these sites. The throwing motion may be broken down into four phases: wind-up, cocking, acceleration, and deceleration (follow-through) [10,11]. At the transition point between the cocking and acceleration phases, significant torsional stresses are applied to the humerus, whereas, during the acceleration phase itself, severe valgus forces are produced at the elbow [11–13]. These valgus forces result in tensile stresses along its medial (ulnar) aspect and compressive forces along its lateral (radial) margin [13]. Details of the specific injuries at these sites are discussed in detail later in this article.

Injuries to the Immature Skeleton

Different types of stress injuries are seen in the developing skeleton. Before closure, the growth plate is less resistant to shear and tensile forces and is not very resistant to rotational and compressive forces [14]. Consequently, the physis is quite susceptible to stress injuries in the younger athlete. Epiphysiolysis is a term that denotes a stress reaction of the physis before its closure, in which there is resorption and widening involving an unfused physis in response to chronic stresses. This type of injury most commonly affects the proximal humeral physis, the medial epicondylar apophysis of the elbow, and the distal radial physis [14–16]. These will be discussed more fully later on.

IMAGING FINDINGS IN OSSEOUS STRESS INJURIES

Radiographs

Conventional radiographs are notoriously insensitive for detecting stress injuries in bone. The sensitivity of initial radiographs, obtained at the time of presentation, has been reported to be as low as 15% and will become positive over time in only 50% of patients [17,18].

The earliest radiographic finding in a stress reaction involving cortical bone is the "gray cortex" sign [19]. This is an area of subtle, ill-defined intracortical lucency, related to the osteoclastic tunneling that occurs in an area of stress damage. This finding is extremely difficult to identify, and most stress reactions are detected somewhat later when periosteal or endosteal new bone formation is evident on radiographs. If the offending activity is continued, the microfractures and osteoclastic tunnels within the area of stress reaction will coalesce into a lucent intracortical fracture line or even a displaced fracture.

Within trabecular bone, the earliest radiographic finding is usually that of a subtle linear or curvilinear focus of sclerosis, related to the microcallus that forms at the sites of trabecular fractures. This finding also is difficult to detect in the early stages, and a high index of suspicion is often needed to do so.

CT

CT is also insensitive in detecting stress injuries in their early stages but can be helpful for identifying a fracture line in an area of probable stress reaction demonstrated on a radionuclide or MRI study [20].

Radionuclide Scanning

Radionuclide bone scanning is extremely sensitive for detecting osseous stress injuries, even in their early stages [21]. Because the radiopharmaceutical is taken up at any area of active bone turnover, the scan will become positive at the stage of accelerated bone remodeling, before the development of clinical symptoms. Studies have demonstrated that as many as 46% of abnormal foci on bone scans are asymptomatic [22].

MRI

MRI is at least as sensitive as radionuclide scanning for detecting these injuries. The earliest MRI findings include marrow edema or periosteal fluid at the site of a stress reaction [23]. In the later stages of the stress injury continuum, a discrete fracture line will be seen. However, the findings must be correlated with clinical information, because a recent study revealed that MRI findings suggesting stress reactions were evident in as many as 43% of asymptomatic runners [24].

MRI exhibits certain advantages over radionuclide scanning: shorter scan time, no ionizing radiation, improved specificity (given the better spatial resolution of MRI), and the capability simultaneously to image bone and soft tissues. One disadvantage is its current inability to screen the entire skeleton, as is possible with radionuclide scanning.

SPECIFIC ANATOMIC SITES

Stress fractures have been reported to occur at multiple sites in the upper extremity. Although numerous athletic activities have been associated with these injuries, the two most common are gymnastics and throwing sports, such as baseball and softball. See Table 1 for a list of stress fracture sites in the upper extremity and the sports associated with injuries at each site. A more detailed discussion of specific injuries follows.

Clavicle, Scapula, and First Rib

The clavicle and scapula connect the upper extremity to the axial skeleton. Although fractures of these bones are most commonly secondary to acute, major

Table 1
Upper extremity stress fractures: sites and associated activities

Site	Activities
Clavicle	Gymnastics, rowing, diving, javelin
Scapula	Golf, trap shooting, cricket, jogging with hand weights
First rib	Pitching, weightlifting, volleyball, basketball
Humerus	
Proximal physis	Baseball
Shaft	Baseball, softball, javelin, shot put, arm wrestling, weightlifting
Medial epicondyle	Baseball
Ulna	
Olecranon tip	Javelin
Posteromedial olecranon	Baseball
Mid-olecranon	Baseball, weightlifting, javelin
Ulnar shaft	Softball, tennis, volleyball, bowling, table tennis, polo, baton twirling
Distal radius	Gymnastics
Wrist	
Scaphoid	Gymnastics, shot put
Hamate	Tennis
Triquetrum	Breakdancing
Metacarpals	Tennis, softball

trauma, stress fractures have been reported to involve both. Although they are not part of the upper extremity proper, stress fractures of the first rib are discussed as well, because these are often secondary to activities involving the upper extremities.

Clavicle

The clavicle is anchored to the shoulder by the acromioclavicular joint and to the axial skeleton by the sternoclavicular joint. The pectoralis major and deltoid muscles tend to pull the clavicle downward, whereas the sternocleidomastoid and trapezius pull upward. Depending on the activity, these opposing forces can result in bending, torsional, and shear forces affecting the clavicle, especially when there are muscular imbalances [25]. Clavicular stress fractures have been reported in athletes participating in gymnastics, diving, rowing, and javelin throwing [25,26]. Osteolysis of the distal clavicle is another stress-related process, often seen in weightlifters (Fig. 1) [27].

Scapula

Like those affecting the clavicle, scapular stress fractures are rare, but they have been reported in a golfer (acromion), a trapshooter (coracoid process), a cricket player (inferolateral border), and a jogger running with hand weights (superior margin) (Fig. 2) [28–31].

First rib

Stress fractures of the first rib have been described in athletes involved in a number of sports, including baseball pitching, basketball, volleyball, weightlifting, and even soccer (related to "heading" the ball) [32]. These injuries are related to the shear forces that develop when the scalene muscles pull the rib

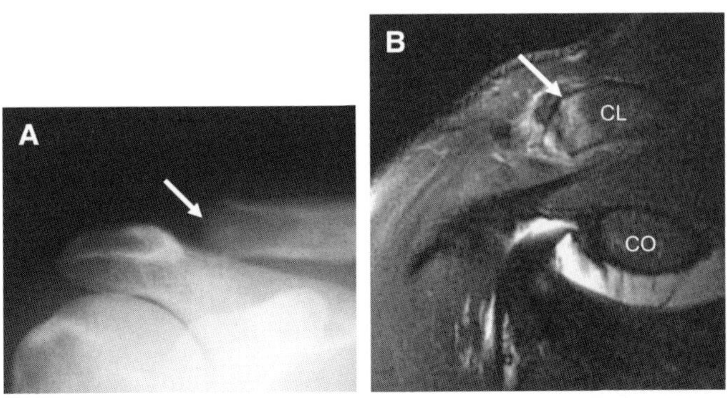

Fig. 1. Distal clavicular osteolysis. (*A*) Anteroposterior radiograph reveals ill-defined, stress-related osteolysis of the distal clavicle (*arrow*). (*B*) Coronal fat-saturated T2-weighted image of the shoulder in a different patient (a young firefighter who also lifted weights) demonstrates increased signal intensity in the distal clavicle (*short arrow*) compatible with stress-related changes. CL, clavicle; CO, coracoid process.

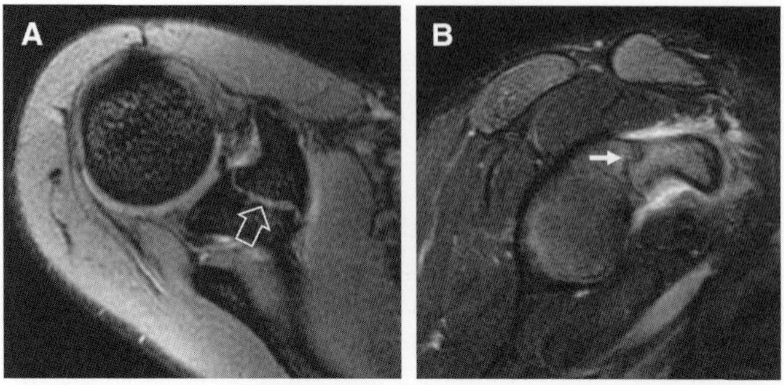

Fig. 2. Stress fracture at base of coracoid process. (*A*) Axial gradient echo image through the shoulder demonstrates a nondisplaced stress fracture at the base of the coracoid process in this trapshooter (*open arrow*). (*B*) Sagittal fat-saturated T2-weighted image displays the fracture (*small arrow*), as well as associated edema in the coracoid process and adjacent soft tissues. (Courtesy of T. Sanders, MD, Charlottesville, VA.)

upward while the serratus anterior muscle pulls the rib caudally. The resulting stress fracture occurs at the level of the groove for the subclavian artery–the site of maximum shear forces (Fig. 3). Notably, in throwers, these fractures tend to involve the first rib on the side of the nondominant arm [33].

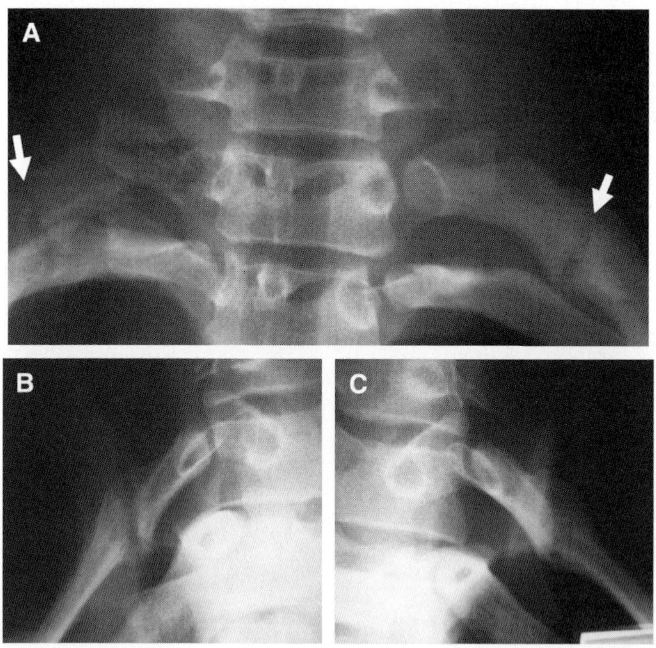

Fig. 3. Bilateral first rib stress fractures. (*A*) Anteroposterior radiograph reveals bilateral stress fractures of the first ribs in this weightlifter (*arrows*). (*B,C*) The fractures are well demonstrated on oblique radiographs.

Humerus

Epiphysiolysis

Also known as "Little Leaguer's shoulder," this is a stress reaction of the unfused proximal humeral physis that is usually seen in young, skeletally immature throwers. This injury is most likely related to the shear stresses that develop during the cocking phase of throwing, which may also lead to humeral retrotorsion [34]. Radiographic findings include widening of the proximal humeral physis relative to the unaffected side. MRI may reveal changes of marrow edema adjacent to the injured physis (Fig. 4) [35].

Shaft fractures

Stress fractures of the humeral shaft have been described in athletes participating in numerous sports, primarily those involving throwing (baseball, softball, javelin, shotput), but also arm wrestling and weightlifting [12,36,37]. Regardless of the sport, these injuries most commonly result in a spiral fracture involving the mid- to distal shaft, often with a large butterfly fragment [13,36].

During the throwing motion, tremendous torsional stresses are applied to the humerus, most notably at the point between the late cocking and early acceleration phases when the external rotators (deltoid, supraspinatus, infraspinatus, and teres minor) are still contracting and the powerful internal rotators

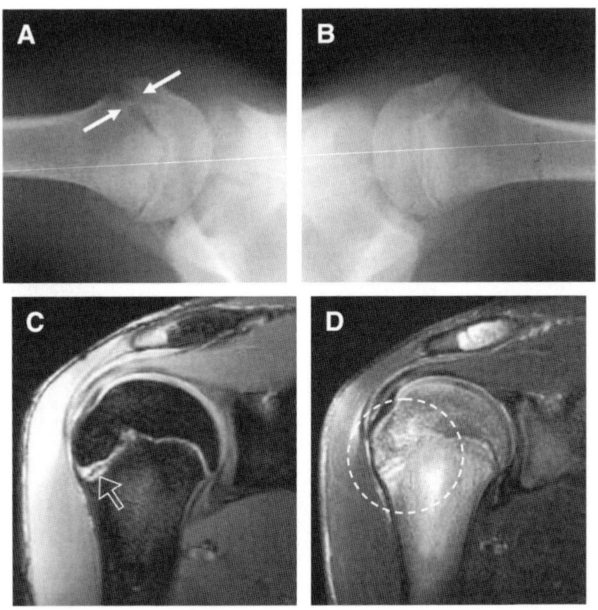

Fig. 4. Proximal humerus epiphysiolysis. (*A,B*) Axillary radiographs of the shoulders in a young baseball pitcher who presented with right shoulder pain demonstrate widening of the proximal humeral physis on the right (*arrows*) compatible with epiphysiolysis. (*C*) The same finding is present on this oblique coronal gradient echo image (*open arrow*). (*D*) Note the associated marrow edema on this fat-saturated T2-weighted image (*dashed circle*).

(pectoralis major, latissimus dorsi, subscapularis) begin to contract in the opposite direction [13]. The forces generated are of such a magnitude that the humerus may fracture as a result of a single throw [38,39].

In arm wrestling, torsional, bending, and axial compressive forces are all exerted on the humerus and may result in a similar fracture [36]. Humeral shaft fractures have also been reported in weightlifters, again most likely resulting from the opposing muscular forces involved in maneuvers such as the bench press [39].

These spiral, often mildly comminuted fractures are evident on radiographs at the junction of the mid- and distal thirds of the humerus (Fig. 5). Earlier diagnosis of a humeral stress fracture has been accomplished using radionuclide imaging [40]; theoretically, MRI should be able to display the changes of early humeral stress reactions as well.

Elbow

Medial epicondyle

Because of the valgus force that occurs at the elbow throughout much of the throwing motion, the medial aspect of the joint experiences significant tensile forces. In the older athlete, the medial (ulnar) collateral ligament is most vulnerable to injury, whereas in the younger thrower, the medial epicondyle apophysis is most often affected. Although the medial epicondyle ossification center may become acutely avulsed, chronic stresses often lead to epiphysiolysis (apophysitis) at this site [41]. Also known as "Little Leaguer's elbow," this is similar to the process that occurs in the proximal humerus and is manifested on radiographs as widening and poor definition of the growth plate [16]. As with the proximal humerus, comparison views of the opposite elbow are often helpful in making the diagnosis (Fig. 6). The identification of marrow edema within

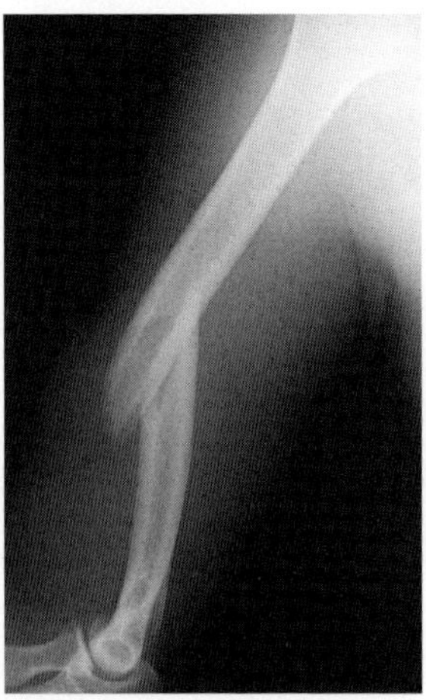

Fig. 5. Humeral shaft fracture. Lateral radiograph of the humerus demonstrates an angulated fracture of its mid- to distal shaft in this patient who sustained the injury while arm wrestling.

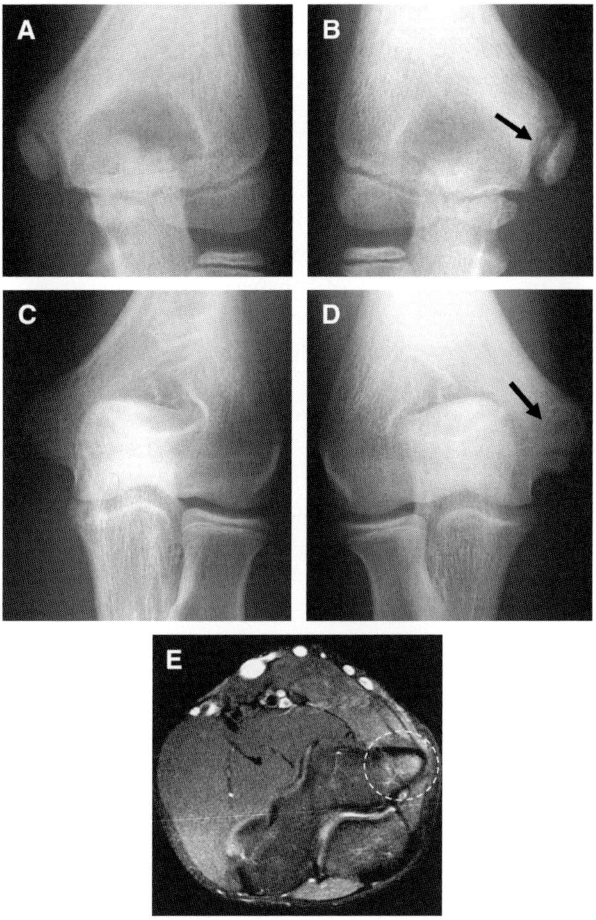

Fig. 6. Medial epicondylar apophysitis. (*A,B*) Anteroposterior radiographs of both elbows in an adolescent baseball pitcher reveal asymmetric widening of the left medial epicondylar growth plate (*arrow*) compatible with apophysitis. (*C,D*) Anteroposterior radiographs in a different adolescent pitcher reveal similar findings in the left medial epicondylar physis, with associated marrow edema (*dashed circle*) identified on the corresponding fat-saturated axial T2-weighted image obtained at that level (*E*).

the apophysis on MRI may allow for earlier diagnosis, before the appearance of radiographic findings.

Olecranon

A stress fracture of the olecranon may occur at one of three sites, resulting from a different mechanism of injury at each.

Proximal tip. A stress fracture of the extreme proximal tip of the olecranon has been reported in javelin throwers and is thought to be due to impingement of the tip against the olecranon fossa at terminal extension of the elbow [42]. This "door-stop" mechanism typically results in a small, triangular-shaped fracture fragment that may be evident on a lateral radiograph (Fig. 7).

Proximal, posteromedial olecranon. MRI in a small group of professional baseball players presenting with posterior elbow pain revealed focal marrow edema at the posteromedial margin of the proximal olecranon (Fig. 8) [43]. Of interest, this edema was seen at the site where other throwing athletes develop posteromedial osteophytes, usually in the setting of medial instability due to ulnar collateral ligament insufficiency. All of the patients in this study demonstrated intact ulnar collateral ligaments, and the authors postulated that this presumed stress reaction resulted from tensile failure of the trabeculae at this site, related to the steady valgus overload produced with throwing. The posteromedial osteophytes seen in patients who have torn or insufficient ulnar collateral ligaments most likely develop from shear forces related to the ulnar subluxation that occurs in those patients.

Mid-olecranon. A transverse or oblique stress fracture through the mid-olecranon has been reported in baseball players, javelin throwers, and weightlifters and is thought to result from repeated, forceful contraction of the triceps musculature (Fig. 9) [15].

Ulnar Shaft

Midshaft fractures of the ulna have been reported in athletes competing in a variety of sports, including softball, tennis, volleyball, bowling, polo, and table tennis, as well as in a baton twirler and in a patient who was using crutches as part of her treatment for osteochondritis dissecans of the opposite knee [44–46]. These diaphyseal fractures are of two different types.

Torsional

This type of mid-diaphyseal fracture is observed in athletes who undergo repetitive alternation between extremes of pronation and supination (eg, the "windmill" pitching mechanism in softball, the two-handed backhand in tennis). The

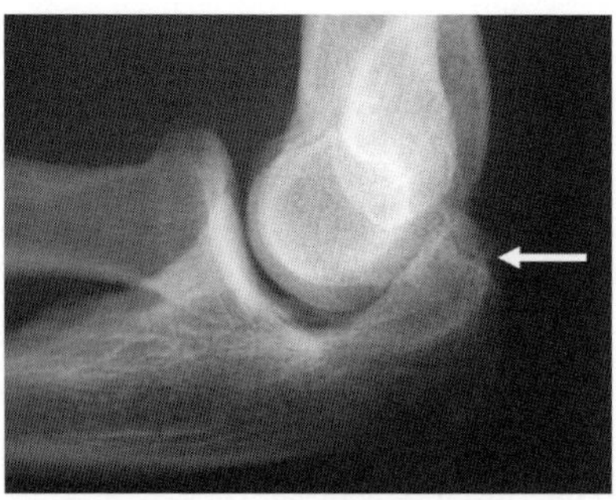

Fig. 7. Fracture at tip of olecranon. Lateral radiograph of the elbow demonstrates a small curvilinear fracture through the extreme tip of the olecranon in this javelin thrower (*arrow*).

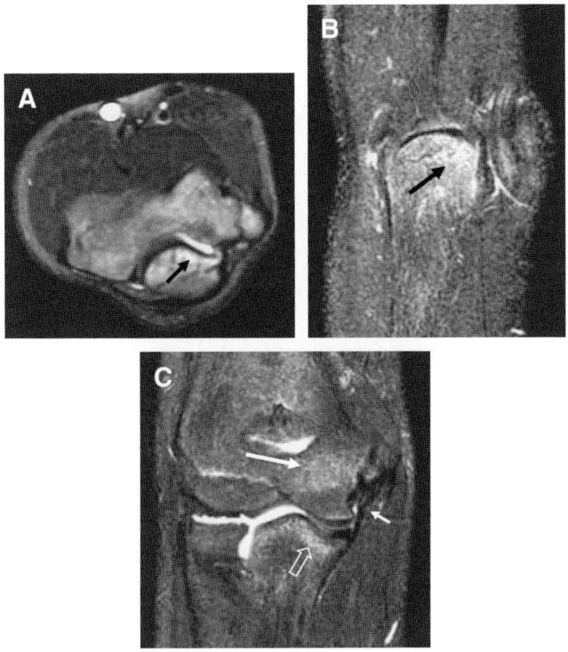

Fig. 8. Focal edema of the posteromedial olecranon (MRI). (*A*) Axial, (*B*) coronal (at the level of the olecranon), and (*C*) coronal (at the level of the ulnar collateral ligament [*short arrow*]) fat-saturated T2-weighted images reveal focal edema in the posterior medial aspect of the olecranon of this 13-year-old baseball pitcher (*arrows*). Note also the marrow edema in the medial epicondylar apophysis (*large arrow*) and coronoid process (*open arrow*).

torsional shear stresses associated with these movements are concentrated in the midshaft of the ulna, presumably because of three factors: this segment is where the cross-sectional area of the bone is smallest, where its cortex is thinnest, and where it assumes a more triangular (rather than circular) shape [44,45].

Bending ("lifting")

Repetitive flexion of the elbow with loading of the forearm but without excessive pronation or supination (eg, in weightlifting, underhand volleyball setting) results in significant bending forces in the forearm [44,45]. The stresses of this type of loading are most concentrated at sites where the bone changes shape rapidly, and this occurs in the proximal and distal thirds of the ulna, where this type of stress fracture is typically found [47].

Distal Radius

Epiphysiolysis

Stress injuries involving the distal radial physis have been described almost exclusively in young gymnasts [14]. This predominance is probably due to a number of factors. Gymnastics is an unusual sport in that the upper extremity is commonly used for weight bearing, which results in compressive forces [5].

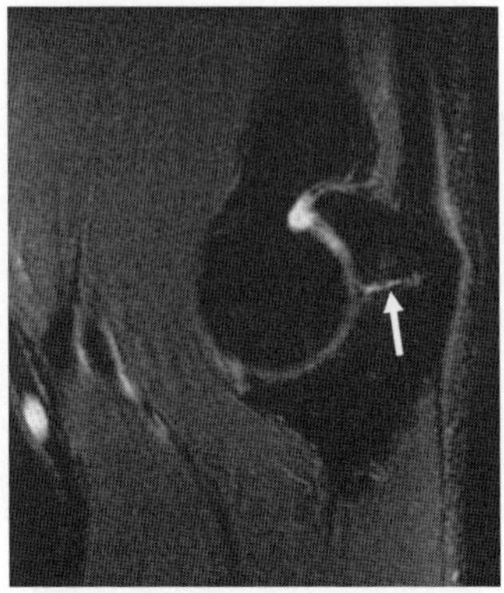

Fig. 9. Mid-olecranon stress fracture (MRI). Sagittal fat-saturated T2-weighted image of the elbow shows a nondisplaced, incomplete stress fracture in the mid-olecranon (*arrow*). (Courtesy of T. Sanders, MD, Charlottesville, Virginia.)

In many events, rotational forces are also involved, leading to additional torsional shear stresses. As with epiphysiolysis at other sites, this injury is manifested as a widening of the distal radial physis on radiographs; because of the nature of the sport, it may be present bilaterally (Fig. 10).

Distal shaft

A case of stress fractures involving the distal radial shafts bilaterally has been reported in a gymnast, although this is an unusual site for a stress injury [48].

Wrist

Scaphoid

Several reports exist of midscaphoid stress fractures in gymnasts, with a similar injury reported in a shot putter as well [49–52]. The mechanism of this injury is

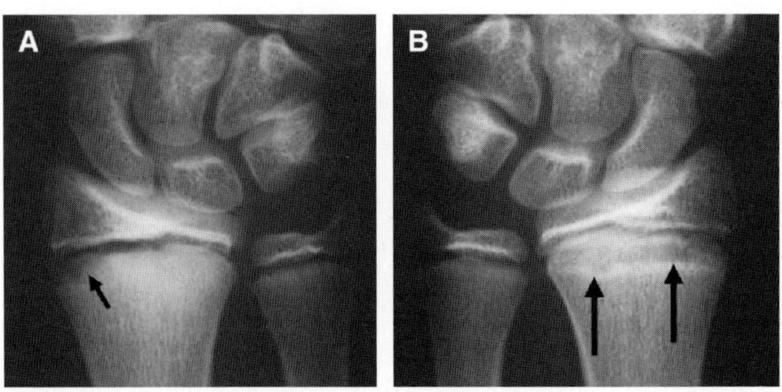

Fig. 10. Distal radial epiphysiolysis. (*A,B*) Anteroposterior radiographs of the wrists reveal widening and poor definition of the distal radial physes. This is more pronounced on the right (*larger arrows*) than on the left (*smaller arrow*).

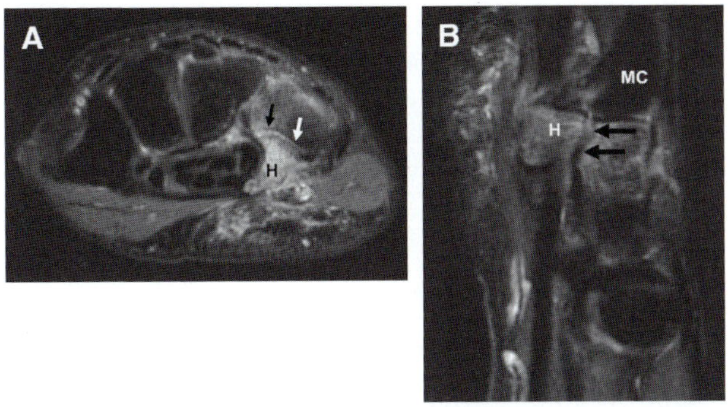

Fig. 11. Hook of hamate fracture (MRI). (*A*) Axial and (*B*) sagittal fat-saturated images of the wrist reveal diffuse marrow edema in the hamate as well as a nondisplaced fracture (*arrows*). H, hook; MC, proximal metacarpal. (Courtesy of T. Sanders, MD, Charlottesville, VA.)

most likely weight bearing (or weightlifting in the case of the shot putter) on a severely dorsiflexed wrist. In this position, the compressive forces attempt to push the scaphoid into palmar flexion, while at the same time the volar extrinsic ligaments of the wrist act to keep the proximal portion of the bone in a more extended position [50,52]. The forces are then concentrated just distal to these ligaments at the level of the midscaphoid, which is where the fractures were observed in these patients.

Other carpal bones

Stress injuries in the other carpal bones are exceedingly rare. A fracture of the hook of the hamate is usually the result of an acute injury, such as the

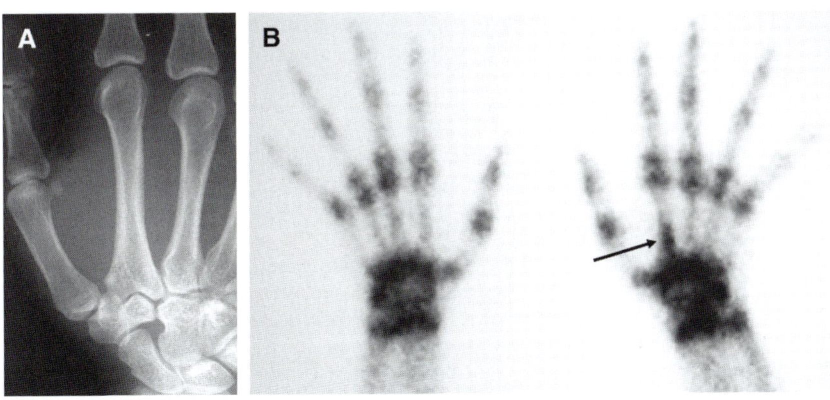

Fig. 12. Second metacarpal stress fracture. (*A*) Anteroposterior radiograph of the hand shows no evidence of osseous injury in this 19-year-old tennis player who presented with right hand pain. (*B*) A follow-up radionuclide bone scan reveals focal abnormal uptake in the proximal aspect of the second metacarpal (*arrow*).

impaction of the hook against a golf club or tennis racquet. However, there has been one reported case of a stress fracture at this site in a tennis player who had recently changed his serving technique (Fig. 11) [53]. A triquetral stress reaction was also reported in a breakdancer, engaged in an activity that places similar stresses on the wrist to those of gymnastics [54].

Metacarpals

Stress fractures of the metacarpals are also extremely uncommon, with only a few case reports in the literature. Two reports exist of second metacarpal stress fractures, both in tennis players (Fig. 12) [55]. Possible factors include the length of this, the longest of the metacarpals, and its restricted range of motion at the second carpometacarpal joint, where it is essentially limited to flexion and extension. A stress fracture involving the proximal aspect of the fifth metacarpal in a softball pitcher was thought to have resulted from strong adduction forces at that site related to gripping the ball [56].

SUMMARY

Although it is much less common than injuries in the lower extremities, an upper extremity stress injury can have a significant impact on an athlete, especially when it is not recognized until it has progressed to a displaced fracture. If an accurate and timely diagnosis is to be made, the clinician must have a high index of suspicion of a stress fracture in any athlete who is involved in a throwing, weightlifting, or upper extremity weight-bearing sport and presents with chronic pain in the upper extremity. Imaging should play an integral role in the work-up of these patients; if initial radiographs are unrevealing, further cross-sectional imaging should be strongly considered. Although a three-phase bone scan is highly sensitive in this regard, MRI has become the study of choice at most centers.

References

[1] Brukner P. Stress fractures of the upper limb. Sports Med 1998;26:415–24.

[2] Burr DB, Martin RB, Schaffler MB, et al. Bone remodeling in response to in vivo microdamage. J Biomech 1985;18:189–200.

[3] Frost HM. Some ABC's of skeletal pathophysiology. V. Microdamage physiology. Calcif Tissue Int 1991;49:229–31.

[4] Uhthoff HK, Jaworski ZFG. Periosteal stress—indirect reactions resembling stress fractures: a radiologic and histologic study in dogs. Clin Orthop 1986;199:284–91.

[5] Sinha AK, Kaeding CC, Wadley GM. Upper extremity stress fractures in athletes: clinical features of 44 cases. Clin J Sport Med 1999;9:199–202.

[6] Jones BH, Harris JMCA, Vih TN, et al. Exercise-induced stress fractures and stress reactions of bone: epidemiology, etiology and classification. Exerc Sport Sci Rev 1989;17:379–422.

[7] Daffner RH, Pavlov H. Stress fractures: current concepts. AJR Am J Roentgenol 1992;159:245–52.

[8] Ahluwalia R, Datz FL, Morton KA, et al. Bilateral fatigue fractures of the radial shaft in a gymnast. Clin Nucl Med 1994;19(8):665–7.

[9] Yoshikawa T, Mori S, Santiesteban AJ, et al. The effects of muscle fatigue on bone strain. J Exp Biol 1994;188:217–33.

[10] Gainor BJ, Piotrowski G, Puhl J, et al. The throw: biomechanics and acute injury. Am J Sports Med 1980;8:114–8.

[11] Marymont JV, Coupe KJ, Clanton TO. Sports-related spontaneous fractures of the humerus. Orthop Rev 1989;18:957–60.
[12] Linn RM, Kriegshauser LA. Ball thrower's fracture of the humerus: a case report. Am J Sports Med 1991;19:194–7.
[13] DiCicco JD, Mehlman CT, Urse JS. Fracture of the shaft of the humerus secondary to muscular violence. J Orthop Trauma 1993;7:90–3.
[14] Carter SR, Aldridge MJ. Stress injury of the distal radial growth plate. J Bone Joint Surg Br 1988;70-B:834–6.
[15] Tullos HS, Erwin WD, Woods W, et al. Unusual lesions of the pitching arm. Clin Orthop Rel Res 1972;88:169–82.
[16] Klingele KE, Kocher MS. Little League Elbow: valgus overload injury in the pediatric athlete. Sports Med 2002;32:1005–15.
[17] Greany RB, Gerber FH, Laughlin RL, et al. Distibution and natural history of stress fractures in US Marine recruits. Radiology 1983;146:339–46.
[18] Nielsen MB, Hansen K, Holmes P, et al. Tibial periosteal reactions in soldiers: a scintigraphic study of 29 cases of lower leg pain. Acta Orthop Scand 1991;62:531–4.
[19] Mulligan ME. The "gray cortex": an early sign of stress fracture. Skeletal Radiol 1995;24: 201–3.
[20] Matheson GO, Clement DB, McKenzie DC, et al. Stress fractures in athletes: a study of 320 cases. Am J Sports Med 1987;15:46–58.
[21] Ammann W, Matheson GO. Radionuclide bone imaging in the detection of stress fractures. Clin J Sports Med 1991;1:115–22.
[22] Matheson GO, Clement DB, McKenzie DC, et al. Scintigraphic uptake of 99m-Tc at non-painful sites in athletes with stress fractures: the concept of bone strain. Sports Med 1987;4:65–75.
[23] Anderson MW, Greenspan A. Stress fractures. Radiology 1996;199:1–12.
[24] Bergman GA, Fredericson M, Ho C, et al. Asymptomatic tibial stress reactions: MRI detection and clinical follow-up in distance runners. AJR Am J Roentgenol 2004;183:635–8.
[25] Abbot AE, Hannafin JA. Stress fracture of the clavicle in a female lightweight rower. A case report and review of the literature. Am J Sports Med 2001;29(3):370–2.
[26] Fallon KE, Fricker PA. Stress fracture of the clavicle in a young female gymnast. Br J Sports Med 2001;35(6):448–9.
[27] Kaplan PA, Resnick D. Stress-induced osteolysis of the clavicle. Radiology 1986;158:130–40.
[28] de Villiers RVP, de Beer J, Koenig J. Scapular stress fracture in a professional cricketer and a review of the literature. S Afr Med J 2005;95:312–5.
[29] Sandrock AR. Another sports fatigue fracture. Stress fracture of the coracoid process of the scapula. Radiology 1975;117:274.
[30] Hall RJ, Calvert PT. Stress fracture of the acromion: an unusual mechanism and review of the literature. J Bone Joint Surg Br 1995;77-B:153–4.
[31] Veluvolu P, Kohn HS, Guten GN, et al. Unusual stress fracture of the scapula in a jogger. Clin Nucl Med 1988;13:531–2.
[32] Matsumoto T, Fujita K, Fujioka H, et al. Stress fracture of the first rib in a soccer player: a rare etiology of shoulder pain. J Shoulder Elbow Surg 2003;12(2):197–9.
[33] Mintz AC, Albano A, Reisdorff EJ, et al. Stress fracture of the first rib from serratus anterior tension: an unusual mechanism of injury. Ann Emerg Med 1990;19:411–4.
[34] Sabick MB, Kim YK, Torry MR, et al. Biomechanics of the shoulder in youth baseball pitchers: implications for the development of proximal humeral epiphysiolysis and humeral retrotorsion. Am J Sports Med 2005;33:1716–22.
[35] Hatem SF, Recht MP, Profitt B. MRI of Little Leaguer's shoulder. Skeletal Radiol Oct 2006;35:103–6.
[36] Whitaker JH. Arm wrestling fractures—a humerus twist. Am J Sports Med 1977;5:67–77.
[37] Joseph TA, Zehr RJ. Spontaneous humeral shaft fracture in a weight lifter. Orthopedics 2000;23:603–5.

[38] Kircher T, Cappuccino A, Torpey BM. Muscular violence as a cause of humeral fractures in pitchers. Contemp Orthop 1993;26:475–80.
[39] Horwitz BR, DiStafano V. Stress fracture of the humerus in a weight lifter. Orthopedics 1995;18:185–7.
[40] Rettig AC, Beltz HF. Stress fracture in the humerus in an adolescent tennis tournament player. Am J Sports Med 1985;13:55–8.
[41] Cain EL, Dugas JR, Wolf RS, et al. Elbow injuries in throwing athletes: a current concepts review. Am J Sports Med 2003;31:621–35.
[42] Hulkko A, Orava S, Nikula P. Stress fractures of the olecranon in javelin throwers. Int J Sports Med 1986;7:210–3.
[43] Schickendantz MS, Ho CP, Koh J. Stress injury of the proximal ulna in professional baseball players. Am J Sports Med 2002;30:737–41.
[44] Fines BP, Stacy S. Stress fracture of the ulna in an adolescent baton twirler. Skeletal Radiol 2002;31(2):116–8.
[45] Fragniere B, Landry M, Siegrist O. Stress fracture of the ulna in a professional tennis player using a double-handed backhand stroke. Knee Surg Sports Traumatol Arthrosc 2001;9(4): 239–41.
[46] Garcia Suarez G, Garcia Garcia J, Perez Carro L. Stress fracture of the ulna associated with crutch use. J Orthop Trauma 2001;15(7):524–5.
[47] Tanabe S, Nakahira J, Bando E, et al. Fatigue fracture of the ulna occurring in pitchers of fast-pitch softball. Am J Sports Med 1991;19:317–21.
[48] Read MRF. Stress fractures of the distal radius in adolescent gymnasts. Br J Sports Med 1981;15:272–6.
[49] Engel A, Feldner-Busztin H. Bilateral stress fracture of the scaphoid. Arch Orthop Trauma Surg 1991;110:314–5.
[50] Manzione M, Pizzutillo PD. Stress fracture of the scaphoid waist. Am J Sports Med 1981;9: 268–9.
[51] Hanks GA, Kalenak A, Bowman LS, et al. Stress fractures of the carpal scaphoid: a report of four cases. J Bone Joint Surg Br 1989;71-A:938–41.
[52] Matzkin E, Singer DI. Scaphoid stress fracture in a 13-year-old gymnast: a case report. J Hand Surg [Am] 2000;25(4):710–3.
[53] Guha AR, Marynissen H. Stress fracture of the hook of the hamate. Br J Sports Med 2002;36:224–5.
[54] Lohman M, Kivisaari L, Partio EK. Stress reaction in the carpal bones caused by breakdancing. Emerg Radiol 2003;10:102–4.
[55] Waninger KN, Lombardo JA. Stress fracture of index metacarpal in an adolescent tennis player. Clin J Sports Med 1995;5:63–6.
[56] Jowett AD, Brukner PD. Fifth metacarpal stress fracture in a female softball pitcher. Clin J Sports Med 1997;7:220–1.

Clin Sports Med 25 (2006) 505–526
CLINICS IN SPORTS MEDICINE
ELSEVIER
SAUNDERS

Imaging of Ulnar-Sided Wrist Pain

Claire A. Coggins, MD
Department of Radiology, Virginia Commonwealth University, Main Hospital, 3rd Floor, Room 3-343, 1250 East Marshall Street, Richmond, VA 23298, USA

Ulnar-sided wrist pain has long been a diagnostic dilemma for both radiologists and hand surgeons. The small size of the anatomic structures, the diversity of disorders that can cause symptoms, and the high rate of asymptomatic findings at the ulnar aspect of the wrist are some of the factors that contribute to the difficulty of diagnosis and management in this region. In fact, ulnar wrist pain has been called the "low back pain of the wrist" [1]. Previous authors have described as many as 44 different entities to consider in the differential diagnosis of ulnar-sided wrist pain. This article focuses on the more common causes of pain in this region, including tears of the triangular fibrocartilage complex (TFCC), disorders of the distal radioulnar joint (DRUJ), tears of the lunotriquetral ligament, disorders of the extensor carpi ulnaris (ECU) tendon, disorders of the pisotriquetral joint, the impingement and impaction syndromes, and ulnar wrist masses.

Anatomy, pathophysiology, and radiographic appearance of the various entities are discussed, including a brief review of treatment options. The goal of this article is to provide a concise approach to the diagnosis and imaging of a difficult but common problem.

IMAGING MODALITIES

Several different imaging modalities can be useful in the evaluation of ulnar-sided wrist pain. Conventional radiographs may demonstrate ulnar variance, carpal alignment, evidence of acute or remote trauma, and degenerative changes. CT is most useful for evaluation of DRUJ subluxation. Conventional arthrography (single compartment or three compartment) can detect complete and partial tears of the TFCC, as well as unidirectional communicating defects between the radiocarpal and midcarpal joints. MRI is useful for evaluation of ligament disruption, cartilage defects, tendon abnormalities, occult fractures, and avascular necrosis. MR arthrography combines the usefulness of conventional arthrography in detecting full-thickness TFCC tears with the ability to visualize marrow, ligaments, and soft tissues [2]. High-resolution MR with a dedicated wrist coil is essential in achieving the spatial resolution and

E-mail address: cacoggins@vcu.edu

0278-5919/06/$ – see front matter
doi:10.1016/j.csm.2006.02.008

sportsmed.theclinics.com

signal-to-noise ratio to evaluate the small structures about the wrist [3]. Skeletal scintigraphy, although sensitive, is not specific and has limited use in evaluation of ulnar wrist pain. Likewise, sonography has limited use in this region and is used primarily for evaluation of ganglia or other masses.

TRIANGULAR FIBROCARTILAGE COMPLEX

The TFCC functions as a cushion for the ulnar carpus, absorbing approximately 20% of the axial load of the wrist, and as a major stabilizer of the DRUJ [4]. Palmer and Werner [5] defined the TFCC as composed of five structures:

Triangular fibrocartilage proper (articular disc) and volar and dorsal radioulnar (RU) ligaments
Ulnocarpal meniscus
Ulnocarpal ligaments
Ulnar collateral ligament (UCL)
ECU tendon sheath

The triangular fibrocartilage proper and volar and dorsal RU ligaments arise from the ulnar border of the sigmoid notch of the radius and insert at the base of the ulnar styloid [4]. The dorsal and volar RU ligaments as well as the peripheral 20% of the articular disc are well vascularized. The inner 80% of the articular disc is avascular, as is its radial attachment [6,7]. On the volar aspect of the wrist, the volar RU ligament extends distally to the lunate and triquetrum as the ulnolunate and ulnotriquetral ligaments, respectively. The UCL extends from the base of the ulnar styloid to the hamate and to the fifth metacarpal base. The ulnocarpal meniscus, or meniscus homologue, is a thickening of the UCL that passes distally to attach to the ulnar aspect of the triquetrum [4,5]. At the dorsal aspect of the wrist, the floor of the ECU tendon sheath passes distally to attach to the triquetrum, hamate, and fifth metacarpal base [8]. The interval between the meniscus homologue, the ulnotriquetral ligament, and the UCL is referred to as the prestyloid recess, which is an extension of the radiocarpal joint (Fig. 1) [9].

Tears of the TFCC can be either traumatic or degenerative. Traumatic injury is usually the result of hyperrotation of the forearm, distraction of the wrist, or axial loading. Traumatic tears of the TFCC tend to occur closer to the radius than degenerative tears (Fig. 2) [4].

Degenerative tears of the TFCC usually result from chronic loading on the ulnar aspect of the wrist and tend to occur in the thinner central portion of the articular disc [4].

In 1978, Mikic [10] evaluated 180 cadaver wrists and demonstrated that TFCC degeneration is directly related to age; statistically, all patients older than 50 have a degenerated TFCC, and many have perforations. Mikic found no TFCC perforations in patients younger than 30. In addition, Viegas and colleagues [11] examined 393 cadaver wrists and found a direct relation between the age of the specimen and the incidence of TFCC tears. In light of these

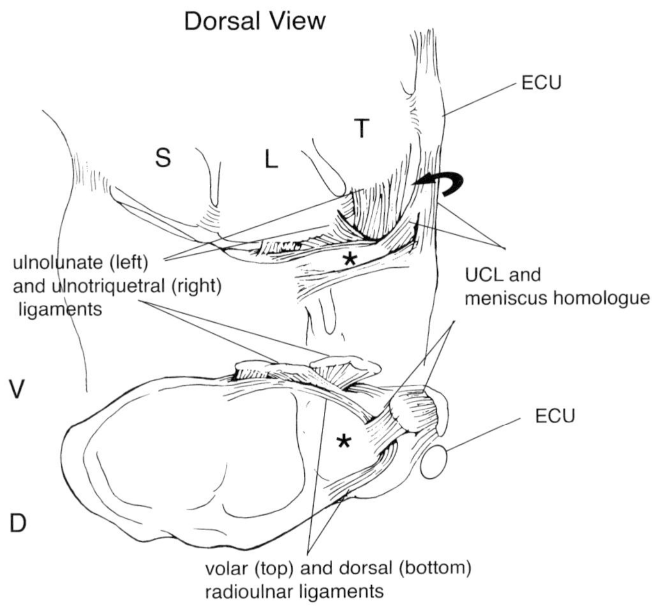

Fig. 1. Triangular fibrocartilage complex. Dorsal view coronal and axial illustrations of the wrist demonstrate the components of the TFCC. The triangular fibrocartilage proper (*asterisks*) and volar and dorsal RU ligaments arise from the ulnar border of the sigmoid notch of the radius and insert at the base of the ulnar styloid. The interval between the meniscus homologue, the ulnotriquetral ligament, and the UCL is referred to as the prestyloid recess (*curved arrow*). D, dorsal; L, lunate; S, scaphoid; T, triquetrum; V, volar.

findings, TFCC tears must be evaluated in the context of the patient's age, symptoms, and clinical examination to determine whether the TFCC tear is actually the cause of the patient's pain or merely an incidental finding.

In 1988, Palmer [4] devised a classification for lesions of the TFCC, with Type I tears being traumatic and Type II tears degenerative (Table 1).

MRI, conventional arthrography, and MR arthrography are the most useful modalities for imaging the TFCC. Conventional arthrography may be useful in excluding complete tears of the TFCC. However, there can be a connection between the radiocarpal and distal RU joints in 7% to 35% of asymptomatic individuals [12,13]. On MRI, the TFCC is best viewed on coronal images, where it is seen as a low T1, low T2 signal intensity structure extending from the ulnar aspect of the distal radius to the base of the ulnar styloid. When degeneration of the TFC is present, there may be intermediate signal intensity within the TFC on short TE images that does not increase on T2 or T2* images [14]. Degeneration can also appear as thinning of the TFC [3]. When a perforation is present, there may be intermediate signal intensity on T1 and proton-density spin-echo images, which increases on T2-weighted and gradient echo images [15]. In partial tears, the signal abnormality extends

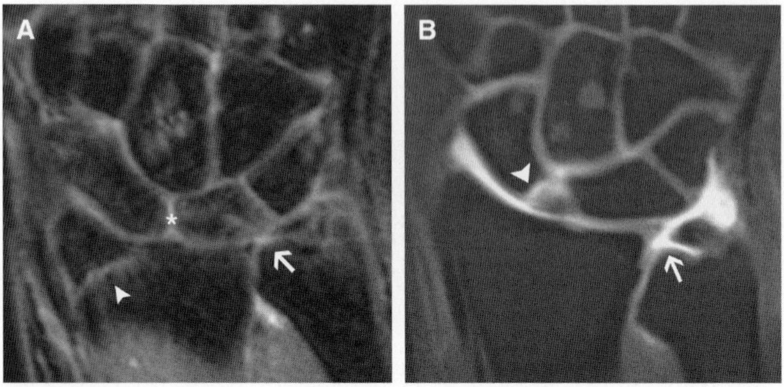

Fig. 2. Traumatic TFCC tears. Coronal fat-suppressed T2-weighted image (*A*) demonstrates a focal tear at the radial aspect of the triangular fibrocartilage (TFC) (*arrow*), representing a traumatic tear in this 42-year-old patient who is status post trauma. The patient also has a radial styloid fracture (*arrowhead*) and a scapholunate ligament tear (*asterisk*). Coronal fat-suppressed T1-weighted image from an MR arthrogram (*B*) demonstrates avulsion of the TFC from the sigmoid notch of the radius (*arrow*), consistent with a Palmer class 1D traumatic tear of the TFC. The patient also has avulsion of the scapholunate ligament, with associated bony avulsion of the scaphoid (*arrowhead*).

only to one articular surface, whereas in complete tears, the signal abnormality extends to both proximal and distal articular surfaces (Fig. 3) [3]. Fluid signal intensity in the DRUJ may be seen with TFC tears, but this is nonspecific and may also be seen with synovitis or DRUJ irritation [15]. The presence of gadolinium in the DRUJ after MR arthrography increases the specificity. However, as mentioned previously, there can be a communication between the radiocarpal and distal RU joints in asymptomatic individuals.

Table 1
Palmer classification for triangular fibrocartilage complex lesions

Class 1: Traumatic	Class 2: Degenerative
1A: Central perforation	2A: TFCC wear
1B: Ulnar avulsion with/without distal ulnar fracture	2B: TFCC wear + lunate and/or ulnar chondromalacia
1C: Avulsion from lunate or triquetrum	2C: TFCC perforation + lunate and/or ulnar chondromalacia
1D: Avulsion from sigmoid notch of radius	2D: TFCC perforation + lunate and/or ulnar chondromalacia + LT ligament tear
	2E: TFCC perforation + lunate and/or ulnar chondromalacia + LT ligament tear + ulnocarpal arthritis

Abbreviation: LT, lunotriquetral.

Adapted from Palmer AK. Triangular fibrocartilage complex lesion: a classification. J Hand Surg [Am] 1989;14(4):596; with permission.

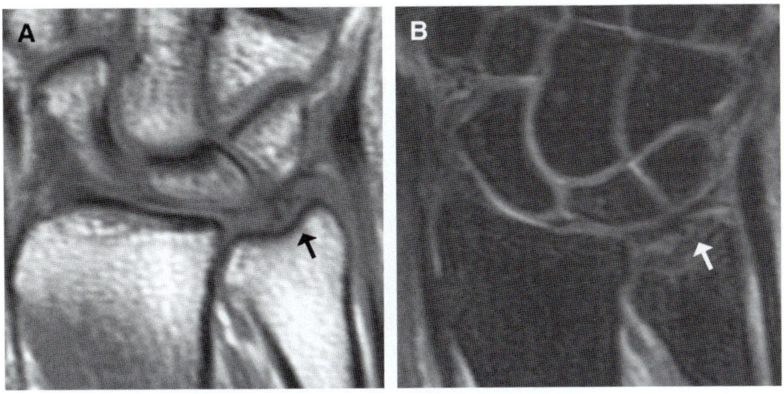

Fig. 3. Partial TFCC tear. Coronal T1-weighted (*A*) and fat-suppressed T2-weighted (*B*) images demonstrate increased T1, increased T2 signal intensity along the undersurface of the triangular fibrocartilage (*arrows*) that does not extend to the distal articular surface, consistent with a partial TFCC tear.

Over the past 20 years, several authors have reported wide variation in sensitivity, specificity, and accuracy of MRI compared with arthroscopy. Sensitivity has ranged from 17% to 100%, specificity from 79% to 93%, and accuracy from 64% to 97% [16–21]. The lower numbers reflect studies evaluating the peripheral TFCC. The peripheral TFCC is difficult to evaluate on conventional MRI because of the loose connective tissue in this region, which can appear hyperintense on T2-weighted images, mimicking a tear. Most recently, Schmitt and colleagues [22] studied 125 patients with MR arthrography and arthroscopic correlation in 2003. They demonstrated a sensitivity of 97.1%, a specificity of 96.4%, and an accuracy of 96.8% for the detection of TFCC lesions. Although more studies of MR arthrography are necessary, MR arthrography may prove to be most useful for evaluating MR problem areas, such as ulnar-sided TFCC tears (Fig. 4).

LUNOTRIQUETRAL LIGAMENT

The lunotriquetral ligament (LTL) is a true ligament in its dorsal and volar aspects and is membranous in the proximal fibrocartilaginous region [23]. The volar portion is the strongest portion of the LTL [24,25]. The dorsal and volar portions attach directly to bone, whereas the membranous portion attaches to hyaline cartilage [15]. The LTL acts as one of the three major stabilizers of the LT joint, along with the volar radiolunotriquetral ligament and the dorsal radiocarpal ligament [26]. The scaphoid imparts a flexion moment, and the triquetrum imparts an extension moment, with a "balanced lunate" suspended between them [23,27]. When there is disruption of the ligamentous attachment between the lunate and triquetrum, the lunate becomes unbalanced and flexes with the scaphoid, leading to a volar intercalated segmental instability (VISI) deformity [23].

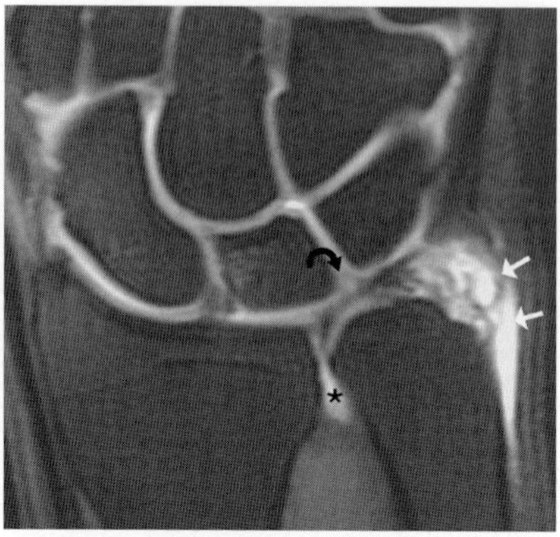

Fig. 4. Ulnar TFCC tear. Coronal fat-suppressed T1-weighted image from an MR arthrogram (radiocarpal joint injection only) demonstrates contrast extravasating into the DRUJ (*asterisk*) and through the ulnar aspect of the TFCC (*arrows*), consistent with an ulnar-sided TFCC tear. Contrast is also noted extending into the midcarpal joint through a torn lunotriquetral ligament (*curved black arrow*).

Tears of the LTL are much less common than scapholunate ligament (SLL) tears, occurring only about one sixth as often [27]. Viegas and colleagues [11] studied 393 cadaveric wrists and found that 36% had disruption of the LTL. Therefore, a finding of LTL disruption is not significant unless it corresponds to the patient's symptoms.

LTL tears can be traumatic or degenerative. Traumatic tears typically result from a fall on a dorsiflexed wrist, forcing the forearm into pronation [28]. Clinically, the patients have point tenderness and experience a painful snap with radial and ulnar deviation. Ballottement and shear tests may be performed to determine whether LT joint instability is present. Both tests involve exerting pressure in opposite directions on adjacent carpal bones [27,29].

The spectrum of LT injury includes partial tear, complete tear, dynamic instability, and static instability. A complete tear of the LTL is not sufficient to cause a VISI deformity. There must also be disruption of one of the secondary restraints of the LT joint (the radiolunotriquetral ligament or the radiocarpal ligament) [22,27]. Viegas and colleagues [30,31] proposed a staging system for ulnar-sided perilunate instability, which covers the spectrum of LT injury:

Stage I: partial or complete LTL disruption (no VISI)
Stage II: complete LTL tear plus disruption of palmar LTLs (dynamic VISI)
Stage III: complete LTL tear plus disruption of palmar LTLs plus disruption of dorsal radiocarpal ligaments (static VISI)

Degenerative tears of the LTL typically occur in association with ulnolunate impaction syndrome (UIS), which is discussed in detail later [32]. Most degenerative perforations occur in the membranous portion of the ligament, while the volar and dorsal portions remain intact.

It is crucial to distinguish whether a torn LTL is traumatic or is part of the ulnolunate impaction syndrome, because the treatments are different (LT joint stabilization or ulnar shortening, respectively) [33,34]. Conventional radiographs are most often normal in stable injuries (partial or complete LTL tears in isolation). Widening of the LT interval is not seen, even in advanced cases. When one or both of the secondary restraints are disrupted in addition to the LTL, there may be a step-off at the LT joint, as well as a VISI deformity (Fig. 5). Conventional radiographs can also demonstrate ulnar variance, which may help differentiate whether the tear is traumatic or is part of the ulnolunate impaction syndrome. Conventional arthrography can demonstrate a communicating defect between the radiocarpal and midcarpal joints. Arthrography can also demonstrate the presence of a TFCC tear. However, TFCC disruption may be seen with both traumatic LTL tears and LTL tears associated with UIS. MRI and MR arthrography have been used for evaluation of the LTL, with great variability in sensitivity and specificity. In 1989, Zlatkin and colleagues [16] proposed three criteria for MR diagnosis of interosseous ligament tears: nonvisualization of the ligament, fluid signal traversing the ligament on T2-weighted images, and morphologic distortion of the ligament. Because nonvisualization of the ligament is a relatively rare manifestation of an LTL tear [15], other findings, such as complete ligamentous disruption or a discrete linear area of high signal traversing the ligament on T2*- or fat-suppressed T2-weighted images, are believed to be more useful signs of LTL disruption (Fig. 6) [18,35–37]. Great variation has been reported in sensitivity and specificity for detection of LTL disruption on MRI compared with arthroscopy, ranging from 40% to 100% and from 33% to 100%, respectively [38]. MR arthrography permits better evaluation of LTL tears, because contrast material

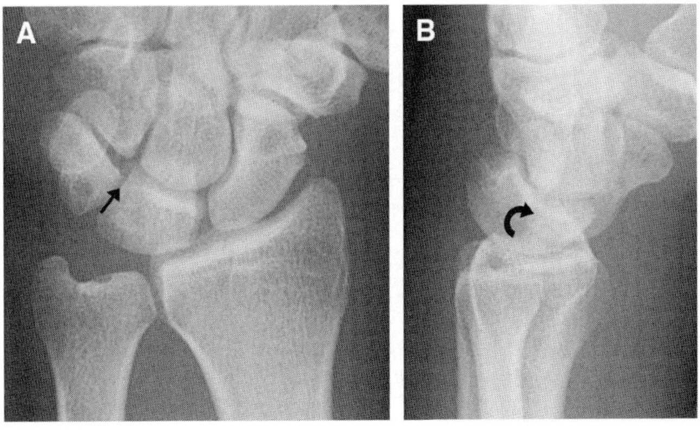

Fig. 5. Traumatic LTL tear with VISI deformity. Frontal radiograph (*A*) in this trauma patient demonstrates a step-off at the lunotriquetral joint (*arrow*). Lateral view (*B*) demonstrates volar tilt of the lunate (*curved arrow*), with a markedly decreased scapholunate angle: findings of a VISI deformity, indicating that the LTL, as well as one or both of the secondary restraints, has been disrupted.

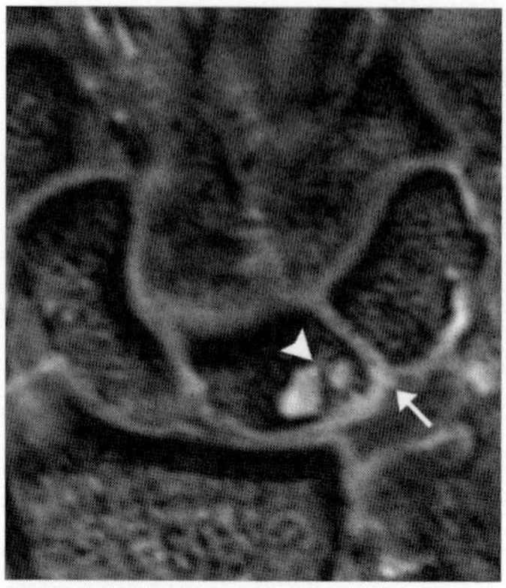

Fig. 6. Degenerative LTL tear. Coronal T2* gradient echo image demonstrates a discrete linear area of high signal traversing the expected location of the LTL (*arrow*). The ligament itself is not visualized. Also noted is cystic change in the ulnar aspect of the lunate (*arrowhead*), indicating a degenerative LTL tear as part of the ulnolunate impaction syndrome.

may be seen crossing the defect from the radiocarpal to the midcarpal joint (Fig. 7) [22,35,39].

DISTAL RADIOULNAR JOINT

The DRUJ is a diarthodial joint consisting of the articulation of the sigmoid notch of the radius with a portion of the distal ulna termed the ulnar seat. The mechanics of the DRUJ allow the distal radius to rotate approximately 150° around a relatively fixed ulnar head [8,40,41]. The contact between the

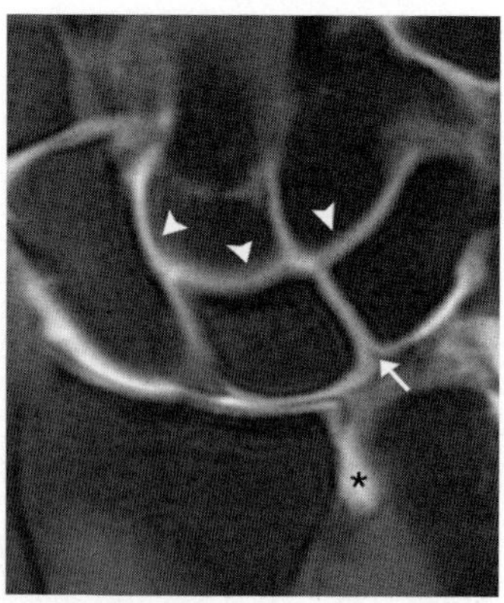

Fig. 7. LTL tear—MR arthrogram. Coronal fat-suppressed T1-weighted image from an MR arthrogram (radiocarpal joint injection only) in the same patient as depicted in Fig. 4 demonstrates gadolinium extending into the midcarpal joint (*arrowheads*) between the lunate and triquetrum (*arrow*). The LTL is not visualized. The scapholunate ligament remains intact. Gadolinium is also seen in the DRUJ (*asterisk*), indicating a TFCC tear.

articular surfaces of the sigmoid notch and the ulnar seat is maximal (approximately 60%) in neutral forearm rotation. In full supination and pronation, the contact decreases to less than or equal to 10% [42]. Therefore, ligamentous joint support is crucial. Stabilizers of the DRUJ include the joint capsule, the interosseous membrane, the TFCC, the floor of the ECU tendon sheath, and the pronator quadratus muscle [43]. The TFCC provides intrinsic support, with the dorsal and volar RU ligaments providing the most stability. The other structures listed provide extrinsic support [44].

Causes of DRUJ pain include osteoarthritis, inflammatory arthritis, infection, chronic instability, and ligamentous laxity. Patients who have DRUJ pathology typically experience pain when the distal ulna and distal radius are pressed together. They may also have crepitus on forearm rotation [8]. Conventional radiographs are of limited use in evaluating the DRUJ. Osteophytes, subchondral changes, and joint space narrowing can be seen in advanced osteoarthritis (Fig. 8). MRI is useful in excluding some causes, such as infection and inflammatory arthritis. However, MRI is suboptimal for evaluation of DRUJ subluxation, because the patient positioning necessary to achieve neutral forearm rotation is difficult in an MR scanner. Therefore, CT is the most useful method for evaluating DRUJ subluxation. Both the symptomatic and asymptomatic wrist should be scanned in neutral rotation, full pronation, and full supination [44]. Three different methods have been proposed for evaluation of DRUJ instability: Mino's criteria, the epicenter method, and the congruity method.

Mino's criteria involve drawing a line through the dorsal ulnar and radial borders of the distal radius and a line through the volar ulnar and radial borders of the distal radius. If the distal ulna moves above or below the lines drawn, there is dorsal or volar incongruity, respectively [45]. Wechsler and colleagues [46] proposed the congruity and epicenter methods [46]. The congruity

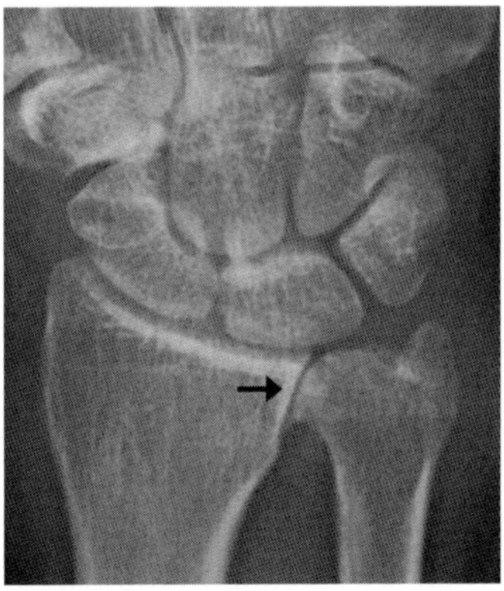

Fig. 8. DRUJ arthritis. Frontal view of the wrist demonstrates joint space narrowing and osteophyte formation involving the DRUJ (*arrow*).

method involves reconstructing the arcs of the ulnar head and sigmoid notch and comparing the congruity of these arcs. The epicenter method involves designating the center of rotation of the DRUJ as a point halfway between the center of the ulnar styloid and the center of the ulnar head. The chord of the sigmoid notch is denoted by drawing a line connecting the dorsal and volar aspects of the medial border of the sigmoid notch. A perpendicular line is then drawn from the epicenter to the chord. If the line intersects the middle half of the chord, the DRUJ position is considered normal. If the line intersects the outer half, there is mild subluxation. If the line is outside the sigmoid chord, there is severe subluxation (Fig. 9) [46].

Chiang and colleagues [44] examined CT scans of 80 wrists in 40 patients who had suspected DRUJ subluxation. CT was performed in neutral rotation, active pronation, and active supination. The authors found the epicenter method to be the most accurate of the three methods, presumably because it takes into account normal translation of the joint in pronation and supination.

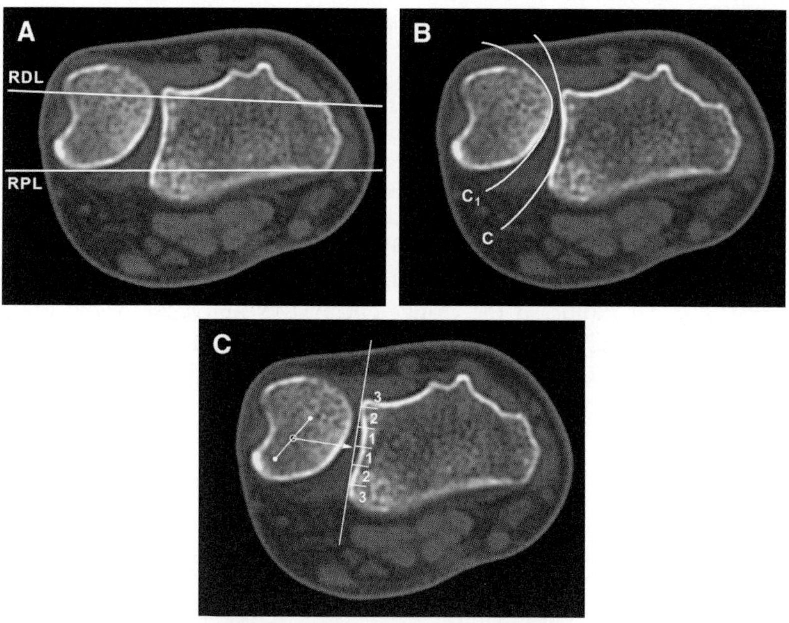

Fig. 9. Methods for evaluating DRUJ subluxation. Three identical axial CT images of the DRUJ in pronation demonstrate the three criteria for evaluating subluxation of the DRUJ. (*A*) Mino's criteria show the distal ulna dorsal to the RDL (radiodorsal line), indicating dorsal incongruity of the DRUJ. RPL, radiopalmar line. (*B*) Congruity method shows incongruity of the distal radial and carpal arcs (C, arc of the sigmoid notch of the radius; C1, arc of the ulnar seat), indicating an incongruous DRUJ. (*C*) Epicenter method. A perpendicular line drawn from the center of rotation of the DRUJ to the sigmoid chord intersects the middle half of the chord, indicating normal DRUJ position. Although (*A*) and (*B*) show incongruity of the DRUJ, (*C*) does not, illustrating the increased specificity of the epicenter method, which takes into account the normal translation of the DRUJ in supination and pronation.

EXTENSOR CARPI ULNARIS TENDON

Disorders of the ECU tendon include subluxation, dislocation, tendinopathy, tenosynovitis, and rupture. The tendon courses through the sixth dorsal compartment, contained within a fixed fibrous tunnel, or subsheath, which extends from the base of the ulnar styloid to the triquetrum. This tunnel is covered by but not adherent to the extensor retinaculum and provides a straight approach to the carpus for the tendon, regardless of the degree of pronation or supination [47]. The mechanism for ECU subluxation or dislocation is typically forearm supination and ulnar deviation of the hand [47]. The subsheath tears, and the patient feels a painful soft snap. MRI shows malposition of the tendon and may show inflammation of the tendon sheath (Fig. 10). Tendinopathy, tenosynovitis, and tendon rupture are all well evaluated on MRI. In tendinopathy, the tendon is typically thickened and may have increased signal intensity on T1- or T2-weighted images [15]. In tenosynovitis, fluid signal intensity is seen within the tendon sheath (Fig. 11). The sixth dorsal compartment is the second most common location of stenosing tenosynovitis in the upper extremity; this is most commonly related to sports requiring repetitive wrist motion [48]. Discontinuity of tendon fibers on MRI is seen with complete rupture of the tendon.

PISOTRIQUETRAL JOINT

Disorders that can affect the pisotriquetral joint (PTJ) include osteoarthritis, inflammatory arthritis, and joint instability. Seven separate structures insert on the pisiform. These are the flexor carpi ulnaris, the flexor retinaculum, the pisohamate ligament, the pisometacarpal ligaments, the abductor digiti minimi muscle, the extensor retinaculum, and the meniscus homolog [49–51]. The pisiform is connected to the triquetrum by a loose fibrous capsule, and disruption of any one of the seven structures listed could lead to PTJ instability [52]. In addition, some surgeries, such as carpal tunnel release and ulnar shortening, predispose to PTJ instability. Clinically, patients who have PTJ disorders present with pain in the hypothenar area, which is reproduced by "rocking" the

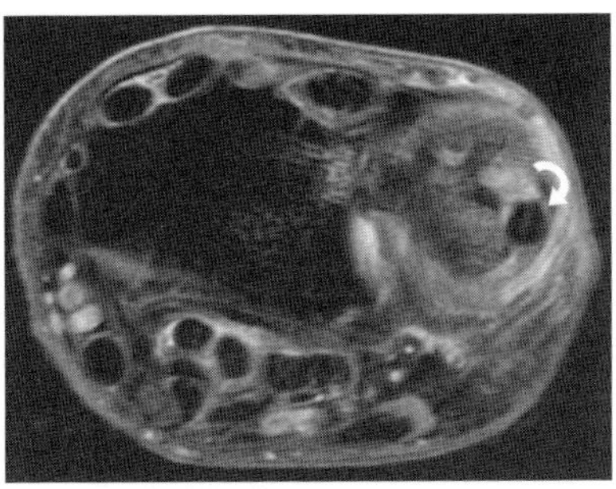

Fig. 10. ECU subluxation. Axial fat-suppressed T2-weighted image demonstrates subluxation of the ECU from its normal position in the dorsal groove of the distal ulna (*curved arrow*). A large amount of associated soft tissue swelling is seen.

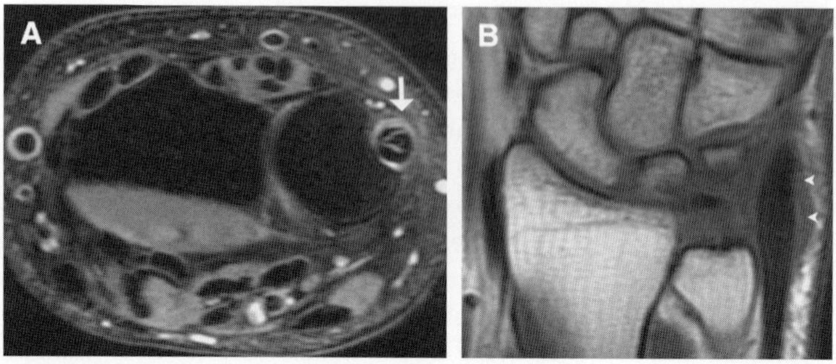

Fig. 11. ECU tendinopathy, tenosynovitis. Axial fat-suppressed T2-weighted image (*A*) demonstrates thickening and abnormal high T2 signal within the ECU (*arrow*). There is also fluid signal surrounding the tendon. Coronal T1-weighted image (*B*) in the same patient demonstrates fusiform swelling of the ECU (*arrowheads*).

pisiform on the triquetrum [47]. Diagnosis is confirmed by direct injection of anesthetic into the PTJ [53].

Conventional radiographs taken in 30° supination may demonstrate joint space narrowing, erosions, or osteophytes. MRI can detect earlier changes, such as subchondral edema and chondromalacia. If the patient's pain is determined to arise from the PTJ, excision of the pisiform has been found to be highly successful in relieving symptoms [47].

THE IMPACTION AND IMPINGEMENT SYNDROMES

Ulnolunate Impaction Syndrome

UIS, also called ulnar impaction syndrome or ulnocarpal abutment, is a degenerative condition related to excessive load-bearing across the ulnar aspect of the wrist. Chronic impaction between the distal ulna and the ulnar carpus leads to a continuum of changes, usually beginning with a degenerative tear of the TFCC, followed by chondromalacia of the lunate, triquetrum, and distal ulna, then a degenerative tear of the LTL, and, finally, osteoarthritis of the ulnocarpal and distal RU joints (Fig. 12) [54–57]. Factors that predispose to UIS are congenital positive ulnar variance, malunion of a distal radial fracture, previous radial head resection (after Essex-Lopresti fracture), and daily activities that cause excessive loading of the ulnar carpus [58].

The normal load distribution across the wrist is 80% across the radial aspect and 20% across the ulnar aspect [1,5,59]. Palmer and colleagues [60] found that minimal changes in ulnar variance changed the normal load distribution drastically. A 2.5-mm increase in ulnar variance increased the ulnar load to 42%, and a 2.5-mm decrease in ulnar variance decreased the ulnar load to 4.3%. Patients who have UIS present with subacute or chronic pain that is worse with activity and is exacerbated by maneuvers that increase ulnar variance, such as forearm pronation, power grip, and ulnar deviation [54,55].

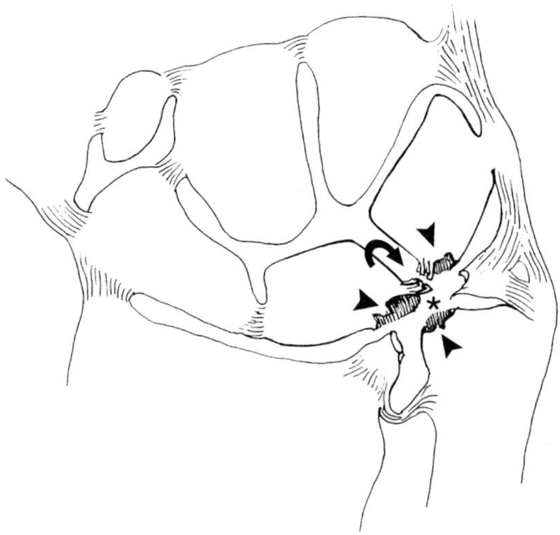

Fig. 12. Ulnolunate impaction syndrome coronal view illustration. Demonstrates the findings in UIS, including central TFCC tear (*asterisk*), chondromalacia of the distal ulna, proximal ulnar aspect of the lunate, proximal radial aspect of the triquetrum (*arrowheads*), and a tear of the LTL (*curved arrow*).

When assessing the distal forearm and wrist for ulnar variance, it is especially important that frontal radiographs be performed with the wrist in neutral forearm rotation, the elbow flexed at 90°, and the shoulder abducted 90° [43]. Radiographs may show positive or neutral ulnar variance as well as subchondral cystic change or sclerosis involving the ulnar head, ulnar aspect of the lunate, or the proximal radial aspect of the triquetrum (Fig. 13). However, conventional radiographs can be normal in early UIS. On MRI, subtle early changes such as cartilage fibrillation, marrow edema, subchondral cystic change, and ligamentous integrity may be visualized (Fig. 14). Ulnar variance cannot be accurately diagnosed on MRI, because the position for a standard frontal view is difficult to duplicate. MR arthrography demonstrates the same changes seen on MRI and can also help to clarify the Palmer classification of a lesion preoperatively. For example, the presence of a TFC perforation can differentiate between a class 2B and a class 2C lesion, and the presence of an LTL or ulnocarpal ligament tear can differentiate between a class 2C and a class 2D lesion [3].

The goal of treatment for UIS is to decrease the load across the ulnar side of the wrist, which can be accomplished using many different surgical procedures. Most procedures focus on ulnar shortening (open or arthroscopic) and attempt to preserve the insertion site of the TFCC onto the base of the ulnar styloid, as well as the integrity of the DRUJ [54]. The choice of surgical procedure depends on the age of the patient, the integrity of the DRUJ, and the cause of the UIS. For example, in patients in whom the cause of the UIS is a malunited distal radial fracture, corrective radial osteotomy may be performed [8]. In patients who have positive or neutral ulnar variance without DRUJ incongruity,

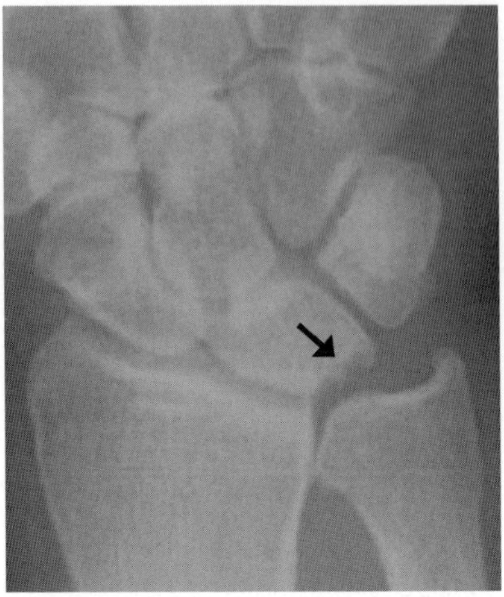

Fig. 13. Ulnolunate impaction syndrome. Frontal radiograph of the wrist demonstrates neutral ulnar variance, subchondral cystic change at the ulnar aspect of the lunate (*arrow*), and early degenerative change of the DRUJ, some of the plain film findings in UIS.

an ulnar shortening osteotomy or a wafer procedure could be performed. Ulnar shortening osteotomy involves resecting bone from the distal ulnar shaft, followed by plate and screw fixation. Wafer procedures (open or arthroscopic) involve excision of the distal 2 to 4 mm of the ulnar head, preserving the ulnar styloid and TFCC attachments. In patients who have UIS and DRUJ

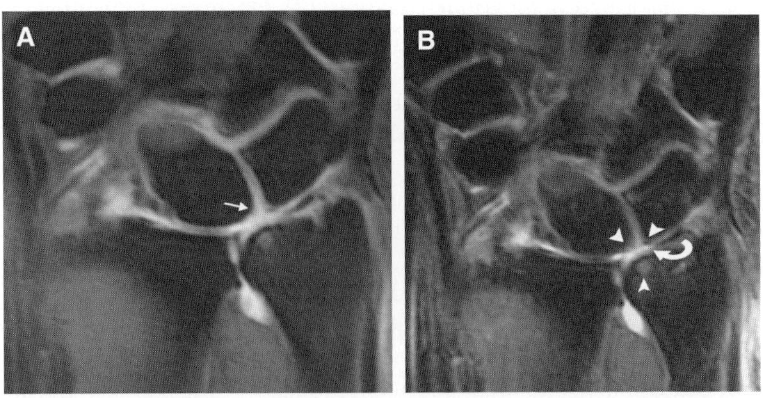

Fig. 14. Ulnolunate impaction syndrome. Coronal fat-suppressed T1-weighted (*A*) and fat-suppressed T2-weighted (*B*) images from an MR arthrogram (radiocarpal joint injection only) demonstrate the full spectrum of MR changes of UIS, including a degenerative tear of the TFCC (*curved arrow*), chondromalacia of the lunate and triquetrum, chondromalacia and cystic change in the distal ulna (*arrowheads*), a degenerative tear of the LTL (*arrow*), and osteoarthritis of the ulnocarpal and distal RU joints.

incongruity, surgical procedures include excision of the distal ulna (Darrach procedure); resection of the ulnar seat, leaving the ulnar shaft and styloid undisturbed (hemiresection-interposition); and DRUJ arthrodesis with creation of a pseudarthrosis proximal to the fusion (Sauve-Kapandji procedure). Potential complications vary by procedure but include nonunion, instability of the ulnar stump, and DRUJ incongruity [8].

Ulnar Styloid Impaction

Ulnar styloid impaction is due to either a long ulnar styloid process or a nonunited styloid process fracture impacting on the proximal triquetrum [38]. Styloid impaction from a long or "parrot-beaked" styloid process can result in chondromalacia of the ulnar styloid and the proximal triquetrum and can lead to LT joint instability (Fig. 15). An ulnar styloid is considered long when its overall length is greater than 6 mm or when the ulnar styloid process index (USPI) is greater than 0.21 ± 0.07 [61]. The USPI is defined as (styloid length − ulnar variance)/width of the ulnar head [62]. Conventional radiographs demonstrate a long styloid or one with a volar or radial curve (Fig. 16) [38]. MRI demonstrates chondromalacia and subchondral changes of the proximal triquetrum and ulnar styloid (Fig. 17). MR arthrography can aid in better evaluation of the TFCC and its ulnar attachments [3]. Therapy for this condition involves resection of all but the proximal 2 mm of the ulnar styloid. The proximal 2 mm is kept intact to preserve the integrity of the TFCC attachments [61].

Ulnar styloid impaction due to ulnar styloid fracture nonunion can result from several different mechanisms, including impaction, DRUJ instability, TFCC injury, irritative loose body, or partial rupture of the ECU tendon

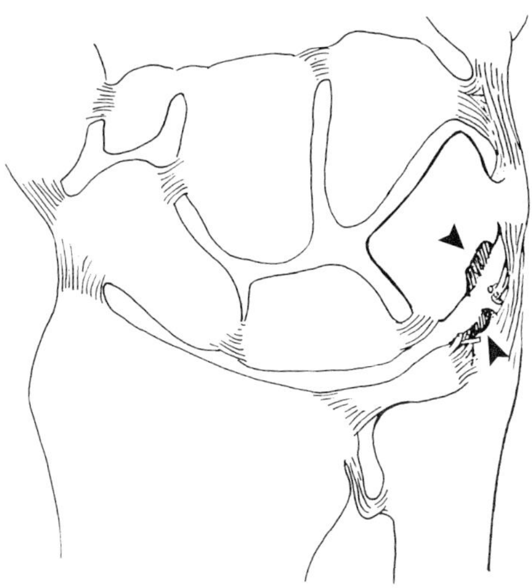

Fig. 15. Ulnar styloid impaction. Coronal view illustration demonstrates chondromalacia and subchondral change involving the tip of a long ulnar styloid and the proximal ulnar aspect of the triquetrum (*arrowheads*).

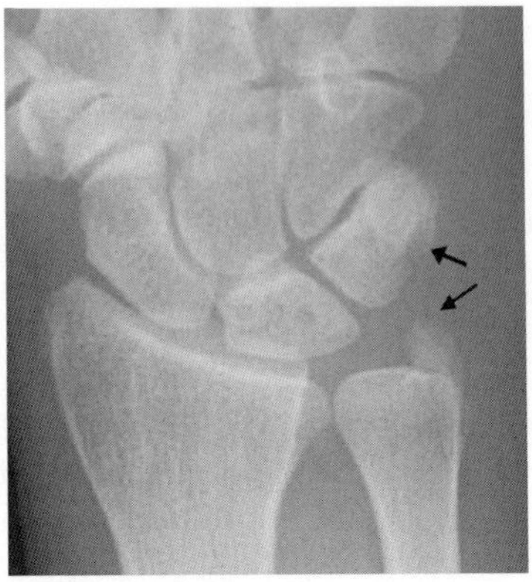

Fig. 16. Ulnar styloid impaction. Frontal radiograph of the wrist demonstrates a curved, or "parrot beak," ulnar styloid, with subchondral changes in both the ulnar styloid and the triquetrum (*arrows*). Soft tissue swelling at the ulnar aspect of the wrist is also seen.

(Fig. 18) [63–69]. Ulnar styloid nonunion is classified as type I or type II. Type I nonunion involves the tip of the ulnar styloid. The TFCC remains intact, and the DRUJ is stable. Type II nonunion involves the base of the ulnar styloid. Hence the TFCC attachment is disrupted, and the DRUJ is unstable [58]. Conventional radiographs demonstrate nonunion of an ulnar styloid fracture and may show subchondral changes in the proximal triquetrum. MRI may show marrow edema, chondromalacia, and ununited bone fragments (Fig. 19). MR arthrography, as mentioned previously, can aid in better evaluation of the ulnar attachments of the TFCC [3]. Treatment depends on the type of nonunion. For a type I nonunion, the bone fragment should be removed. For type II, the ulnar styloid, along with the TFCC, should be fixed to the distal ulna [58].

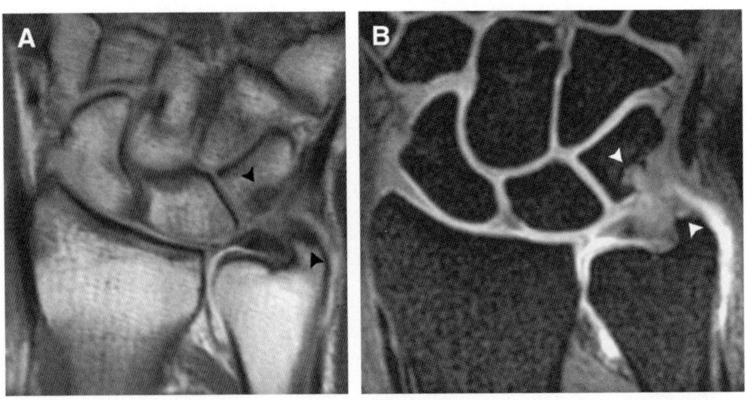

Fig. 17. Ulnar styloid impaction. Coronal T1-weighted (*A*) and 3D spoiled gradient echo fat-suppressed (*B*) images demonstrate a long ulnar styloid (8 mm), with subchondral change involving the tip of the styloid and the ulnar aspect of the triquetrum (*arrowheads*).

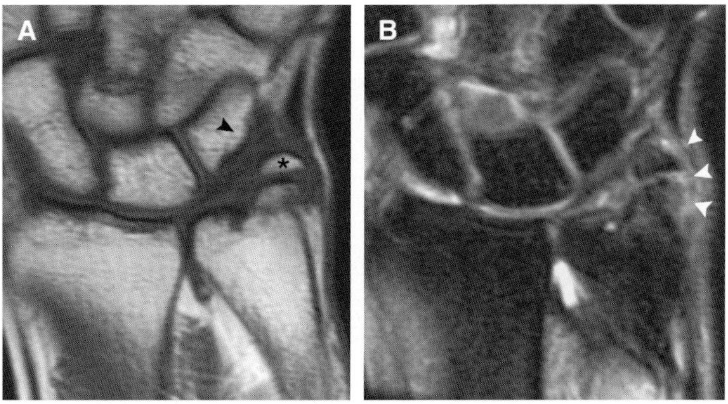

Fig. 18. Ulnar styloid impaction with styloid nonunion. Coronal T1-weighted (*A*) and fat-suppressed T2-weighted (*B*) images demonstrate a type 2 styloid nonunion (*asterisk*), with subchondral change in the ulnar aspect of the triquetrum (*black arrowhead*), subchondral change and marrow edema in the distal ulna and in the styloid fragment (*white arrowheads*), and surrounding soft tissue edema.

Hamatolunate Impaction

The normal lunate has one distal articular facet, where it articulates with the capitate. Approximately 44% to 73% of the population has a second facet at the ulnar side of the lunate, which articulates with the proximal pole of the hamate (Fig. 20) [11]. This type of lunate has been called a type II lunate [70–72]. In a study of cadaveric wrists, Viegas and colleagues [11] found that the

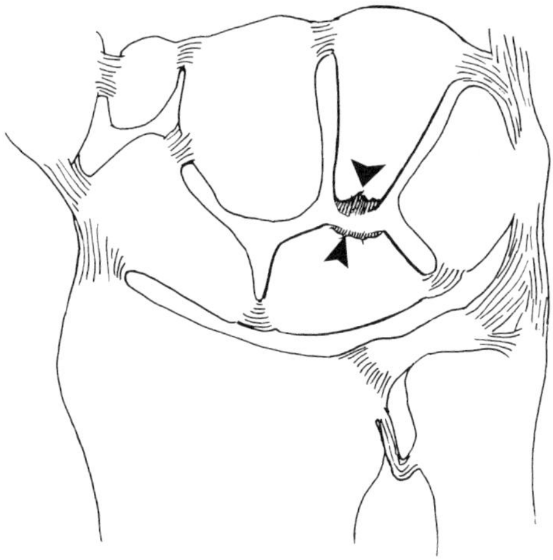

Fig. 19. Hamatolunate impaction. Coronal view illustration demonstrates an additional articular facet at the ulnar aspect of the lunate (type II lunate), with chondromalacia and subchondral change at the facet of the lunate and the proximal pole of the hamate (*arrowheads*).

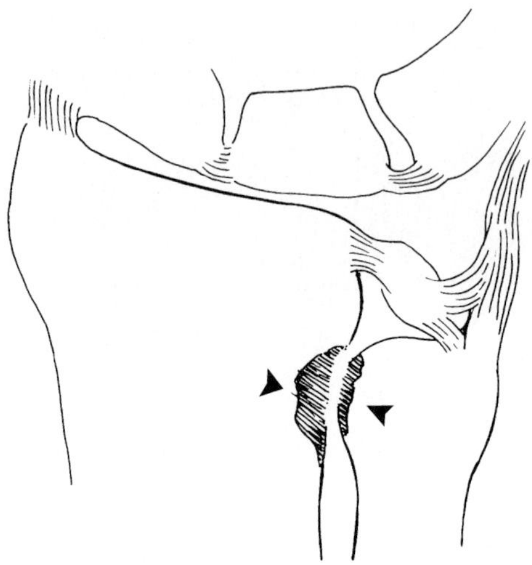

Fig. 20. Ulnar impingement. Coronal view illustration demonstrates a short ulna impinging on the distal radius proximal to the sigmoid notch, forming a painful pseudarthrosis. Scalloping of the cortex and subcortical changes can be seen in both the distal radius and ulna (*arrowheads*).

incidence of arthrosis at the proximal pole of the hamate was 38.2% in the cadaver population with a type II lunate, compared with 1.8% in those with a type I lunate. In the same study, the authors found that the proximal pole of the hamate is one of the most frequent sites of cartilage damage in the wrist. This finding is most likely due to the disruption of the second carpal arc that occurs in patients with a type II lunate [73]. During forced ulnar deviation, the hamate "jumps" over this disruption, leading to increased load on the proximal pole of the hamate [11]. Many of these lesions are clinically silent, and correlation must be made with a patient's symptoms. A type II lunate may be seen on conventional radiographs with a reported accuracy of 64% to 72% [74]. MRI and MR arthrography with a midcarpal joint injection may show chondromalacia of the proximal pole of the hamate, subchondral changes, and marrow edema [38,75].

Ulnar Impingement Syndrome

Ulnar impingement syndrome is a condition that develops when a short ulna impinges on the distal radius proximal to the sigmoid notch [76,77]. The short ulna may be congenital, due to premature fusion of growth plates, or a result of prior surgery (eg, Darrach ulnar shortening surgery, Madelung corrective surgery, surgery for rheumatoid arthritis) [55,76]. The short ulna impinges on the distal radius, forming a painful pseudarthrosis, which is aggravated by pronation and supination (Fig. 21) [54]. Conventional radiographs demonstrate a short ulna abutting the distal radius, with scalloping of the cortex of the distal radius proximal to the sigmoid notch [77]. MRI can aid in earlier diagnosis, with detection of marrow edema and subcortical marrow changes.

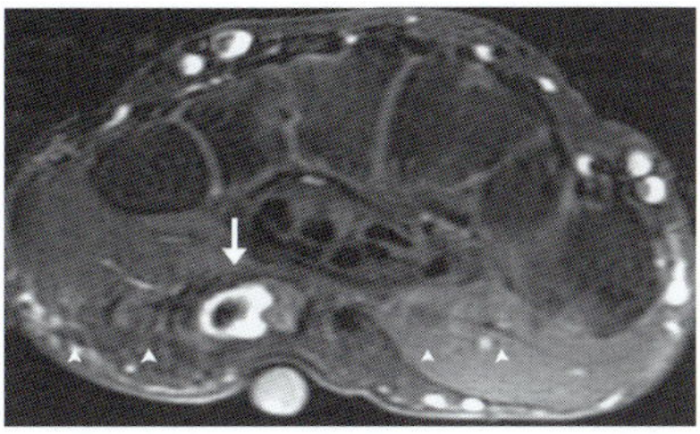

Fig. 21. Ulnar artery aneurysm. Axial fat-suppressed T1-weighted image after administration of intravenous gadolinium demonstrates an enhancing mass in Guyon's canal with associated central flow void (*arrow*) and marked pulsation artifact (*arrowheads*), representing an ulnar artery aneurysm.

ULNAR WRIST MASSES

Guyon's canal is a fascial tunnel that is bounded dorsally by the pisohamate ligament, volarly by forearm fascia and expansions from the flexor carpi ulnaris, medially by the pisiform, and laterally by the hook of the hamate. The canal extends approximately 4 cm from the proximal aspect of the pisiform to the level of the hamate. The ulnar nerve, ulnar artery, and (in some patients) veins pass through Guyon's canal [15]. Any mass in this region could cause compression of the deep motor branch of the ulnar nerve. Masses that have been described in this region include ganglia, anomalous muscles, lipomas, and ulnar artery aneurysms [15].

SUMMARY

Along with clinical history and physical examination, imaging is vital to narrowing down the differential diagnosis in ulnar-sided wrist pain. Treatments vary widely, depending on the cause of the pain, and differentiating the various entities is crucial. Conventional radiographs, conventional arthrography, CT, MRI, and MR arthrography are all useful modalities that are often used in concert to help guide diagnosis and treatment.

Acknowledgments

The author would like to thank D. Laurie Persson for his excellent original illustrations used in this review.

References

[1] Palmer AK. The distal radioulnar joint. Orthop Clin North Am 1984;15:321.
[2] Steinbach LS, Palmer WE, Schweitzer ME. Special focus session. MR arthrography. Radiographics 2002;22(5):1223–46.
[3] Cerezal L, Abascal F, Garcia-Valtuille R, et al. Wrist MR arthrography: how, why, when. Radiol Clin North Am 2005;43(4):709–31.
[4] Palmer AK. Triangular fibrocartilage complex lesion: a classification. J Hand Surg [Am] 1989;14(4):594–606.
[5] Palmer AK, Werner FW. The triangular fibrocartilage complex of the wrist: anatomy and function. J Hand Surg [Am] 1981;6(2):153–62.
[6] Chidgey LK. The distal radioulnar joint: problems and solutions. J Am Acad Orthop Surg 1995;3:95–109.

[7] Thiru-Pathi RG, Ferlic DC, Clayton ML, et al. Arterial anatomy of the triangular fibrocartilage of the wrist and its surgical significance. J Hand Surg [Am] 1986;11(2):258–63.
[8] Deitch MA, Stern PJ. Ulnocarpal abutment: treatment options. Hand Clin 1998;14(2): 251–63.
[9] Nagle DJ. Arthroscopic treatment of degenerative tears of the triangular fibrocartilage. Hand Clin 1994;10(4):615–24.
[10] Mikic ZD. Age changes in the triangular fibrocartilage of the wrist joint. J Anat 1978;126(2):367–84.
[11] Viegas SF, Patterson RM, Hokanson JA, et al. Wrist anatomy: incidence, distribution, and correlation of anatomic variations, tears and arthrosis. J Hand Surg [Am] 1993;18(3):463–75.
[12] Harrison MO, Freiberger RH, Ranawat CS. Arthrography of the rheumatoid wrist joint. AJR Am J Roentgenol 1971;112(3):480–6.
[13] Kessler I, Silberman Z. Experiment study of the radiocarpal joint by arthrography. Surg Gynecol Obstet 1961;112:33–40.
[14] Kang HS, Kindynis P, Brahme SK, et al. Triangular fibrocartilage and intercarpal ligaments of the wrist: MR imaging–cadaveric study with gross pathologic histologic correlation. Radiology 1991;181(2):401–4.
[15] Steinbach LS, Smith DK. MRI of the wrist. Journal of Clinical Imaging 2000;24(5):298–322.
[16] Zlatkin MB, Chao PC, Osterman AL, et al. Chronic wrist pain: evaluation with high-resolution MR imaging. Radiology 1989;173(3):723–9.
[17] Golimbu CN, Firooznia H, Melone CP, et al. Tears of the triangular fibrocartilage of the wrist: MR imaging. Radiology 1989;173(3):731–3.
[18] Schweitzer ME, Brahme SK, Hodler J, et al. Chronic wrist pain: spin-echo and short tau inversion recovery MR imaging and conventional MR arthrography. Radiology 1992;182(1): 205–11.
[19] Potter HG, Asnis-Ernberg L, Weiland AJ, et al. The utility of high-resolution magnetic resonance imaging in the evaluation of the triangular fibrocartilage complex of the wrist. J Bone Joint Surg Am 1997;79(11):1675–84.
[20] Oneson SR, Timins ME, Scales LM, et al. MR imaging diagnosis of triangular fibrocartilage pathology with arthroscopic correlation. AJR Am J Roentgenol 1997;168(6):1513–8.
[21] Haims AH, Schweitzer ME, Morrison WB, et al. Limitations of MR imaging in the diagnosis of peripheral tears of the triangular fibrocartilage of the wrist. AJR Am J Roentgenol 2002;178(2):419–22.
[22] Schmitt R, Christopoulos G, Meier R, et al. Direct MR arthrography of the wrist in comparison with arthroscopy: a prospective study on 125 patients. Rofo 2003;175(7):911–9.
[23] Shin AY, Battaglia MJ, Bishop AT. Lunotriquetral instability: diagnosis and treatment. J Am Acad Orthop Surg 2000;8(3):170–9.
[24] Berger RA. The gross and histologic anatomy of the scapholunate interosseous ligament. J Hand Surg [Am] 1996;21(2):170–8.
[25] Ritt MJ, Bishop AT, Berger RA, et al. Lunotriquetral ligament properties: a comparison of three anatomic subregions. J Hand Surg [Am] 1998;23(3):425–31.
[26] Buterbaugh GA, Brown TR, Horn PC. Ulnar-sided wrist pain in athletes. Clin Sports Med 1998;17(3):567–83.
[27] Reagan DS, Linschied RL, Dobyns JH. Lunotriquetral sprains. J Hand Surg [Am] 1984;9(4): 502–14.
[28] Ambrose L, Posner MA. Lunate-triquetral and midcarpal joint instabilities. Hand Clin 1992;8(4):653–68.
[29] Kleinman WB, Graham TJ. Distal ulnar injury and dysfunction. In: Peimer CA, editor. Surgery of the hand and upper extremity. New York: McGraw-Hill; 1996. p. 667–710.
[30] Viegas SF, Patterson RM, Peterson PD, et al. Ulnar-sided perilunate instability: an anatomic and biomechanic study. J Hand Surg [Am] 1990;15(2):268–78.
[31] Viegas SF. Ulnar-sided wrist pain and instability. AAOS Instructional Course Lectures 1998;47:215–8.

[32] Weiss LE, Taras JS, Sweet S, et al. Lunotriquetral injuries in the athlete. Hand Clin 2000;16(3):433–8.

[33] Milch H. Cuff resection of the ulna for malunited Colles' fracture. J Bone Joint Surg 1941;23: 311–3.

[34] Darrow JC, Linscheid RL, Dobyns JH, et al. Distal ulnar recession for disorders of the distal radioulnar joint. J Hand Surg [Am] 1985;10(4):482–91.

[35] Kovanlikaya I, Camil D, Cakmakci H, et al. Diagnostic value of MR arthrography in detection of intrinsic carpal ligament lesion: use of cine-MR arthrography as a new approach. Eur Radiol 1997;7(9):1441–5.

[36] Zlatkin MB, Rosner J. MR imaging of ligaments and triangular fibrocartilage complex of the wrist. Magn Reson Imaging Clin N Am 2004;12(2):301–31.

[37] Smith DK. MR imaging of normal and injured wrist ligaments. Magn Reson Imaging Clin N Am 1995;3(2):229–48.

[38] Cerezal L, del Pina F, Abascal F. MR imaging findings in ulnar-sided wrist impaction syndromes. Magn Reson Imaging Clin N Am 2004;12(2):281–99.

[39] Braun H, Kenn W, Schneider S, et al. Direct MR arthrography of the wrist: value in detecting complete and partial defects of intrinsic ligaments and the TFCC in comparison with arthroscopy. Rofo 2003;175(11):1515–24.

[40] Ekenstam F, Hagert CG. Anatomical studies of the geometry and stability of the distal radioulnar joint. Scand J Plast Reconstr Surg 1985;19(1):17–25.

[41] Ray RD, Johnson RJ, Jameson RM. Rotation of the forearm—an experimental study of pronation and supination. J Bone Joint Surg 1951;33A(4):993–6.

[42] Ekenstam F. Osseous anatomy and articular relationships about the distal ulna. Hand Clin 1998;14(2):161–4.

[43] Loftus JB, Palmer AK. Disorders of the distal radioulnar joint and triangular fibrocartilage complex: an overview. In: Lichtman DM, Alexander AH, editors. The wrist and its disorders. Philadelphia: WB Saunders; 1997. p. 385–414.

[44] Chiang CC, Chang MC, Lin CFJ, et al. Computerized Tomography in the diagnosis of subluxation of the distal radioulnar joint. Chin Med J (Engl) 1998;61(12):708–15.

[45] Mino DE, Palmer AK, Levinsohn EM. The role of radiography and computerized tomography in the diagnosis of subluxation and dislocation of the distal radioulnar joint. J Hand Surg [Am] 1983;8(1):23–31.

[46] Wechsler RJ, Wehbe MA, Rifkin MD, et al. Computed tomography diagnosis of the distal radioulnar subluxation. Skeletal Radiol 1987;16(1):1–5.

[47] Taleisnik J. Pain on the ulnar side of the wrist. Hand Clin 1987;3(1):51–68.

[48] Hajj AA, Wood MB. Stenosing tenosynovitis of the extensor carpi ulnaris. J Hand Surg [Am] 1986;11(4):519–20.

[49] Harris HA. The pisiform bone. Nature 1944;153:715.

[50] Williams PL, Warwick R. The carpus. In: Pick TP, Howden R, editors. Gray's anatomy. 36th edition. Edinburgh (Scotland): Churchill Livingstone; 1980. p. 162–3.

[51] Weston WJ, Kelsey CK. Functional anatomy of the pisicuneiform joint. Br J Radiol 1973;46(549):692–4.

[52] Paley D, McMurtry RY, Cruickshank B. Pathologic conditions of the pisiform and pisotriquetral joint. J Hand Surg [Am] 1987;12(1):110–9.

[53] Coyle MP Jr, Carroll RE. Dysfunction of the pisotriquetral joint: treatment by excision of the pisiform. J Hand Surg [Am] 1985;10(5):703–7.

[54] Friedman SL, Palmer AK. The ulnar impaction syndrome. Hand Clin 1991;7(2):295–310.

[55] Hodge JC, Yin Y, Gilula LA. Miscellaneous conditions of the wrist. In: Gilula LA, Yin Y, editors. Imaging of the wrist and hand. Philadelphia: Saunders; 1996. p. 523–46.

[56] Escobedo EM, Bergman AG, Hunter JC. MR imaging of ulnar impaction. Skeletal Radiol 1995;24(2):85–90.

[57] Imaeda T, Nakamura R, Shionoya K, et al. Ulnar impaction syndrome: MR imaging findings. Radiology 1996;201(2):495–500.

[58] Cerezal L, del Pinal F, Abascal F, et al. Imaging findings in ulnar-sided wrist impaction syndromes. Radiographics 2002;22(1):105–21.
[59] Palmer AK, Werner FW. Biomechanics of the distal radioulnar joint. Clin Orthop 1984;187:26–35.
[60] Palmer AK, Glisson RR, Werner FW. Relationship between ulnar variance and triangular fibrocartilage complex thickness. J Hand Surg [Am] 1984;9(5):681–3.
[61] Topper SM, Wood MB, Ruby LK. Ulnar styloid impaction syndrome. J Hand Surg [Am] 1997;22(4):699–704.
[62] Garcia-Elias M. Soft-tissue anatomy and relationships about the distal ulnar. Hand Clin 1998;14:165–76.
[63] Burgess RC, Watson HK. Hypertrophic ulnar styloid nonunions. Clin Orthop 1988;228: 215–7.
[64] Cheng SL, Axelrod TS. Management of complex dislocations of the distal radioulnar joint. Clin Orthop 1997;341:183–91.
[65] Lindau T, Adlercreutz C, Aspenberg P. Peripheral tears of the triangular fibrocartilage complex cause distal radioulnar joint instability after distal radial fractures. J Hand Surg [Am] 2000;25(3):464–8.
[66] Lindau T, Hagberg L, Adlercreutz C, et al. Distal radioulnar joint instability is an independent worsening factor in distal radial fractures. Clin Orthop 2000;376:229–35.
[67] Melone CP Jr, Nathan R. Traumatic disruption of the triangular fibrocartilage complex: pathoanatomy. Clin Orthop 1992;275:65–73.
[68] Palmer AK. Triangular fibrocartilage disorders: injury patterns and treatment. Arthroscopy 1990;6(2):125–32.
[69] Reeves B. Excision of the ulnar styloid fragment after Colles' fracture. Int Surg 1966;45(1): 46–52.
[70] Burgess RC. Anatomic variations of the midcarpal joint. J Hand Surg [Am] 1990;15(1): 129–31.
[71] Viegas SF, Wagner K, Patterson R, et al. Medial (hamate) facet of the lunate. J Hand Surg [Am] 1990;15(4):564–71.
[72] Viegas SF. The lunatohamate articulation of the midcarpal joint. Arthroscopy 1990;6(1): 5–10.
[73] Peh WC, Gilula LA. Normal disruption of carpal arcs. J Hand Surg [Am] 1996;21(4): 561–6.
[74] Sagerman SD, Hauck RM, Palmer AK. Lunate morphology: can it be predicted with routine x-ray films? J Hand Surg [Am] 1995;20(1):38–41.
[75] Pfirrmann CW, Theumann NH, Chung CB, et al. The hamatolunate facet: characterization and association with cartilage lesions: magnetic resonance arthrography and anatomic correlation in cadaveric wrists. Skeletal Radiol 2002;31(8):451–6.
[76] Bell MJ, Hill RJ, McMurtry RY. Ulnar impingement syndrome. J Bone Joint Surg Br 1985;67(1):126–9.
[77] McKee MD, Richards RR. Dynamic radio-ulnar convergence after the Darrach procedure. J Bone Joint Surg Br 1996;78(3):413–8.

ELSEVIER
SAUNDERS

Clin Sports Med 25 (2006) 527–542

CLINICS IN SPORTS MEDICINE

Injuries of the Fingers and Thumb in the Athlete

Jeffrey J. Peterson, MD*, Laura W. Bancroft, MD

Department of Radiology, Mayo Clinic, 4500 San Pablo Road, Jacksonville, FL 32224, USA

Hand injuries are common in athletes, accounting for up to 9% of all sports injuries [1]. Injuries to the hand are common in athletes, probably because the hand is characteristically in front of the athlete in most sports and frequently absorbs the initial contact. Furthermore, the hand is used most sports in one way or another. In many competitive team sports, the fingers and thumb are the areas most often injured [1]. Sports-related injuries to the hand can be debilitating and sideline athletes of all levels for considerable time periods. Severe hand injuries may even have a lasting effect on long-term function of the hand and wrist.

Although the hand is the most active portion of the upper extremity, it is the least well protected and therefore at high risk for injury during sports activity [2]. Sports-related hand injuries range from apparently minor problems to those whose severity is immediately apparent, such as a fracture or dislocation of a finger. Finger and thumb injuries usually result from accidents and therefore are difficult to prevent. Depending on the sport, the percentage of injuries involving the hand can vary greatly. Finger and thumb injuries are common in sports that have a high risk for falling, such as skiing, biking, in-line skating, and gymnastics [1]. Football also results in a high percentage of hand and wrist injuries, accounting for 15% of all injuries [3].

IMAGING TECHNIQUES

Imaging evaluation of sports-related injuries should begin with radiographs [4]. Radiographs can be obtained rapidly and are cost efficient. Radiographs can be obtained of the entire hand; if pathology is limited to the digits, dedicated radiographs of the fingers and thumb may be obtained. The initial radiographic examination should include three views: posteroanterior (PA), lateral, and oblique [4]. Lateral views of the digits require isolation from the adjacent digits [4]. Proper positioning is critical to obtaining quality radiographs. Meticulous attention to proper positioning is necessary, and radiographs with suboptimal positioning should be repeated.

*Corresponding author. *E-mail address*: peterson.jeffrey@mayo.edu (J.J. Peterson).

0278-5919/06/$ – see front matter
doi:10.1016/j.csm.2006.02.001

sportsmed.theclinics.com

CT remains the best modality for evaluation of the bony architecture. CT is able to assess for subtle fractures that may not be evident on radiographs and can also be useful to assess fracture healing better than conventional radiographs [4]. Multidetector CT scanners allow high-quality multiplanar reformatted images. Three-dimensional (3D) reformatted and volume-rendered images allow 3D visualization of the osseous structures, which can be useful for surgical planning. Collimation and slice thickness should be minimized, typically between 0.5 and 1.0 mm, to optimize multiplanar and 3D reconstructions. Narrow slice thickness allows isotropic viewing, with creation of multiplanar reformatted images with the same resolution as the original sections.

MRI is the preferred modality for evaluating the soft tissue structures about the fingers and thumb, such as the ligaments and tendons [5]. Osseous abnormalities can also be evaluated well with MRI. Innovations in MRI continue to improve, allowing higher-quality imaging with smaller fields of view (FOV). These innovations include improved gradient strength and speed, specialized coils providing favorable signal-to-noise ratios, larger bore magnets, and higher field strength magnets. Coil selection is critical to quality imaging of the fingers and thumb. Dedicated wrist coils allow excellent imaging of the proximal hand. Dedicated small upper extremity or elbow coils allow excellent versatility in positioning and provide excellent signal-to-noise ratio, even for small FOV. Small extremity coils allow precise positioning of the hand within the center of the coil and are large enough to be used to image several digits in cases of more diffuse hand injuries. Digit coils or small loop coils allow for small FOV imaging, which is optimal for evaluation of individual joints and digits.

FRACTURES

Sports-related fractures of the hand are common. Fractures of the metacarpals or phalanges result from rotation, bending, direct blows, indirect forces, or any combination of these forces [5]. There are several osseous injuries that are seen commonly in athletic injuries. Radiographic detection and characterization of fractures are vitally important, because this guides treatment for the clinician. Characterization of fractures includes the location and direction of the fracture line, the presence or absence of comminution, displacement of the fracture, articular involvement, and associated soft tissue injury. Fractures often are divided into extra-articular and intra-articular fractures. Nondisplaced extra-articular fractures often can be treated with buddy taping or splinting, whereas intra-articular fractures often require surgical treatment [5]. Displaced fractures of the hand have a tendency to angulate volarly because of attachments of the interosseous muscles. Marginal fractures or avulsion fractures involving the metacarpals or phalanges can be sentinels of more serious associated soft tissue injuries [5].

PHALANGEAL FRACTURES

Phalangeal fractures are problematic, in that an isolated fracture can affect the function of the entire hand [4]. Digital function can be impaired by the fracture deformity and by associated soft tissue injuries [4]. There are many variations of phalangeal fractures involving various locations. Fractures involving the shaft may be transverse, oblique, spiral, or comminuted [6]. Displacement and angulation of phalangeal fractures are common and typically result from a combination of two main factors: the mechanism of injury and the deforming forces placed on the fractured bone. The mechanism of injury determines the nature of the fracture. A direct blow to the finger often results in a transverse or comminuted fracture, whereas a twisting injury of the digit often results in an oblique or spiral fracture [4]. Oblique or spiral fractures may also be associated with malrotation. No malrotation is acceptable for phalangeal fractures, because this leads to overlap and malalignment of the digit. Displaced or malrotated fractures should be reduced either by closed or open techniques. Acceptable reduction is less than 6 mm of shortening, less than 15 degrees of angulation, and no rotational deformity [4]. Nondisplaced phalangeal fractures can be treated conservatively. Nondisplaced fractures result in less than 10 degrees of angulation and have no rotational deformity [4]. Nondisplaced phalangeal fractures often can be treated with buddy taping and splinting with good results.

Injuries of the terminal tuft of the phalanges are not uncommon in sports (Fig. 1). These injuries often occur from a crushing force, often when a finger is stepped on by an opponent's cleats [4]. The middle finger or thumb is most commonly affected, because they tend to be more exposed than other digits [4]. Most tuft fractures are stable; however, injury of the tuft often includes injury to the nail or nail bed. A subungual hematoma should be evacuated if greater than 50% of the nail plate is involved [4]. The nail may need to be removed entirely and often takes many months or longer to regenerate.

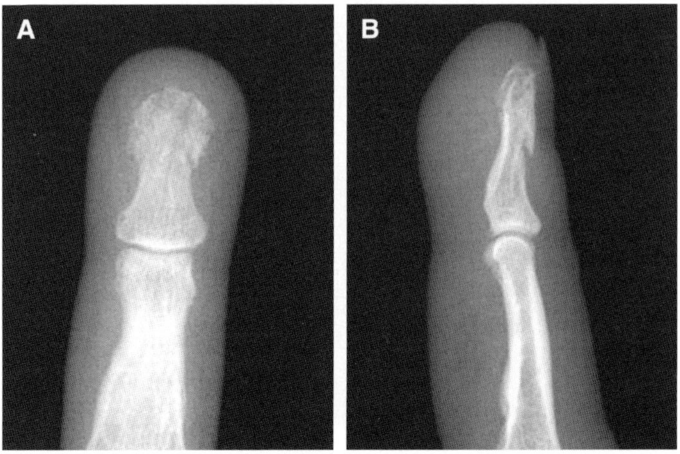

Fig. 1. Terminal tuft fracture. PA (*A*) and lateral (*B*) radiographs of the long finger depict a comminuted fracture of the third distal phalanx. The finger was crushed by an opponent's cleat while playing softball and was associated with a small subungual hematoma.

Interphalangeal (IP) dislocations are common injuries in athletes (Fig. 2) and are often reduced on the sidelines and then taped or splinted. Any injury with a force significant enough to cause joint dislocation almost assuredly results in ligamentous injury or tear. Most IP joint dislocations involve the proximal interphalangeal (PIP) joint [6]. The PIP joint is susceptible especially to forced abnormal motion produced in ball sports and in sports resulting in axial loading of the digit [6]. Most IP joint dislocations are dorsal, with dorsal dislocation of the middle phalanx and disruption of the volar plate [7]. Volar or lateral dislocations also occur but are less common. Urgent reduction is necessary and is often performed by the athlete or the coach, hence the term "coach's finger" [7]. Reduction often is achieved by traction and flexion of the middle phalanx [7]. Once reduced, the digit should be placed in a splint [6]. Associated fractures also must be treated appropriately.

MALLET FINGER

The terminal portion of the extensor mechanism of the finger crosses the dorsal aspect of the distal interphalangeal (DIP) joint. This extensor mechanism is responsible for active extension of the DIP joint. Mallet finger injury is caused by a flexion force on the tip of the finger while the DIP joint is extended [8]. This force results in tearing of the extensor tendon or an avulsion fracture at the tendinous attachment on the dorsal lip of the distal phalangeal base (Fig. 3) [8]. With mallet finger, the active extension power of the DIP joint is lost and the joint rests in an abnormally flexed position. The classic mechanism of injury is an extended finger struck on the tip by a softball, baseball, basketball

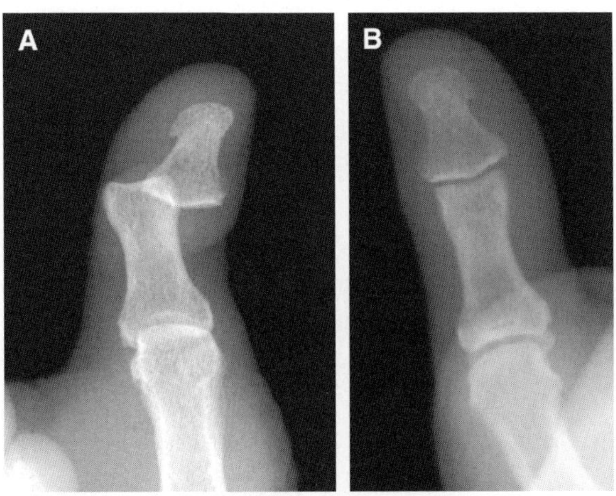

Fig. 2. IP joint dislocation of the thumb sustained while playing flag football. (*A*) PA radiograph of the thumb demonstrates complete dislocation of the IP joint. (*B*) Reduction radiograph was obtained after reduction was performed with traction in the emergency room. No fracture fragments were identified.

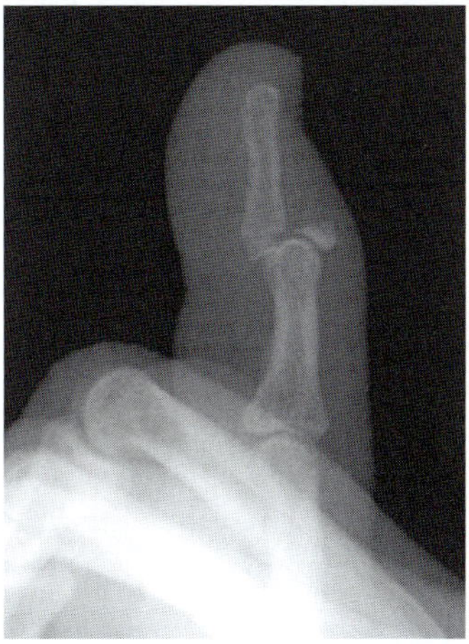

Fig. 3. Mallet finger. Lateral radiograph of the index finger depicts a distracted, intra-articular fracture of the dorsal base of the second distal phalanx at the attachment of the distal extensor tendon. Operative repair was performed secondary to the large size of the fragment and the displacement at the fracture site.

or volleyball [8]. The middle finger or long finger is most commonly injured, although any digit can be involved, including the thumb. Patients present with pain and swelling of the digit with inability to actively extend the DIP joint, although passive extension is possible.

Radiographs are helpful in identifying a small avulsion fracture at the extensor tendon attachment on the base of the distal phalanx. Nonoperative treatment is preferred if the avulsion fragment is small or if there is no osseous involvement [7]. Treatment typically consists of splinting the DIP joint in extension for 6 to 8 weeks [7]. Operative therapy is reserved for severe injuries or fractures involving greater than one third of the articular surface of the DIP joint [7,8]. Operative repair also can be considered for failure of conservative therapy, whereby there is persistent subluxation despite splinting.

Unfortunately, patients with mallet finger often do not present for immediate medical attention. Fractures tend to heal within weeks, and old osseous injuries without significant functional deficits are best left alone [8]. The injury often remodels over time, even in the presence of continued volar subluxation, and rarely leads to significant functional deficit. Late osteoarthritis of the DIP joint following a mallet finger injury is uncommon.

JERSEY FINGER

Another common sports injury involving the hand is jersey finger. Jersey finger is the term used to describe disruption of the flexor digitorum profundus (FDP) tendon from the volar aspect of the distal phalangeal base [7]. This disruption occurs when tackling and attempting to grab someone by the jersey [7]. The finger is pulled or forced into extension while the DIP is being flexed.

The ring finger is involved in up to 75% of cases, although any digit may be injured [7]. Patients clinically present with localized tenderness and pain with swelling and inability to flex the DIP joint [7]. Pain or fullness proximally along the course of the flexor tendon may occur, because there may be tendinous retraction after rupture [7]. Radiographs may depict an avulsion fracture of the volar aspect of the distal phalangeal base at the site of attachment of the FDP.

In contrast to mallet finger, early surgical referral is the treatment of choice for jersey finger [7], especially in the acute setting. Full functional outcome is likely with early surgical intervention, and best results are seen with intervention within 7 to 10 days [7]. In the chronic setting, the functional impairment fortunately is minimal or negligible, and benign neglect often is the treatment of choice [7]. Operative intervention is an option but is less successful with chronic deformities than with acute injuries (Fig. 4).

FLEXOR TENDON TEARS

Flexor tendon tears of the fingers commonly result from sports-related injuries. Treatment of flexor digitorum profundus or flexor digitorum superficialis (FDS) tendon injuries depends on the degree of injury. Often flexor tendon tears are difficult to diagnose clinically. MRI provides a noninvasive method to identify the site of tear, the degree of retraction of the torn fibers, and other associated soft tissue injuries (Fig. 5).

Types of flexor tendon injuries include tenosynovitis, partial tear, and rupture. Flexor tendon tenosynovitis is not infrequently seen with MRI of the finger in athletes. Tenosynovitis is an inflammatory response within the tendon sheath that often is related to repetitive stress [9]. Patients present with pain and swelling along the palmar surface of the digit, and sometimes have extension into the

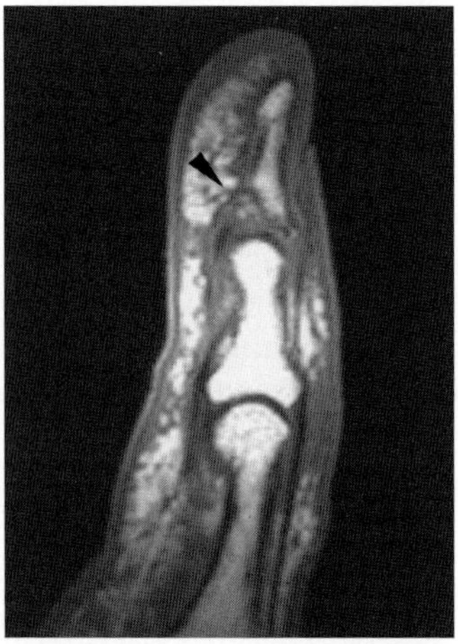

Fig. 4. Jersey finger. Sagittal MR image of the index finger depicts a nondisplaced fracture at the base of the distal phalanx at the attachment of the flexor digitorum profundus (*arrowhead*).

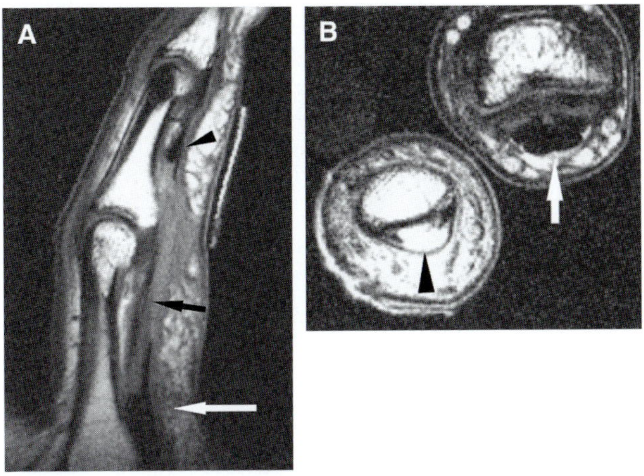

Fig. 5. Flexor digitorum superficialis and profundus tendon tears. (*A*) Sagittal MR image depicts the torn remnants of the flexor digitorum profundus (*black arrowhead*) and the flexor digitorum superficialis (*black arrow*) tendons. The torn flexor tendons are retracted proximally at the level of the proximal phalangeal base (*white arrow*). (*From* Berquist TH, Peterson JJ, Bancroft LW, et al. Trauma. In Berquist TH, editor. MRI of the hand and wrist. Philadelphia: Lippincott; 2003. p. 85; with permission) (*B*) Axial MR image depicts absence of both the flexor digitorum superficialis and profudus tendons (*black arrowhead*) at the level of the middle phalanx compatible with complete tears. Note the adjacent intact flexor tendons (*white arrow*) in the adjacent digit.

palm or forearm. Passive flexion of the finger typically is normal, but active flexion is limited [9]. MRI depicts increased signal within the tendon sheath on fluid-sensitive sequences with enhancement on post-gadolinium images.

Partial tear or rupture of the flexor tendons may occur anywhere along the course of the tendons, and may present with inability to flex one or both of the IP joints, depending on the site of rupture. Pain or fullness proximally along the course of the flexor tendon may be seen, because the torn flexor tendon may retract proximally after rupture. Jersey finger is often used to describe disruption of the flexor digitorum profundus from the volar base of the distal phalanx, as described previously. This disruption occurs when the finger is pulled or forced into extension while the DIP is being flexed [7]. Volar plate injury occurs with rupture of the FDS tendon at the PIP joint. This rupture has a similar mechanism of injury as jersey finger, with forced PIP hyperextension during active PIP flexion. Volar plate injuries also may be associated with avulsion fractures at the base of the middle phalanx (Fig. 6). Patients present with inability to actively flex the PIP joint, although passive extension is possible [7].

BOUTONNIERE DEFORMITY

Another uncommon injury involving the finger is the boutonniere deformity (Fig. 7). Normally, the central slip of the extensor tendon of the finger inserts

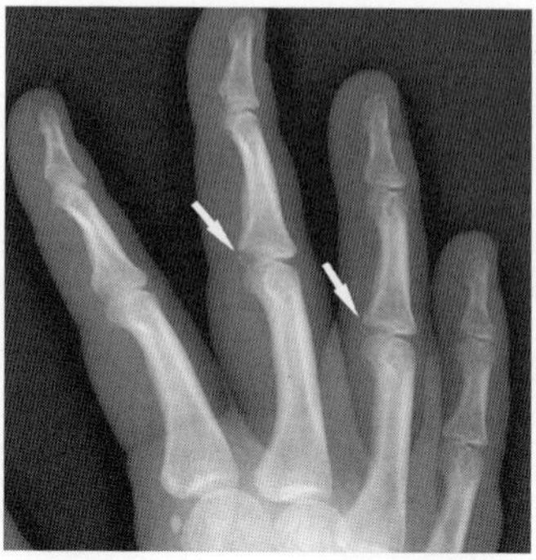

Fig. 6. Volar plate injury. Oblique radiograph of the hand demonstrates fractures of the volar bases of the third and fourth middle phalanges (*arrows*) at the attachments of the flexor digitorum superficialis tendons. Fractures were sustained while playing football.

on the middle phalanx [8]. With forced flexion of the PIP joint or volar dislocation of the PIP joint, disruption of this central slip of the extensor tendon can occur [8]. The lateral bands of the extensor tendon at the PIP joint are initially dorsal to the joint. With chronic disruption of the central band, however, the lateral bands retract and displace laterally and volarly, resulting in the characteristic boutonniere deformity. Injury is usually caused by a blow to the dorsum of the middle phalanx while the athlete is actively extending the finger, forcing the PIP joint into flexion [8]. Splinting of the digit in full extension for 6 to 8 weeks is the typical treatment for boutonniere deformity; however, surgical treatment may be necessary for severe or chronic injury [7].

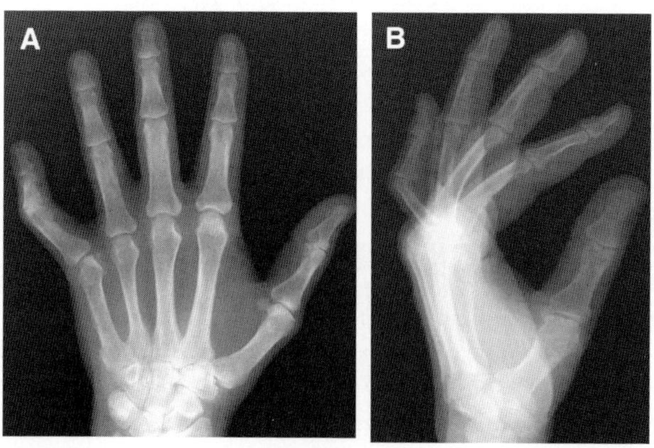

Fig. 7. Boutonniere deformity. Softball player injured his finger while sliding into a base. PA (*A*) and lateral (*B*) radiographs of the hand depict the characteristic fixed flexion deformity of the PIP joint with mild hyperextension of the DIP joint, compatible with boutonniere deformity.

FLEXOR TENDON PULLEY SYSTEM INJURY

Another finger injury that can occur in athletes is disruption of the flexor tendon pulley system. The flexor tendons pass through fibro-osseous canals from the heads of the metacarpals to the DIP joints, known as the flexor tendon pulley system (Fig. 8) [10,11]. The fibro-osseous canals of the pulley system are composed of focally thickened areas of the flexor tendon sheaths that are lined by synovium [10]. The pulleys accurately track the flexor tendons and keep them close to the bone during flexion and extension [10,11]. They also provide a fulcrum to transfer the linear force of the muscle and tendon into the rotation and torque needed to flex the distal phalanx [10]. The flexor tendon pulley system is composed of five annular pulleys and three cruciform pulleys [10]. An intact pulley system is crucial for proper flexion of the digits, and the A2 pulley is most important to flexor tendon function [10]. Injury typically initiates at the A2 pulley followed by the A3 and A4 pulleys. The A1 pulley rarely is injured [10]. Flexor tendon pulley injuries are seen in rock climbers and athletes in other sports that result in forced extension of a flexed finger [11].

MRI can diagnose ruptures of the A2 and A4 pulleys (Fig. 9). The diagnosis of pulley rupture can be made by direct visualization of the torn pulley; however, diagnosis more commonly is made with indirect signs [10]. Visualization

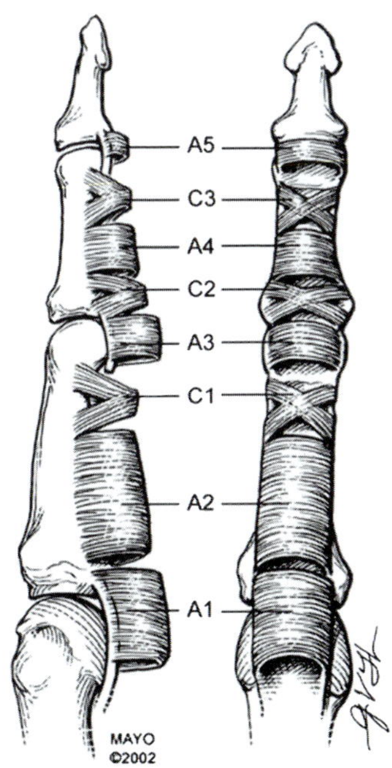

Fig. 8. The flexor tendon pulley system, with five annular and three cruciform pulleys. (*From* Berquist TH, Peterson JJ, Bancroft LW, et al. Trauma. In Berquist TH, editor. MRI of the hand and wrist. Philadelphia: Lippincott; 2003. p. 80; with permission)

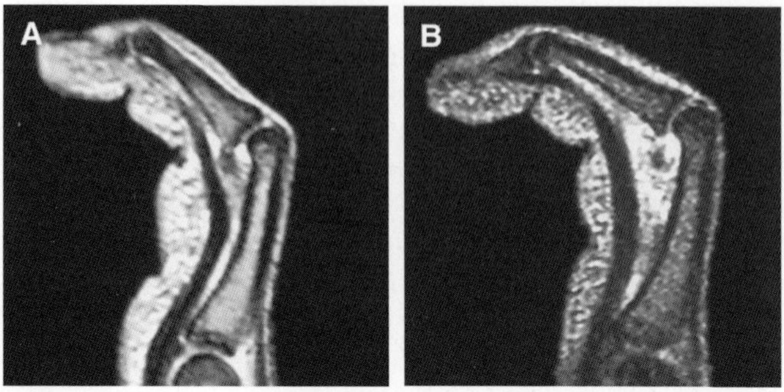

Fig. 9. Flexor tendon pulley injury. Sagittal T1-weighted (*A*) and T2-weighted (*B*) MR images of the finger in a rock climber with pulley injuries. Imaging reveals a bowstring sign with displacement of the flexor tendons away from the PIP joint in flexion, indicating rupture of the A2 and A3 flexor tendon pulleys.

of a gap between the bone and the flexor tendon with the finger in flexion allows diagnosis of pulley rupture. This gap is referred to as the bowstring sign. Disruption of the A2 pulley can be made with imaging of the finger in flexion by detecting a bowstring deformity of the flexor tendon, which extends to the base of the proximal phalanx [10].

METACARPAL FRACTURE

Metacarpal fractures account for up to one third of all hand fractures [4]. The most common fracture of the hand is fracture of the fifth metacarpal, accounting for approximately 50% of all metacarpal fractures and 20% of all fractures of the hand [4,10]. The mechanism of injury is either a direct blow to the hand or an indirect force from torsion or bending of the distal finger [10]. Dorsal apex angulation is common with metacarpal fractures. The more distal the fracture, the greater the degree of angulation that can be tolerated. Metacarpal fractures involving the ring and middle fingers inherently are more stable than those involving the index and fifth fingers, because there is dual support from the deep transverse intermetacarpal ligaments on the radial and ulnar sides [10].

Metacarpal fractures can be subdivided into distal fractures, fractures of the metacarpal neck, metacarpal shaft fractures, fractures of the metacarpal base, and fractures involving the base of the thumb. Distal metacarpal fractures by definition are intra-articular and therefore require urgent attention [5]. Most result from axial loading of the metacarpal by the tension exerted by the collateral ligaments [5]. Because distal metacarpal fractures are intra-articular fractures, they often are associated with soft tissue injuries, such as disruption of the collateral ligaments of the MCP joints.

Metacarpal neck fractures most commonly involve the fifth digit and are referred to as boxer's fractures (Fig. 10). These fractures usually result from

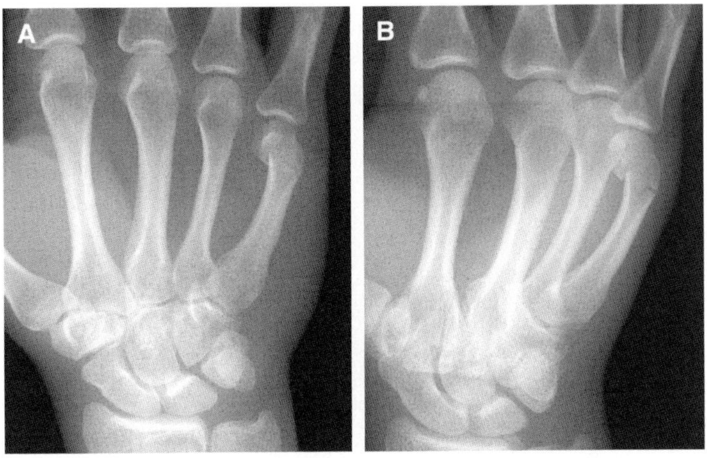

Fig. 10. Boxer's fracture. PA (*A*) and oblique (*B*) radiographs depict a fracture of the fifth metacarpal neck with volar angulation of the distal fragment. This fracture was treated conservatively with splinting with adequate results.

punching a hard object, such as a wall or another person [10]. The fracture occurs just below the metacarpal head and the metacarpal head is displaced in a volar direction. The distal fifth metacarpal takes the brunt of the impact and breaks through the narrowest area near the neck, typically resulting in apex dorsal angulation or displacement at the fracture site [4]. Casting or splinting is helpful to avoid further instability and to promote healing with stability at the fracture site. Apex dorsal angulation up to 40 degrees is acceptable for nonoperative management [7]. Fractures in this location often heal with residual apex dorsal angulation, which typically is not problematic. Fractures that are markedly comminuted or angulated occasionally may require open reduction and internal fixation.

Metacarpal shaft fractures are not uncommon sports injuries (Fig. 11). Their propensity for displacement is related directly to the extent of surrounding muscle and periosteal damage that occurred at the time of injury [5]. Rotation of a metacarpal shaft fracture is a great concern, because even a small degree of rotation can create a substantial degree of deformity at the fingertip [5]. Most fractures of the metacarpals and phalanges are low energy and result in simple fracture patterns that can be treated conservatively [10]. Minimally displaced, transverse or oblique, midshaft fractures are treated most frequently with closed reduction. Greater deformity is tolerated in the fourth and fifth fingers versus the second and third fingers [10]. Up to 50 degrees of apex dorsal angulation is tolerated in the fourth and fifth metacarpals, although only 30 degrees is tolerated in the second and third metacarpals [10]. Open reduction is reserved for high-energy trauma, fractures with excessive angulation, or multiple fractures.

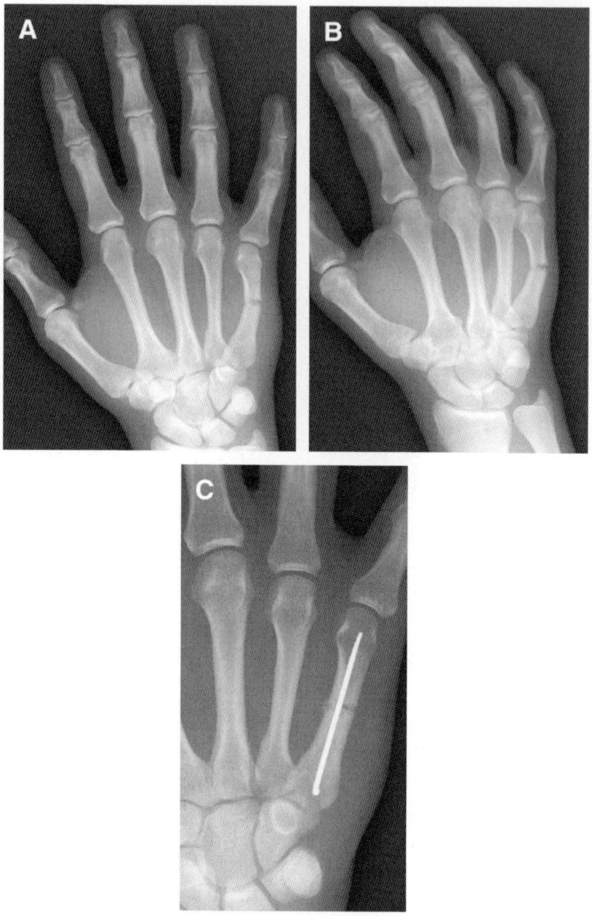

Fig. 11. Fifth metacarpal fracture in a wrestler. PA (*A*) and oblique (*B*) radiographs of the hand depict a transverse fracture of the mid fifth metacarpal shaft. Note the degree of angulation at the fracture site and abnormal apposition of the fourth and fifth digits. (*C*) The fracture was treated surgically with open reduction and pin fixation.

Fractures of the metacarpal base should be evaluated carefully for involvement of the adjacent carpometacarpal (CMC) joint, which occurs commonly [5]. Fractures of the metacarpal base occurring most commonly involve the fourth and fifth metacarpals. Fractures in this location often are reduced easily, but have a tendency to re-subluxate and often are treated operatively with percutaneous pinning [5].

BENNETT FRACTURE

An important subset of metacarpal injuries involves the base of the thumb. These injuries result from an axial load applied to the thumb [5]. The most common is the Bennett fracture, named after Edward Hallaran Bennett, MD, who first described the fracture pattern in 1882 [12]. The original description was that of a fracture involving the base of the first metacarpal; however, the current definition of a Bennett fracture is an intra-articular fracture or dislocation involving the base of the first metacarpal (Fig. 12) [7]. With these fractures, the small fragment of the first metacarpal continues to articulate with the trapezium [10], whereas the remainder of the first metacarpal shaft is retracted laterally by the action of the abductor pollicis longus muscle [10]. The mechanism is classically an axial load to the flexed and adducted thumb [7]. Injuries such as this commonly occur in throwing athletes, such as a quarterback who strikes an object (eg, a helmet or the ground) on followthrough [7]. Early diagnosis and treatment are imperative to prevent loss of function of the first carpometacarpal joint [13]. Bennett fractures are unstable fractures, and unless properly recognized and treated this intra-articular fracture subluxation may result in an unstable arthritic first CMC joint [10]. Bennett fractures are treated most commonly with closed reduction with a thumb cast and immobilization of the first CMC joint. Open or closed reduction combined with internal fixation frequently is required [5]. If the fracture involves less than 20% of the articular surface, closed reduction with pinning generally is adequate. For fractures with more than 1 mm of articular incongruity after closed reduction, open reduction and fixation are indicated [4].

ROLANDO FRACTURE

A Rolando fracture is similar to a Bennett fracture, except it results in a comminuted intra-articular fracture of the base of the first metacarpal (Fig. 13) [7]. The fracture was originally described as Y-shaped, with a three-fragment fracture that extended to the CMC joint surface [14]. Today the eponym is used widely for any comminuted intra-articular fracture at the base of the thumb [7]. The

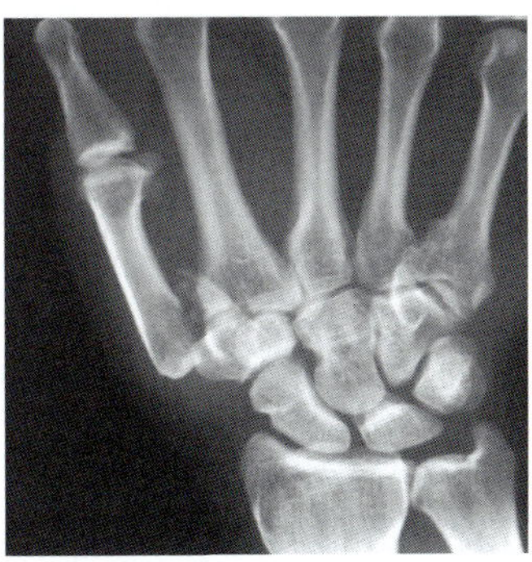

Fig. 12. Bennett fracture. PA radiograph depicts an intra-articular fracture involving the base of the thumb. A small fragment of the first metacarpal remains with the trapezium, whereas the remainder of the first metacarpal is displaced radially by the action of the abductor pollicis longus muscle.

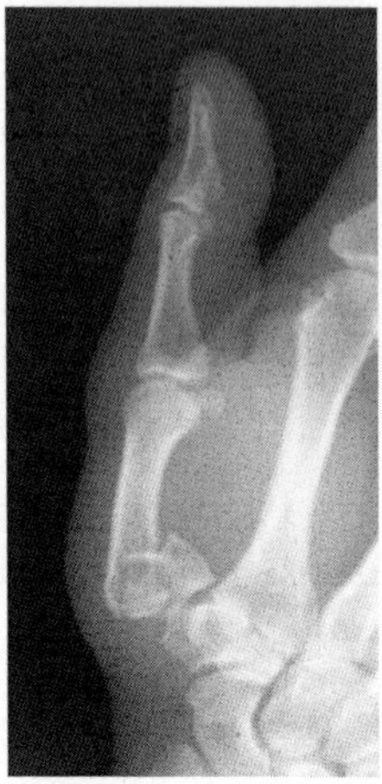

Fig. 13. Rolando fracture. Comminuted intra-articular fracture of the first metacarpal base was sustained by this athlete while making a football tackle.

Rolando fracture occurs secondary to axial loading that crushes the articular surface of the first metacarpal. The Rolando fracture can be associated with significant posttraumatic arthritis if there is significant incongruity at the articular surface of the base of the first metacarpal. Marked decrease in hand function can result if proper fixation is not achieved; therefore, significant joint incongruity requires operative reduction [7].

GAMEKEEPER'S THUMB

Another common athletic injury involving the base of the thumb is disruption of the ulnar collateral ligament (UCL) of the first MCP joint as a result of an acute radial or valgus stress on the thumb [15]. Injury can occur in the form of an avulsion fracture, an isolated ligament tear, or combined fracture and ligament rupture [15]. The historical eponym refers to Scottish gamekeepers who repeatedly dispatched small animals by using their thumbs to push forcefully on the back of the animals' heads, breaking their necks [15]. Today this injury commonly is referred to as skier's thumb, because it is seen most commonly in snow skiers. Skier's thumb results from a fall while holding a ski pole, causing forced abduction and extension of the thumb [7].

Radiographs may depict a small avulsion fracture fragment at the ulnar aspect of the base of the first metacarpal, at the attachment of the UCL (Fig. 14). Stress radiographs may demonstrate instability and widening of the ulnar aspect of the first MCP articulation, with greater than 30 degrees difference between the stress and neutral positions [7,14]. MRI or MR arthrography may be helpful in cases of suspected gamekeeper's thumb by accurately depicting the osseous and soft tissue structures about the MCP joint, including the UCL and other ligaments and tendons (Fig. 15) [16]. If the fracture fragment is

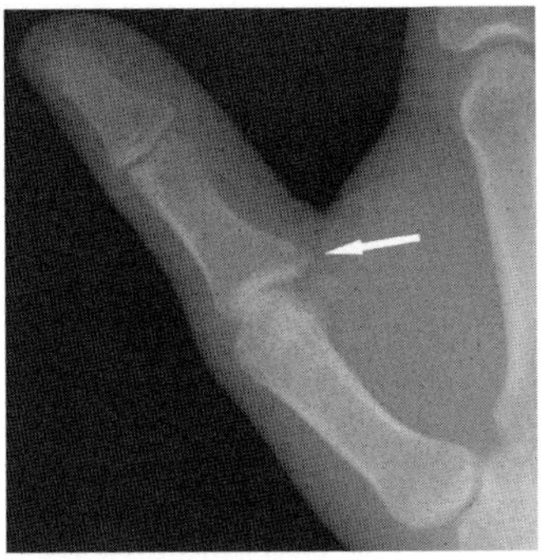

Fig. 14. Gamekeeper's thumb. Middle-aged patient injured his finger in a skiing accident. PA radiograph of the hand shows a small avulsion fracture of the ulnar aspect of the base of the first proximal phalanx at the distal attachment of the ulnar collateral ligament (*arrow*).

nondisplaced, conservative therapy with splinting of the thumb may lead to healing and restoration of stability in select patients [7,14]. Surgical repair is preferable in most patients, however [14].

Stener lesion is an abnormality occasionally seen with gamekeeper's thumb, in which there is an abnormal folded position of the torn end of the ulnar collateral ligament superficial to the adductor aponeurosis [17]. Spontaneous ligament healing is inhibited by the interposition of the thumb extensor mechanism between the torn fragments of the ulnar collateral ligament [15]. Stener lesion is suspected when the MCP joint is grossly unstable, or when there is a persistent

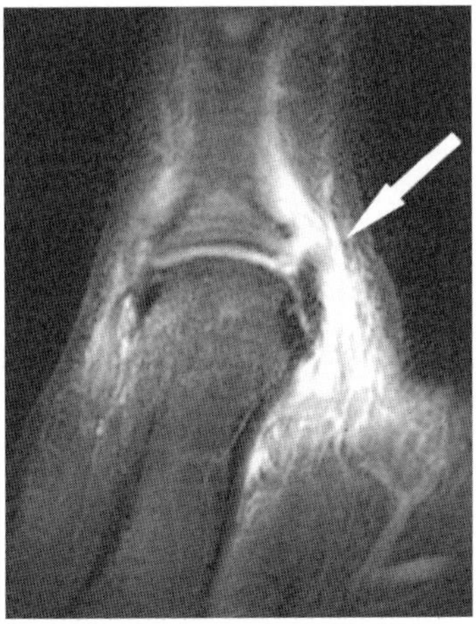

Fig. 15. Ulnar collateral ligament tear of the first MCP joint. Short tau inversion recovery (STIR) image of the first MCP joint using a digit or small loop coil precisely depicts rupture of the ulnar collateral ligament (arrow) at its attachment on the base of the first proximal phalanx.

firm mass on the ulnar aspect of the first metacarpal head. Stener lesions have been reported to occur in up to 29% of patients with UCL injuries [16]. MRI can demonstrate both the UCL and the extensor aponeurosis and can depict Stener lesions accurately [6]. If a Stener lesion is present, only operative intervention allows apposition and healing of the traumatically displaced ligament in an anatomic position [15].

SUMMARY

In conclusion, injuries of the fingers and thumb in the athlete are common. Mallet finger, jersey finger, boutonniere deformity, Bennett and Rolando fractures, and gamekeeper's thumb are just a few of the injuries that can occur in athletes. A thorough understanding of the mechanism of injury, osseous and soft tissue abnormalities, imaging features, and treatment is important in the care of athletes. Prompt and accurate diagnosis is important and may help minimize outcomes of malunion, posttraumatic arthritis, and debility.

References

[1] Rettig AC. Epidemiology of hand and wrist injuries in sports. Clin Sports Med 1998;17:401–6.
[2] Patel D, Dean C, Baker RJ. The hand in sports: an update on the clinical anatomy and physical examination. Prim Care 2005;32:71–89.
[3] Rettig AC. Athletic injuries of the wrist and hand. Part I: traumatic injuries of the wrist. Am J Sports Med 2003;31:1038–48.
[4] Lee SG, Jupiter JB. Phalangeal and metacarpal fractures of the hand. Hand Clin 2000;16:323–32.
[5] Walsh JJ. Fractures of the hand and carpal navicular bone in athletes. South Med J 2004;97:762–5.
[6] Morgan WJ, Slowman LS. Acute hand and wrist injuries in athletes: evaluation and management. J Am Acad Orthop Surg 2001;9:389–400.
[7] Hong E. Hand injuries in sports medicine. Prim Care 2005;32:91–103.
[8] Aronowitz ER, Leddy JP. Closed tendon injuries of the hand and wrist in athletes. Clin Sports Med 1998;17:449–67.
[9] Rettig AC. Wrist and hand overuse syndromes. Clin Sports Med 2001;20:591–611.
[10] Rosner JL, Zlatkin MB, Clifford P, et al. Imaging of athletic wrist and hand injuries. Semin Musculoskelet Radiol 2004;8:57–79.
[11] Gabl M, Rangger C, Lutz M, et al. Disruption of the finger flexor pulley system in elite rock climbers. Am J Sports Med 1998;26:651–5.
[12] Bennett EH. Fractures of the metacarpal bones. Dublin Med Sci J 1882;73:72–5.
[13] Palmer RE. Joint injuries of the hand in athletes. Clin Sports Med 1998;17:513–31.
[14] Rolando S. Fracture of the base of the first metacarpal and a variation that has not yet been described. 1910. Clin Orthop Rel Res 1996;327:4–8.
[15] Harper MT, Chandnani VP, Spaeth J, et al. Gamekeeper thumb: diagnosis of ulnar collateral ligament injury using magnetic resonance imaging, magnetic resonance arthrography and stress radiography. J Magn Reson Imaging 1996;6:322–8.
[16] Spaeth HJ, Abrams RA, Bock GW, et al. Gamekeeper thumb: differentiation of nondisplaced and displaced tears of the ulnar collateral ligament with MR imaging. Work in progress. Radiology 1993;188:553–6.
[17] Stener B. Displacement of the ruptured ulnar collateral ligament of the metacarpophalangeal joint. J Bone Joint Surg Am 1962;44B:869–79.

Clin Sports Med 25 (2006) 543–568
CLINICS IN SPORTS MEDICINE
ELSEVIER SAUNDERS

Imaging of Sports Injuries of the Upper Extremity in Children

Kathleen H. Emery, MD[a,b,*]

[a]Department of Radiology, Cincinnati Children's Hospital Medical Center, 3333 Burnet Avenue, Cincinnati, OH 45229, USA
[b]University of Cincinnati Medical Center, Department of Radiology, 234 Goodman Street, Cincinnati, OH 45219, USA

Because sports have become a more integral part of extracurricular activity in children, and because the intensity of competition and training has escalated, it is not surprising that the incidence of acute and repetitive musculoskeletal injuries in the skeletally immature athlete have increased significantly. These injuries tend to occur in patterns distinctly different from those seen in the skeletally mature athlete. The unique anatomy of the growing musculoskeletal system results in altered responses when exposed to similar stresses [1–4]. Concomitant with the increasing frequency of injuries has been an enhanced awareness of these unique injury patterns among those responsible for the care of these young athletes.

Much of the literature regarding upper extremity sports injuries in the skeletally immature athlete has focused on those related to throwing and gymnastics, though virtually any sport in which the upper extremity is exposed to acute or repetitive stress can result in symptoms that may bring the child to clinical attention [1]. Most of the injuries encountered result from chronic overuse, though acute traumatic injury patterns may be seen in the child athlete. The author focuses attention more on the effects of chronic stress in the child athlete. As such, a recurring theme is the unique vulnerability of the growth plate in the growing skeleton with overuse syndromes [1–4]. This article is not intended as an exhaustive review of upper extremity injuries in young, skeletally immature athletes. Instead, it focuses on the more commonly encountered injuries of the shoulder, elbow, and wrist and the role imaging plays in their diagnosis and management.

IMAGING MODALITIES

Conventional radiography remains the primary and often times the only imaging modality necessary for evaluating sports injuries of the upper extremity.

*Department of Radiology, Cincinnati Children's Hospital Medical Center, 3333 Burnet Avenue, Cincinnati, OH 45229. *E-mail address*: kathleen.emery@cchmc.org

0278-5919/06/$ – see front matter
doi:10.1016/j.csm.2006.02.003

sportsmed.theclinics.com

MRI has become a vital tool for diagnosis and follow-up of many sports-related musculoskeletal injuries regardless of the athlete's age. MRI has no known side effects at FDA-approved field strengths and possesses an unparalleled level of soft tissue contrast and multiplanar imaging capability that underlies its unique role in delineating radiographically occult injuries. In the skeletally immature athlete, these vulnerable structures include the growing physis, musculotendinous units, ligaments, and marrow spaces. The accuracy of MRI in detecting abnormalities in these structures hinges on meticulous attention to all details of the study. Distracting techniques, such as video goggles, have proven effective in allowing acquisition of diagnostic nonsedated MRI examinations even in young children [5,6]. The use of dedicated surface coils, tailored protocols with high resolution imaging parameters (thin slices, small field of view, and large imaging matrices), and appropriate imaging sequences to highlight normal anatomy and pathology are critical. Standard high-resolution T1 images generally are best for demonstrating normal anatomy. Proton density and T2 fast spin echo and 3D gradient echo sequences provide pathology detection and highlight cartilage (growth plates, unossified epiphyseal cartilage, and hyaline articular cartilage). The benefit of the increased signal-to-noise achieved at higher field strengths (3 tesla) is being exploited to enhance visualization of these structures [7,8].

CT generally is reserved for defining the details of complex bony injuries not evaluated adequately by standard conventional radiographs or MRI. CT does have significant radiation dose which should be a consideration for use in any patient, though particularly in children of younger ages. These concerns have been addressed in the medical literature and have heightened awareness of the potential risks [9]. As a result, radiologists and CT scan manufacturers have taken steps to reduce radiation exposure associated with CT scanning with modifications in design of the scanners and the protocols used in scanning [10]. Nonetheless, the benefit of a medically indicated CT scan far outweighs any potential risk.

SHOULDER

Acute Injuries

Fractures

Acute fractures about the shoulder region in the child or adolescent athlete are not uncommon, and most frequently involve the clavicle, either as the result of a direct blow or indirectly during a fall on an outstretched hand [2]. Most of these injuries are diagnosed readily on conventional radiographs, and rarely require additional advanced imaging. Scapular fractures are uncommon and may occur as the result of direct trauma in collision sports [2]. Avulsion fractures of the growth centers of the coracoid and glenoid have been associated with indirect trauma [2]. These injuries may be more challenging to diagnose on conventional radiographs and when suspected can be significantly easier to see on MRI.

Glenohumeral dislocation

Traumatic glenohumeral dislocations tend to occur in collision sports, particularly football and hockey. Nearly 40% of shoulder dislocations occur in patients under the age of 22 [11]. Shoulder dislocation in patients under the age of 10 is exceedingly rare, however, with only 8 of 500 patients (1.6%) in the largest reported series of shoulder dislocations being under 10 years of age [12].

Recurrent dislocations and glenohumeral instability have been reported in 48% to 100% of patients, with the highest incidence generally seen in athletes who return to sports activity and patients with open physes [12–15]. The 100% recurrence was in a population of 21 children who were not compliant with physiotherapy after immobilization [14]. Identification of a Hill-Sachs defect on radiography is associated with a significantly higher incidence of recurrence, 82% versus 50% recurrence without a Hill-Sachs defect [12]. Initial treatment following closed reduction of an anterior dislocation has been controversial, though the literature suggests no effect on recurrence rate with immobilization of the joint over use of a sling until comfortable followed by physical therapy [14–17]. MRI and arthroscopic studies performed within 8 to 10 days in young patients with traumatic anterior dislocation have demonstrated anterior inferior labral injury with detachment and an effusion in virtually all patients [18,19]. Athletes restricted from full activity and sports participation have better outcomes given that ligament and capsular healing take 6 weeks to 3 months [17,20]. Even with recurrent dislocation, on prolonged follow-up of 10 years up to 22% of shoulders may stabilize spontaneously [16].

Surgical treatment of instability ultimately is required in 40% to 50% of children and adolescents to improve functional outcome [13,16,21]. Indications for surgery include irreducible instability (soft tissue interposition), displaced greater tuberosity fractures, and unstable glenoid rim fractures [11].

Imaging of glenohumeral macroinstability. Nearly all glenohumeral dislocations occur anteriorly with the arm abducted and externally rotated and are apparent immediately on clinical examination. Posterior dislocations are as rare in children as they are in adults [2]. Conventional radiographs are the initial imaging examination. With classic anterior dislocation, the humeral head is displaced inferomedially and superimposed over the lower aspect of the glenoid on the anteroposterior (AP) radiograph (Fig. 1A). A straight AP view of the shoulder provides an oblique view of the glenohumeral joint, which is tilted anteriorly approximately 40° [22]. Lesser degrees of subluxation may be difficult to evaluate on this view. With slight internal rotation of the humerus, the posterolateral aspect of the humeral head is displayed optimally to evaluate for Hill-Sachs defect. A true AP view (Grashey view) better profiles in the glenohumeral joint by tilting the x-ray beam approximately 40° laterally [22]. Other structures, however, are not as well evaluated on this view as on the standard AP view including the acromion, distal clavicle, and the acromioclavicular joint. The axillary view provides a tangential image of the glenohumeral joint from below but requires the arm to be abducted with the x-ray beam projected through

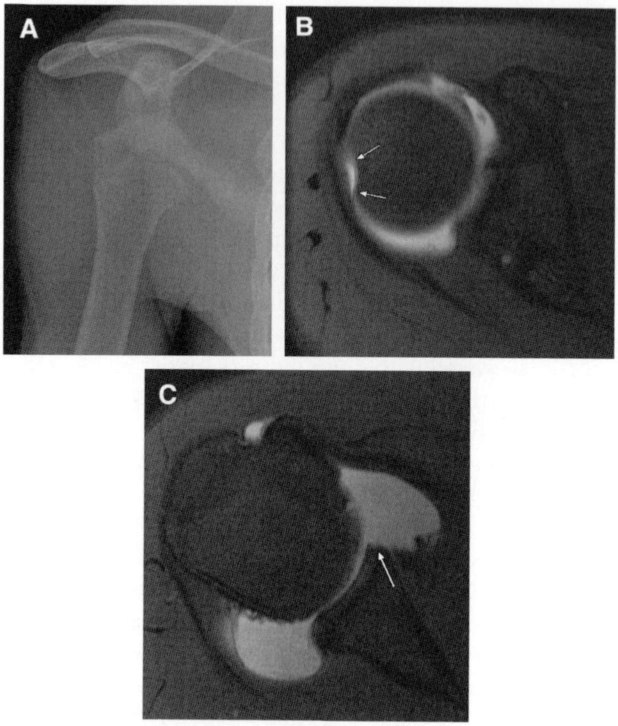

Fig. 1. A 15-year-old male with acute anterior glenohumeral dislocation. Radiograph (*A*) demonstrates obvious inferomedial displacement of the right humeral head. MR arthrogram performed 9 days later shows the Hill Sachs lesion of the humeral head (*B, arrow*) and the cartilaginous Bankart defect of the anteroinferior labrum (*C, arrow*).

the shoulder 15° to 30° medially from distal to proximal [22]. This requirement may limit the use of this view in patients with limited mobility or acute injury. There are other methods for obtaining an axillary-type view that may be tolerated better in this patient population [23]. A scapular Y view projects the humeral head over the glenoid fossa and is accomplished by tilting the x-ray beam along the plane of the scapula [22]. This view does not require abduction of the arm and often is tolerated better in the acutely injured patient. It is adequate for evaluating traumatic dislocations, but is of limited use for detecting subtle subluxation or details of bony anatomy.

With acute anterior dislocation, the posterolateral aspect of the humeral head impacts on the anteroinferior rim of the glenoid. This impact may create a visible depression in the humeral head (Hill-Sachs defect) seen in 38% to 90% of patients [11,12,16]. An avulsion fracture of the anteroinferior glenoid rim (Bankart fracture) has been described in approximately 5% to 8% of patients and greater tuberosity fractures of the humerus are reported in 12% to 15%

of shoulder dislocations [12,16]. These findings may be detected more readily on postreduction radiographs.

In patients with recurrent instability more detailed imaging is necessary. In the 1980s, CT arthrography was the modality of choice for imaging of the glenoid labrum in cases of instability [24,25]. Although CT provides excellent spatial resolution, the use of ionizing radiation is a drawback. The soft tissue contrast achieved with CT is inferior to that of MRI and more recent studies have documented the superiority of MRI and MR arthrography over CT arthrography for evaluation of glenohumeral instability (see Fig. 1) [26]. MR arthrography provides capsular distension and separation of intra-articular structures that is lacking in conventional MRI in the absence of a joint effusion. These are major factors in why MR arthrography has come to be the modality of choice in imaging of recurrent glenohumeral instability in the younger, athletic population [26–28]. This technique has an overall reported sensitivity of 91% for detection of labral pathology [27] and 91% accuracy for partial rotator cuff tears [29]. Although the arm typically is in neutral position for this study, additional imaging of the shoulder with the arm in an abducted, externally rotated position places the anterior band of the inferior glenohumeral ligament under stress and pushes contrast along the undersurface of the rotator cuff (Fig. 2). This phenomenon has been reported to increase the sensitivity of detection of anterior labral pathology (the most common of type of labral injury in younger athletes) to 96% [30] and improve detection of undersurface partial tears of the rotator cuff [31,32]. A detailed discussion of the various types and classification of labral tears on MRI is beyond the scope of this article [33].

Chronic Repetitive Injuries

Cumulative stress accounts for most shoulder injuries in skeletally immature athletes. Most of these repetitive microtrauma injuries are seen with greater

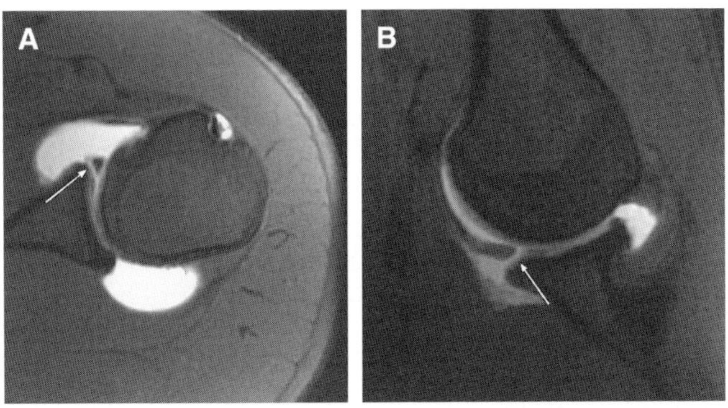

Fig. 2. A 17-year-old wrestler who suffered a dislocation with spontaneous relocation. Radiographs were unremarkable. Axial fat suppressed T1 weighted image (*A*) from shoulder arthrogram shows a cartilaginous and bony Bankart lesion with the detached anterior band of the inferior glenohumeral ligament (*arrow*) best seen on the abducted externally rotated view (*B*).

frequency during the mid to late teen years because the shoulder is subjected to progressively higher stresses with increasing muscular development and strength characteristic of athletes in this age group. Chronic overuse injuries from repetitive motion have been described most commonly in baseball players, though any sport requiring overhead activity, including football, swimming, tennis, and volleyball, may cause similar types of injuries [1]. The patterns of injury vary with the nature of the stress. In baseball, the force is more explosive over a shorter period of time, whereas in swimming the force is gentler and more dynamic but sustained over longer periods of time [34].

Little League shoulder

The term *Little League shoulder* refers to epiphysiolysis of the proximal humeral growth plate. The inciting force seems to be the excess rotational stress applied to the physis during throwing as the shoulder is forcibly internally rotated and adducted from an externally rotated abducted position [35]. The injury is seen almost exclusively in 13- to 16-year-old baseball players (most frequently pitchers) who typically present with gradual onset of pain most frequently localized in the lateral aspect of the proximal humerus, which is aggravated with throwing [36]. The physis is responsive to hormonal influences and is known to diminish in strength with increases in testosterone [37] making it an area vulnerable to injury in this age group.

Widening of the proximal humeral physis is the most common radiographic finding in Little League shoulder, though this may be subtle and require comparison views of the contralateral humerus. There may be associated fragmentation, sclerosis, demineralization, and cystic change (Fig. 3). These more chronic radiographic findings support the concept of gradual repetitive microtrauma as the underlying etiology in the development of this condition [36]. Because MRI is exquisitely sensitive to the normal and abnormal growth plate

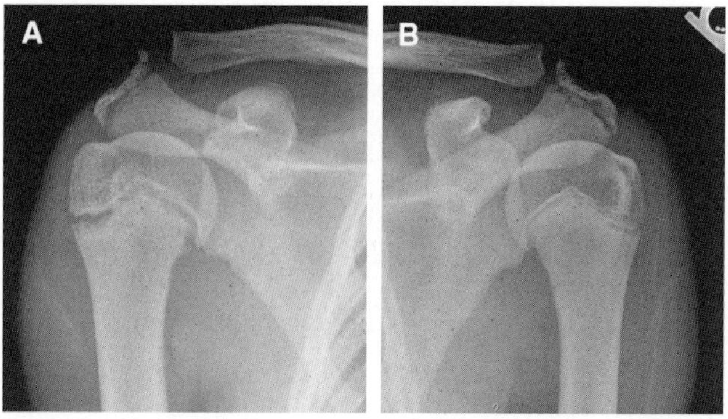

Fig. 3. Little League shoulder. Adolescent pitcher with shoulder pain and findings of Little League shoulder on the right (*A*) with widening and fragmentation of the proximal humeral growth plate. Asymptomatic left humerus (*B*) for comparison.

[38–41] one would predict that it would readily depict the physeal injury and mirror findings described in other growth plate injuries. Findings of chronic growth plate injury include physeal widening with intraphyseal clefts and loss of definition of the zone of provisional calcification (Fig. 4A,B) [41]. Because the diagnosis usually is apparent clinically and changes identified on radiography, however, there are no published reports describing the MR findings.

Little League shoulder usually is a benign self-limiting condition that responds to rest with discontinuation of all throwing for an average of 3 months followed by a gradual return to throwing with emphasis on proper mechanics [36,42]. Because the chronic radiographic changes may take several months to remodel, resolution of symptoms (and not normal radiographs) is the primary determinant of timing for the gradual resumption of throwing [36].

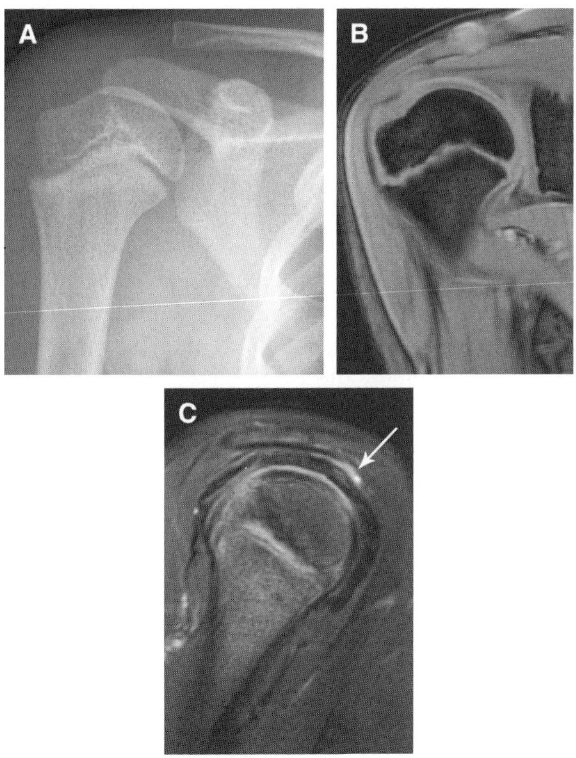

Fig. 4. Proximal humeral physeal stress injury and rotator cuff tendonitis. A 7-year-old gymnast with right shoulder pain. Radiograph (*A*) shows mild irregular widening of the proximal humeral growth plate confirmed on coronal gradient echo images (*B*). Sagittal T2 MRI (*C*) illustrates thickening of the rotator cuff with surrounding high T2 signal fluid consistent with tendonitis or partial tear.

Rotator cuff/impingement/microinstability

Rotator cuff tears are encountered most commonly in middle-aged and elderly patients. This injury is rare in children and adolescents with less then 1% of rotator cuff tears occurring in patients under the age of 20 years [43,44]. The rotator cuff is stronger and more elastic in the younger athlete lacking the degenerative changes typically seen in the older population [42]. A recent series by Tarkin and colleagues [44] described four adolescent patients with rotator cuff tears (two supraspinatus and two subscapularis) that were incurred during vigorous participation in athletic competition. Although not seen in their patients, this injury may be associated with greater or lesser tuberosity avulsions in the skeletally immature patient in whom the physis tends to be the weak link [2].

More commonly, rotator cuff pathology in the skeletally immature athlete is manifested as tendonitis or strain of the rotator cuff as the result of repetitive microtrauma [2]. Those athletes actively participating in sports involving overhead arm motion, including baseball, swimming, and tennis, are predisposed to this injury. Rotator cuff and subacromial bursa impingement occur much less commonly in the skeletally immature athlete than in adults. Because the supraspinatus tendon, greater tuberosity, long head of the biceps, and subacromial bursa pass beneath the coracoacromial arch the repetitive mechanical contact can lead to acute and chronic inflammation of the rotator cuff, which may progress to scarring, tendonitis, and possible tear if left untreated [2]. Primary impingement can occur as the result of a tight coracoacromial arch (anatomic variation in shape and slope of the acromion or pathologic spurring) or simple overuse. Younger athletes can develop secondary rotator cuff impingement in the setting of an anatomically normal coracoacromial arch. Repetitive microtrauma associated with overhead sports has been shown to lead to structural changes in the tendon, ligament, and capsule [45]. Secondary rotator cuff muscle weakness and biomechanical imbalance can result and cause subtle upward migration of the humeral head predisposing to secondary impingement [2]. Additionally, younger patients have a higher incidence of inherent multidirectional laxity of the shoulder requiring greater reliance on the dynamic stability afforded by the rotator cuff musculature. With repetitive stress, the muscles become fatigued and impingement may occur secondary to this multidirectional instability [2]. Clinical assessment for uni- or multidirectional instability is critical in the young athlete with shoulder pain suggesting impingement so that both issues can be addressed therapeutically [2].

Patterns of glenohumeral instability can be divided by the direction of glenohumeral translation. Anterior instability is the most common and is associated with excess repetitive external rotation during overhead motion. In addition to rotator cuff impingement against the coracoacromial arch superiorly, the cuff may be pinched against the posterosuperior glenoid rim causing internal impingement [45]. Posterior instability is less common, and has been associated with the throwing athlete during deceleration and follow-through stages [2]. These patients are more likely to develop a posterior labral tear rather than rotator cuff abnormalities. Multidirectional instability (more than one direction) more commonly occurs in sports requiring repetitive shoulder abduction and external rotation, such as competitive swimming (especially with the butterfly stroke) and gymnastics [1].

Imaging of the rotator cuff

Conventional radiographs in the setting of suspected rotator cuff damage in the child athlete are usually normal. Conventional arthrography has been replaced by MRI as the imaging modality of choice for evaluating the rotator cuff [46]. The four muscles and their respective tendons that compose the rotator cuff (the supraspinatus superiorly, the infraspinatus posterior superiorly, the teres minor posterior inferiorly, and the subscapularis anteriorly) are well visualized on MRI [23]. The normal tendon appears dark in signal intensity on all pulse sequences in young patients. With tendinopathy, intermediate T2 signal (less than fluid) is seen within a tendon that may also be mildly thickened (Fig. 4C) [33]. Partial-thickness tears may occur along the articular or bursal surface, and manifest as fluid signal on T2-weighted images extending part way through the thickness of the tendon superiorly or inferiorly (Fig. 5) [29,47]. A full-thickness tear appears as fluid signal extending completely through the tendon superiorly to inferiorly. A complete tear disrupts the tendon totally (superior to inferior and anterior to posterior) resulting in musculotendinous retraction and possible superior subluxation of the humeral head [33]. Subscapularis tendon tears are less common and may be more difficult to see, but frequently are associated with biceps tendon abnormalities [48].

Cystlike changes in the humeral head are associated with rotator cuff abnormalities [49]. The cause of these cysts is not clear and possible theories include secondary effects of impaction or traction or even a reversible cause, such as a vascular or inflammatory cause [50]. Although internal impingement of the

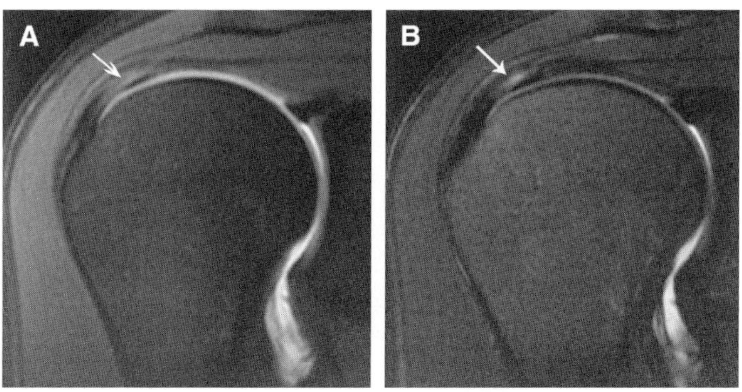

Fig. 5. Partial rotator cuff tear. A 15-year-old male athlete with shoulder pain on abduction. Coronal fat suppressed T1 image (*A*) and T2 image (*B*) from an MR arthrogram demonstrate high signal contrast within a thinned supraspinatus tendon (*arrow*).

cuff between the humeral head and posterior glenoid is less common than superior impingement, a constellation of findings has been described including undersurface tears of the posterior cuff, along with cystic changes in a more posterior aspect of the humeral head than is typically seen in other rotator cuff abnormalities and posterosuperior labral abnormalities (signal change or altered morphology) [50]. The overall reported sensitivity and specificity of MRI in detection of rotator cuff tears ranges from 84% to 100% [29,46,47]. Detection of partial thickness tears on the articular side is enhanced with the use of direct MR arthrography and additional imaging in the abducted externally rotated (ABER) position [29,31,32].

ELBOW

Acute Injuries

Medial epicondyle avulsion is the most common acute fracture seen in the adolescent throwing athlete [51]. Acute valgus stress with violent flexor–pronator muscle contraction creates a tensile force of a magnitude that exceeds the strength of the medial epicondylar apophysis resulting in apophyseal avulsion [52]. Similar repetitive lower-magnitude forces cause chronic changes of the apophyseal growth plate. The athlete experiences acute medial elbow pain and inability to continue playing. Radiographs usually demonstrate a minimally displaced avulsion with variable physeal widening or epicondylar rotation (Fig. 6) [52]. The findings may be sufficiently subtle to warrant comparison views of the asymptomatic elbow or stress views (manual or gravity stress) [53] of the symptomatic elbow. Ulnar collateral ligament (UCL) rupture has a similar presentation, though this injury is much less likely in an adolescent in whom the medial epicondylar physis is the weak point rather than the ligament. Associated UCL rupture is unlikely in the setting of epicondylar avulsion

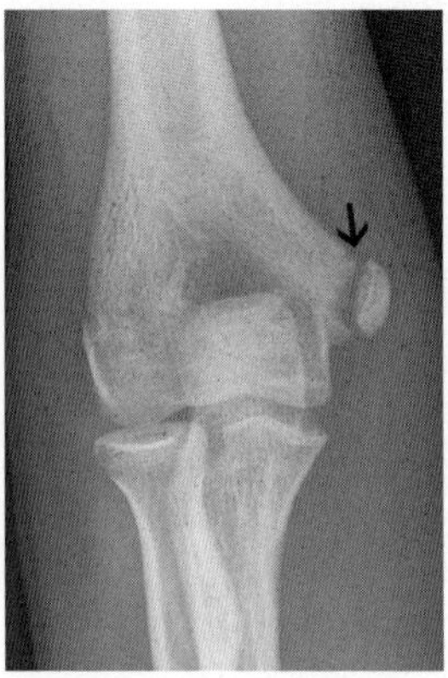

Fig. 6. Type I medial epicondyle avulsion fracture.

[52]. Rarely, the fragment displaces into the joint, which occurs more frequently in the setting of elbow dislocation [54]. Fracture classification is based on patient age and fragment size [53]: Type I in children under age 14 with a large fragment (usually the entire apophysis), Type II in patients 15 years and older with a large fragment, and Type III in those aged 15 years or older with a small fragment (more likely to occur as the physis fuses). Treatment is somewhat controversial with regard to acceptable fragment displacement (3–5 mm versus 2 mm) for determining conservative versus operative therapy and what should be accepted in athletes with greater demands for high-level functioning of the elbow [52].

Cross-sectional imaging usually is not necessary for diagnosis and management of this injury. We have found MRI to be helpful for problem solving in select cases in which radiographs may be confusing or for defining associated injuries.

Chronic Injuries

Little League elbow

Little League elbow was initially described in 1960 in two Little League baseball pitchers presenting with medial elbow pain and abnormal radiographs of the medial epicondyle of the humerus, documented as separation and fragmentation [55]. More recently, it is has been used as a nonspecific description of a group of pathologic entities in and about the elbow joint in young overhead athletes whose elbows are exposed to the stress patterns that have been well described with the throwing motion [3,56]. The stresses include tension overload on the medial elbow restraints (medial epicondyle, common flexor tendon, and UCL), compression overload on the lateral articular surface (capitellum and radial head), posteromedial shear forces on the posterior articular surface, and extension overload on the lateral restraints (lateral ligaments and lateral epicondyle) [3]. The same motion is common to the tennis serve, football pass, and javelin throw, so these injuries are not limited to the baseball player [3]. Similar stresses have also been described in gymnasts whose elbows become weight-bearing joints in various routines and are subject to similar injuries [57]. We focus on the medial tension and lateral compression injuries as posterior extension and shear injuries are much less common [3].

In the skeletally immature athlete with medial elbow pain and suspected repetitive medial tension injury, there usually is tenderness over the medial epicondyle with soft tissue swelling [3]. As around any joint in the immature skeleton, the physeal plate is the weakest link and the most likely site of injury. Radiographs may demonstrate overgrowth, separation, and fragmentation of the medial epicondyle compared with the nondominant arm. Similar findings may be seen in a significant number of athletes without symptoms (nearly 50% in one study) and the radiographic changes are believed to represent a physiologic response to repetitive traction stress [58]. MRI should show abnormal physeal widening but is usually not necessary in the younger patient in this setting because the injury is treated conservatively. With inadequate treatment and repeated valgus stress on the elbow, there may be nonunion of the medial epicondyle. In the older adolescent athlete nearing skeletal maturity, MRI may prove useful in distinguishing other causes of medial elbow pain that should be considered, including UCL injury and medial epicondylitis (Fig. 7) [59].

UCL injury is a much less frequent cause of medial elbow pain in the child athlete with open physes [1]. It is more common after the growth plates have closed. The patient complains of medial elbow pain that is increased during the late cocking and acceleration stages of throwing [1]. Valgus instability may be demonstrated on physical examination. Radiographs usually are normal but may show heterotopic calcification in UCL tears [60]. Valgus stress views may be obtained to determine stability of the elbow joint [1]. Most tears involve the anterior bundle of the UCL proximally and are depicted on MRI as irregularity, laxity, poor definition, and abnormal increased T1 and T2 signal in and around the ligament [59]. The hemorrhage or edema found in the UCL at arthroscopy correlate with these signal alterations and likely are because of repeated microtears that can weaken or disrupt the ligament [59]. Before

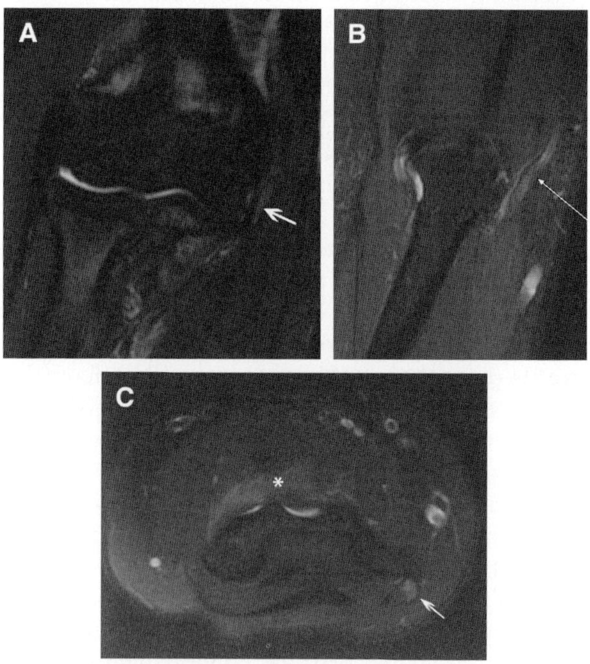

Fig. 7. Ulnar collateral ligament strain and ulnar neuropathy. A 14-year-old female softball catcher with dominant arm elbow pain and tingling. Coronal T2 image (*A*) shows fluid around the anterior bundle of the UCL (*arrow*). Coronal (*B*) and axial (*C*) relatively T2-weighted images show the abnormal thickening and high signal in the ulnar nerve (*arrows*) and edema in the brachialis muscle (*).

physeal fusion, the epicondylar insertion of the UCL has slightly higher T2 and T1 signal than the mature ligament, believed related to high elastin composition and low type 1 collagen content at the enthesis. This phenomenon must be taken into account when interpreting the UCL in young patients [61]. Full-thickness tears should demonstrate discontinuity of the ligament. Partial-thickness UCL tears can be more challenging. One study found MRI to be only 57% sensitive and 100% specific for surgically proven partial-thickness tears [62]. Sensitivity for detecting partial-thickness tears may be enhanced with intra-articular saline and MR arthrography, with one study showing sensitivity of 86% for detecting partial-thickness tears [63]. Partial-thickness undersurface tear of the anterior band of the UCL at the ulnar attachment creates a characteristic T sign originally described on CT arthrography [62]. This sign is created because there is leakage of contrast around the detached portion of the UCL and within the intact superficial fibers and joint capsule [62]. Chronic tears should show abnormal thickening of the ligament.

Medial epicondylitis is a pathologic condition of the common flexor tendon related to microscopic or macroscopic avulsion injury of the tendon at its medial epicondylar insertion. It is seen occasionally in late adolescence or early adulthood and occurs much less commonly than lateral epicondylitis, but should be considered in the differential of medial elbow pain with repetitive valgus stress. The common flexor tendon lies just superficial to the UCL, and MRI demonstrates tendon thickening with increased T1 and T2 signal and peritendinous edema in cases of medial epicondylitis [64,65]. The common mechanism of injury and close spatial proximity of the common flexor tendon and UCL help explain the frequency of coexisting injury in these structures (Fig. 8) [66].

Ulnar nerve compression is the most common neuropathy at the elbow. Although the nerve may be compressed at several sites, compression usually occurs at the cubital tunnel as the nerve passes behind the medial epicondyle [67]. In the athlete with repeated elbow flexion (as in repetitive throwing) the size of the cubital tunnel is compromised by the taut, stretched arcuate ligament (bordering the dorsal aspect of the tunnel) and medial bulging of the UCL and joint capsule [67]. The nerve is stretched against the medial epicondyle and may even sublux. The athlete with ulnar neuritis may have paresthesias along the ulnar aspect of the hand or elbow pain, sometimes with diminished hand function. On MR images, the ulnar nerve usually is conspicuous because it is surrounded by fat. With ulnar neuritis, the nerve often is thickened and of increased signal on T2-weighted images (Fig. 7) [67]. Edema in the denervated flexor carpi ulnaris and flexor digitorum profundus also may be seen.

The most recognized lateral compression injuries of the elbow in skeletally immature athletes involve the capitellum and include Panner disease and osteochondritis dissecans (OCD). The two disorders may represent different stages of the same process, specifically disordered endochondral ossification of the capitellum [68], though they affect different age groups and have different clinical outcomes [3,69,70].

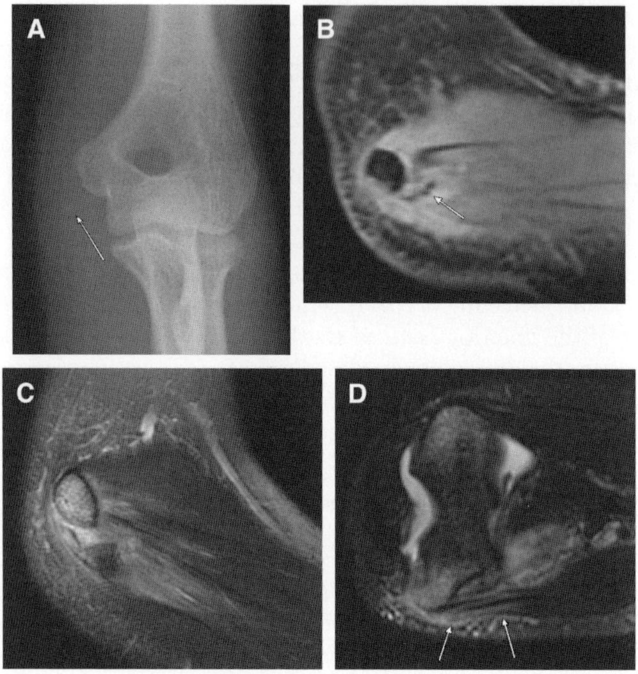

Fig. 8. Partial medial epicondyle avulsion and common flexor tendon tear in an adolescent gymnast. Radiograph (*A*) shows soft tissue swelling and a subtle bone fragment below the medial epicondyle (*arrow*). Sagittal gradient echo MR image (*B*) also shows the small dark bone fragments (*arrow*). Sagittal (*C*) and axial (*D*) T2-weighted images better demonstrate the abnormal increased signal in the partially torn common flexor tendon (*arrows*).

Panner disease is considered a benign, self-limiting osteochondrosis or necrosis of the capitellum typically affecting the dominant elbow of boys between the ages of 7 and 12 years during the active phase of capitellar ossification. The presentation is that of dull elbow pain and swelling in the dominant arm exacerbated by activity [68,69]. Radiographically there is fragmentation of the capitellar ossification center with intermixed areas of rarefaction and sclerosis involving all or part of the capitellum. Healing can be observed radiographically with conservative management [3]. MRI usually is not indicated but if performed reveals partial or complete replacement of the normal fatty marrow signal in the capitellum with diminished T1 and increased T2 signal (Fig. 9) [71]. The overlying cartilage should be unaffected and osteochondral loose body formation does not occur.

OCD of the capitellum is seen in slightly older patients, usually boys aged 12 to 15, in whom capitellar ossification is nearly complete. Baseball players and gymnasts are prone to this injury. The anterolateral aspect of the capitellum is the common location. Studies have shown that the blood supply to this area

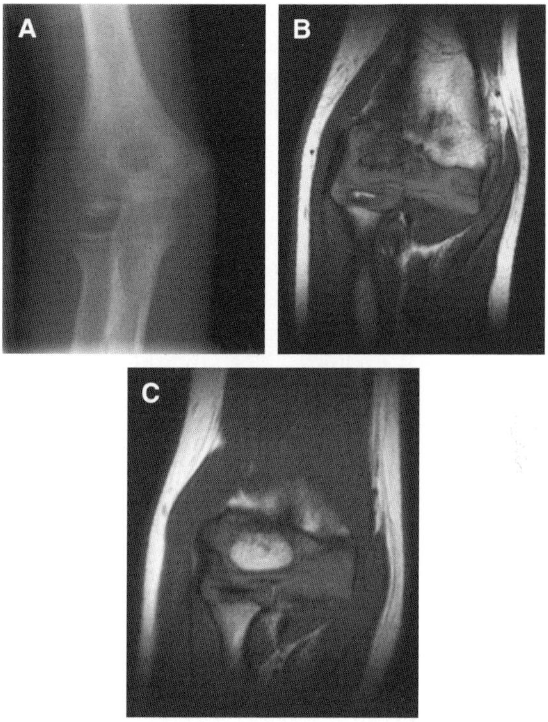

Fig. 9. Panner disease in an 8-year-old male. AP Radiograph (*A*) shows the abnormal fragmentation and rarefaction of the capitellar ossification center. Coronal T1 image (*B*) shows abnormal low signal replacement of fatty marrow as compared with a normal capitellum (*C*).

consists of end arterioles that are not connected to adjacent metaphyseal vessels [72]. Additionally, the central aspect of the radial head is considerably stiffer than the adjacent capitellum [73]. The combination of ischemia and articular cartilage biomechanical differences may explain the development of capitellar OCD in the setting of repeated lateral compression forces. Genetic predisposition also may play a role [74]. Osteochondral lesions of the trochlea have been reported but are much less common [3].

The clinical presentation is that of an adolescent athlete with lateral elbow pain and swelling. Elbow locking is a late finding. Radiographically, there may be little or no change in the capitellum in the early stages of OCD, and routine radiographs have limited sensitivity for detection of OCD and intra-articular loose bodies. Subchondral flattening may be the earliest finding and can be difficult to appreciate on standard radiographs; it may be more apparent on anteroposterior radiographs with 45-degree elbow flexion [75]. Comparison views of the asymptomatic elbow may be helpful. With repeated trauma there is progression to focal cystic rarefaction, fragment formation, and eventual articular defect with loose body formation [70,75]. Routine radiography is unreliable for detecting intra-articular loose bodies and assessing lesion stability; both are paramount for determining clinical management because once the lesion is unstable or loose it is unable to unite [69,75,76]. In one study of 15 patients with OCD confirmed by MRI or surgery, only 7 of 15 lesions were identified prospectively by radiography and only 10 of 15 on retrospective review. Of the 7 proven intra-articular loose bodies in these 15 patients, 3 were seen prospectively whereas only 4 were seen on the retrospective reading [77].

At least one report of sonography for assessing capitellar OCD suggests it may facilitate assessment of lesions though it is operator dependent, requiring pretest knowledge of clinical history, physical examination findings, and radiographic results for maximal usefulness [78]. In addition, reactive synovitis or elbow contracture limits sonographic evaluation [78]. MRI does not have these limitations and is exquisitely sensitive for detecting OCD lesions even in the earliest stages in which only diminished T1 signal at the capitellar surface is seen without T2 signal abnormality (Fig. 10) [79]. At this stage, conservative management often results in healing [69,76]. With more advanced lesions, associated increased T2 marrow signal either in a peripheral ring around the lesion or uniformly throughout the lesion is identified [80] with possible cyst formation at the bone-fragment interface with loose in situ fragments. Approximately 50% of patients have long-term elbow symptoms even with activities of daily living that appear associated with advanced or large lesions and osteoarthritic change regardless of type of therapy [81]. This finding implies that early detection of smaller lesions could afford a better prognosis.

It is critical to assess the integrity of the articular cartilage and fragment viability and to detect loose fragments. Articular cartilage assessment of the elbow is more challenging than in larger joints like the knee, and known variants may create pitfalls in diagnosis. The most recognized is the pseudodefect of the capitellum, which is a normal groove between the rounded capitellum and the lateral epicondyle [82]. An early report from 1992 suggested that intravenous contrast showed promise for determining viability of lesions and loose bodies [83] in a small group of patients (N = 3). Fragment enhancement suggested viability and good blood supply [83]. There have not been subsequent reports providing confirmation and the author's experience with gadolinium for OCD in the knee did not find supportive evidence for administering IV gadolinium [84]. Although MRI was more sensitive than radiography for elbow loose body detection in one study of 13 children with three loose bodies [80], a larger study in 26 adults with mechanical symptoms (locking or catching) found that neither CT arthrography nor MRI performed better than radiography in detecting loose bodies [85]. It is unclear whether the difference in these results may have related to differences in the histologic composition or bony content of the loose bodies (which was not described fully in either study) and patient selection. It is known that intracapsular fat pads and synovial folds can mimic loose bodies on MRI [82]. Gadolinium MR arthrography of the elbow has been shown to have sensitivity and specificity similar to CT

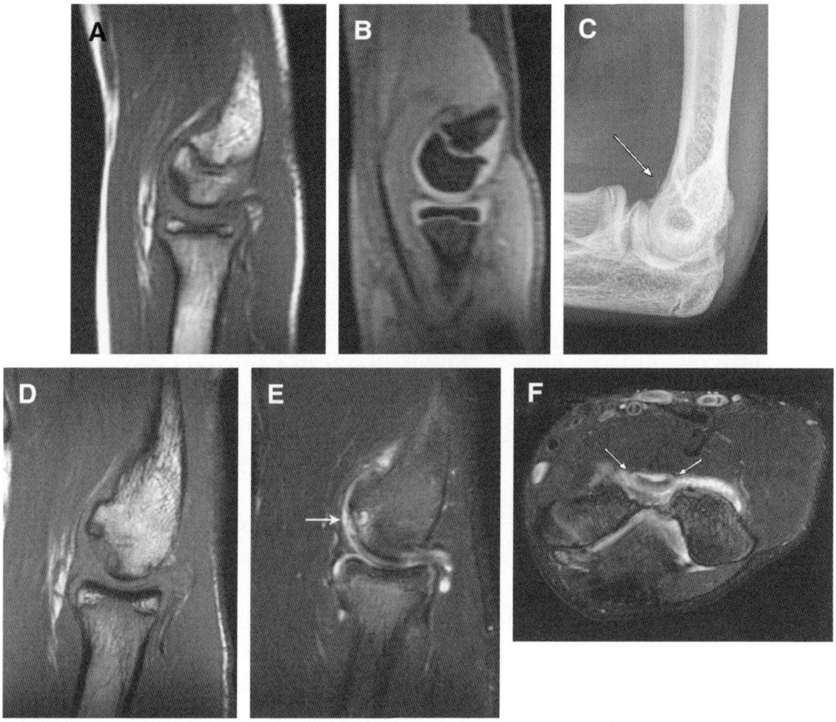

Fig. 10. Capitellar OCD with progression to loose body formation. At age 12 the radiographs were normal but T1 sagittal MR image (*A*) shows the scalloped area of abnormal decreased marrow signal in the subchondral bone with intact overlying cartilage on the sagittal gradient echo sequence (*B*). The patient returned 2 years later at age 14 with a possible loose body (*arrow*) on lateral radiograph of the elbow (*C*). Sagittal T1 image (*D*) at that time shows the progression of the lesion with disrupted overlying articular cartilage (*arrow*) on the sagittal T2 image (*E*), and axial T2 image (*F*) confirms the intra-articular loose body (*arrows*) in the anterior joint space that was removed arthroscopically.

arthrography (78% and 95%, and 87% and 94%, respectively) in overall detection of articular cartilage lesions of the elbow in a recent study of 26 cadaver elbows [86]. Although MR arthrography of the knee in OCD has shown improved accuracy for articular cartilage assessment and fragment separation over MRI without intra-articular contrast [87], the potential role of MR arthrography for evaluation of articular cartilage integrity and loose body detection in OCD of the elbow has yet to be studied in a controlled fashion.

Lateral epicondylitis occurs as the result of repeated microtrauma to the lateral epicondylar apophysis and extensor tendon (mainly the extensor carpi radialis) with repetitive wrist extension and is seen most frequently in those participating in racquet sports [1]. Although this condition is more common than medial epicondylitis, it is encountered more frequently in adults. As at other growth centers in the skeletally immature athlete, the growth plate is the weakest area, not the extensor origin, and repetitive trauma results in an apophysitis rather than extensor tendonitis that would be seen in the older athlete. The diagnosis is made clinically with pain that is localized over the lateral epicondyle and extensor origin. Radiographs may show widening or fragmentation of the apophysis. MRI usually is not indicated but if performed mirrors those findings described in medial epicondylitis [65].

WRIST

Acute Injuries

Most acute injuries in the pediatric wrist are fractures of the distal radius that may involve the growth plate [4]. These usually are apparent on conventional radiographs and may occur in the setting of athletic competition as the result of a fall on an outstretched hand [4]. Distal radial fractures usually heal uneventfully but on rare occasions may be associated with injury of the triangular fibrocartilage (TFC) (Fig. 11) or scapholunate ligament (Fig. 12), both of which are uncommon injuries in children [88,89]. Fifty-two percent of the patients in one review of 29 skeletally immature patients who had surgically proven TFC tears had sustained a distal radial fracture at the time of the original injury, and 86% had coexisting pathology including ulnar styloid nonunion, distal radioulnar joint instability, ulnocarpal impaction, and intercarpal ligament tears [89]. All three children in a recent report of scapholunate ligament injury had sustained a distal radial fracture [88]. All of these injuries were diagnosed surgically. Gymnasts, who have a significantly higher incidence of ulna plus variance (see later discussion of gymnast wrist) and ulnocarpal abutment, are at risk for developing TFC abnormalities. There are no published series reporting the efficacy of MRI in children for diagnosis of TFC and scapholunate ligament injuries. Most TFC tears that are related to trauma are peripheral rather than central tears that tend to be degenerative [90]. One adult study evaluating MRI (both indirect arthrograms and unenhanced studies) found only 17% sensitivity, 79% specificity, and 64% accuracy for diagnosing peripheral TFC tears [91]. Direct MR arthrography was shown by Zanetti and colleagues to improve the diagnostic performance of MRI for detecting TFC and intercarpal ligament injuries in an adult population [92].

Of the carpal bones, the scaphoid is the most frequently fractured [93]. A fracture may not be visible on initial radiographs but should be suspected when there is tenderness localized to the anatomic snuff box. Secondary radiographic signs (dorsal swelling and an obliterated scaphoid fat stripe) may be lacking in children [94]. Wrist immobilization and follow-up radiographs are the standard. Early MRI was shown in a study of 18 skeletally immature patients with suspected scaphoid fracture (10 of whom ultimately had proven fractures, eight of which were radiographically occult initially) to have a negative predictive value of 100% [95]. It is unclear that the information influences patient management, however, and thus MRI has not become a standard part of the diagnostic algorithm of suspected scaphoid fractures in children.

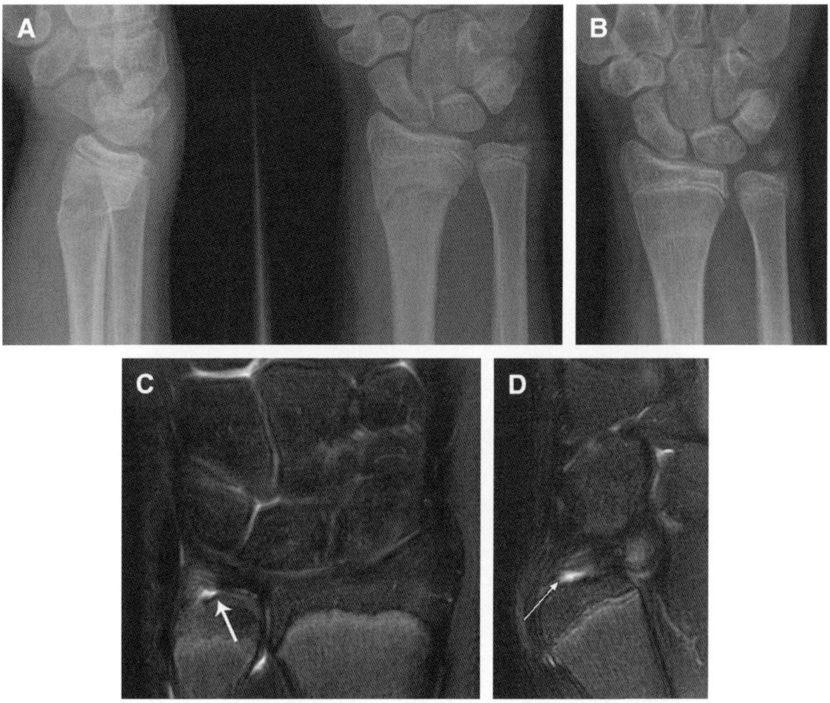

Fig. 11. Possible peripheral TFC tear. This adolescent female had suffered a distal radial fracture with ulnar styloid avulsion (*A*) with subsequent probable fibrous nonunion of the styloid at follow-up (*B*). She complained of persistent ulnar-sided wrist pain and coronal (*C*) and sagittal (*D*) T2 images at 3 tesla show high signal near the peripheral ulnar attachment of the TFC (*arrow*) (not surgically confirmed).

Chronic Injury

Gymnast wrist

Wrist pain is a common complaint in the elite and nonelite skeletally immature gymnast, occurring in approximately two thirds of patients [96,97]. Stress injury of the distal radius has become a well-recognized cause of wrist pain that has been observed predominantly in adolescent gymnasts and weightlifters whose wrists are subjected to repeated dorsiflexion and excessive axial compression loading [98,99]. Pain is increased with weight bearing and dorsiflexion of the wrist and there may be focal tenderness over the radial condyle [99]. Radiographs of the wrist may be normal, but reported findings include subtle or apparent distal radial growth plate widening (partial or complete), osseous fragmentation within the widened growth plate, and metaphyseal sclerosis and flaring that overlap with the findings seen in rickets (Fig. 13) [96,99,100]. Abnormal radiographic appearance of the growth plate was seen in approximately 25% of symptomatic and 10% of asymptomatic adolescent gymnasts

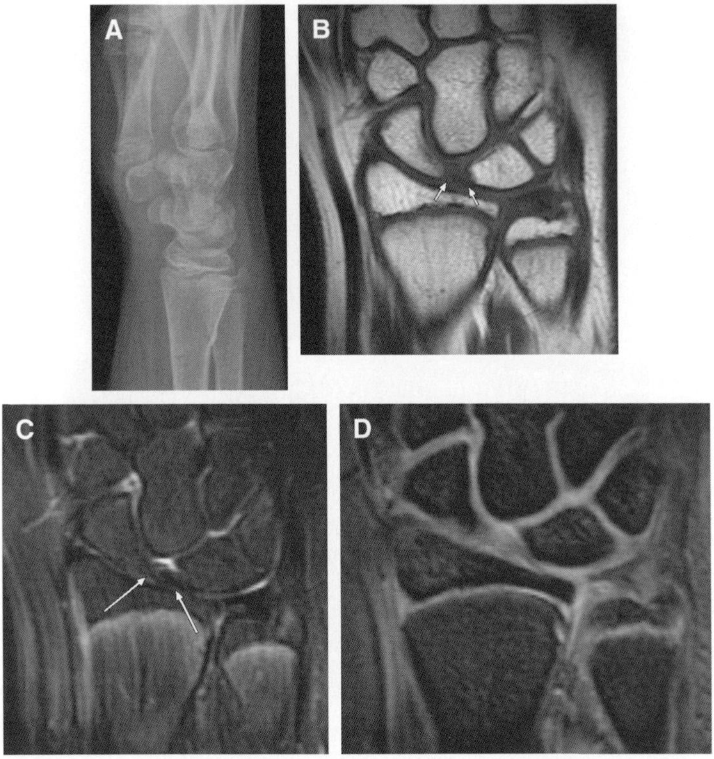

Fig. 12. Probable scapholunate ligament tear. A 13-year-old football player who suffered a hyperextension injury and radial fracture (*A*). After fracture healing he had persistent pain and the MRI shows abnormal widening of the scapholunate distance (*arrows*) on T1 (*B*) with abnormal irregular ligament thickening and surrounding high T2 signal (*arrows*) on coronal T2 (*C*) and gradient echo (*D*) images.

in one large study of 261 Chinese gymnasts [96]. Although similar changes occasionally can be seen in the distal ulna, much more common is the finding of positive ulnar variance that seems to have increasing frequency with greater duration of training [96,98] and is believed to be a secondary finding to the localized growth disturbance of the distal radius.

The MRI findings include growth plate widening with metaphyseal irregularity and extension of cartilage signal (intermediate on T1-weighted and high on T2-weighted images) into the metaphyses (Fig. 14). This finding may have a band-like appearance paralleling the growth plate or run perpendicular to the growth plate and appear as focal tongues [101]. Although initially these focal high T2 signal cartilage tongues were interpreted as fractures [101], they more likely reflect prior or ongoing disruption of endochondral ossification from a metaphyseal insult [40,102]. MRI is more sensitive than radiography in detecting this stress injury. One study of 92 wrists in 47 symptomatic gymnasts who had radiographs and MRI reported 12 of 17 wrists

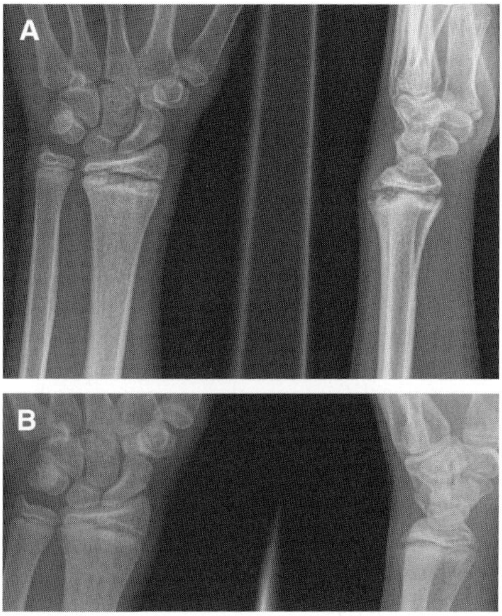

Fig. 13. Gymnast wrist in a 12-year-old gymnast. Initial radiographs (*A*) show the abnormal physeal widening, fragmentation, and metaphyseal flaring that is largely resolved on follow-up radiographs 1 year later (*B*).

that were radiographically normal had abnormalities on MRI [101]. Despite this, radiographs are usually the only imaging indicated in the clinical setting, with conservative treatment of rest (with or without immobilization) followed by rehabilitation being standard. Most patients respond to this regimen with those having more subtle or no radiographic abnormalities likely to have

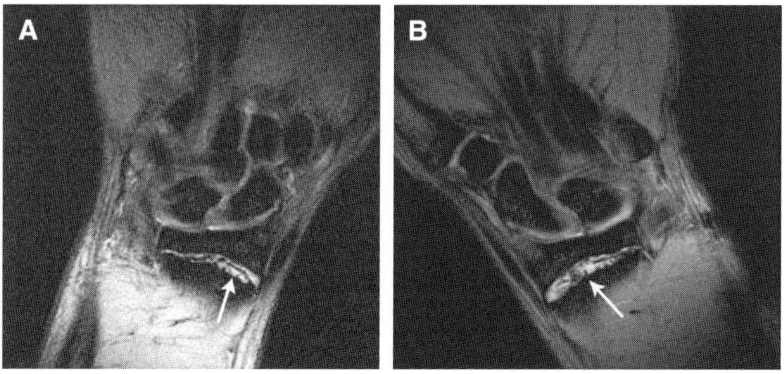

Fig. 14. Bilateral gymnast wrist. A 14-year-old female gymnast with bilateral wrist pain. Coronal gradient echo images (*A, B*) show the abnormally widened distal radial physis bilaterally (*arrows*) with mixed high signal cartilage and dark signal bone fragmentation. (Courtesy of T. Sanders, MD, Keswick, VA.)

more rapid recovery [99]. Premature growth plate fusion is a rare complication [99]. If pain persists after 6 to 9 weeks, MRI or arthrography may be indicated to look for triangular fibrocartilage or ligament abnormality [103].

SUMMARY

The immature musculoskeletal system responds in unique ways to the high-level acute and repetitive stresses involved in sports participation. The unique vulnerability of the physis, particularly in the peri-adolescent period when the level of athletic competition tends to escalate, and the greater ligamentous laxity seen in children figure prominently in the differences in upper extremity injuries encountered in the skeletally immature compared with the skeletally mature athlete. After thorough clinical evaluation, radiography is the initial mainstay of imaging in this setting. MRI is exquisitely sensitive for visualizing the nonosseous structures not readily evaluated by radiography and plays a prominent role in diagnosis and management of these injuries.

References

[1] Chen FS, Diaz VA, Loebenberg M, et al. Shoulder and elbow injuries in the skeletally immature athlete. J Am Acad Orthop Surg 2005;13(3):172–85.
[2] Curtis RJJ. Skeletal injuries: shoulder injuries. In: Stanitski CL, DeLee JC, Drez D, editors. Pediatric and adolescent sports medicine. Philadelphia: W.B. Saunders; 1994. p. 175–215.
[3] Bradley JP. Upper extremity: elbow injuries in children and adolescents. In: Stanitski CL, DeLee JC, Derz D, editors. Pediatric and adolescent sports medicine. Philadelphia: W.B. Saunders; 1994. p. 242–61.
[4] Lovallo JL, Simmons BP. Hand and wrist injuries. In: Stanitski CL, DeLee JC, Drez D, editors. Pediatric and adolescent sports medicine. Philadelphia: W.B. Saunders; 1994. p. 262–78.
[5] Harned 2nd RK, Strain JD. MRI-compatible audio/visual system: impact on pediatric sedation. Pediatr Radiol 2001;31(4):247–50.
[6] Khan JJ, Donnelly LF, Koch BL, et al. Evaluation of a program to reduce the frequency of sedation for MRI and CT in children less than seven years of age. Presented at the Annual Meeting of the Society for Pediatric Radiology. New Orleans, May 4–7, 2005.
[7] Gold GE, Han E, Stainsby J, et al. Musculoskeletal MRI at 3.0 T: relaxation times and image contrast. AJR Am J Roentgenol 2004;183(2):343–51.
[8] Gold GE, Suh B, Sawyer-Glover A, et al. Musculoskeletal MRI at 3.0 T: initial clinical experience. AJR Am J Roentgenol 2004;183(5):1479–86.
[9] Brenner D, Elliston C, Hall E, et al. Estimated risks of radiation-induced fatal cancer from pediatric CT. AJR Am J Roentgenol 2001;176(2):289–96.
[10] Donnelly LF, Emery KH, Brody AS, et al. Minimizing radiation dose for pediatric body applications of single-detector helical CT: strategies at a large children's hospital. AJR Am J Roentgenol 2001;176(2):303–6.
[11] Cleeman E, Flatow EL. Shoulder dislocations in the young patient. Orthop Clin North Am 2000;31(2):217–29.
[12] Rowe CR. Prognosis in dislocations of the shoulder. J Bone Joint Surg Am 1956;38-A(5): 957–77.
[13] Deitch J, Mehlman CT, Foad SL, et al. Traumatic anterior shoulder dislocation in adolescents. Am J Sports Med 2003;31(5):758–63.
[14] Marans HJ, Angel KR, Schemitsch EH, et al. The fate of traumatic anterior dislocation of the shoulder in children. J Bone Joint Surg Am 1992;74(8):1242–4.

[15] Simonet WT, Cofield RH. Prognosis in anterior shoulder dislocation. Am J Sports Med 1984;12(1):19–24.
[16] Hovelius L, Augustini BG, Fredin H, et al. Primary anterior dislocation of the shoulder in young patients. A ten-year prospective study. J Bone Joint Surg Am 1996;78(11):1677–84.
[17] Henry JH, Genung JA. Natural history of glenohumeral dislocation—revisited. Am J Sports Med 1982;10(3):135–7.
[18] Baker CL, Uribe JW, Whitman C. Arthroscopic evaluation of acute initial anterior shoulder dislocations. Am J Sports Med 1990;18(1):25–8.
[19] Speer KP. Anatomy and pathomechanics of shoulder instability. Clin Sports Med 1995;14(4):751–60.
[20] Clayton ML, Weir GJ Jr. Experimental investigations of ligamentous healing. Am J Surg 1959;98:373–8.
[21] Lawton RL, Choudhury S, Mansat P, et al. Pediatric shoulder instability: presentation, findings, treatment, and outcomes. J Pediatr Orthop 2002;22(1):52–61.
[22] Merrill V. Shoulder girdle. In: Ballinger PW, editor. Merrill's atlas of radiographic positions and radiologic procedures. St. Louis: Mosby; 1995. p. 126–47.
[23] Sanders TG, Morrison WB, Miller MD. Imaging techniques for the evaluation of glenohumeral instability. Am J Sports Med 2000;28(3):414–34.
[24] Wilson AJ, Totty WG, Murphy WA, et al. Shoulder joint: arthrographic CT and long-term follow-up, with surgical correlation. Radiology 1989;173(2):329–33.
[25] Singson RD, Feldman F, Bigliani L. CT arthrographic patterns in recurrent glenohumeral instability. AJR Am J Roentgenol 1987;149(4):749–53.
[26] Chandnani VP, Yeager TD, DeBerardino T, et al. Glenoid labral tears: prospective evaluation with MRI imaging, MR arthrography, and CT arthrography. AJR Am J Roentgenol 1993;161(6):1229–35.
[27] Jbara M, Chen Q, Marten P, et al. Shoulder MR arthrography: how, why, when. Radiol Clin North Am 2005;43(4):683–92.
[28] Magee T, Williams D, Mani N. Shoulder MR arthrography: which patient group benefits most? AJR Am J Roentgenol 2004;183(4):969–74.
[29] Meister K, Thesing J, Montgomery WJ, et al. MR arthrography of partial thickness tears of the undersurface of the rotator cuff: an arthroscopic correlation. Skeletal Radiol 2004;33(3):136–41.
[30] Cvitanic O, Tirman PF, Feller JF, et al. Using abduction and external rotation of the shoulder to increase the sensitivity of MR arthrography in revealing tears of the anterior glenoid labrum. AJR Am J Roentgenol 1997;169(3):837–44.
[31] Tirman PF, Bost FW, Steinbach LS, et al. MR arthrographic depiction of tears of the rotator cuff: benefit of abduction and external rotation of the arm. Radiology 1994;192(3):851–6.
[32] Lee SY, Lee JK. Horizontal component of partial-thickness tears of rotator cuff: imaging characteristics and comparison of ABER view with oblique coronal view at MR arthrography initial results. Radiology 2002;224(2):470–6.
[33] Sanders TG, Miller MD. A systematic approach to magnetic resonance imaging interpretation of sports medicine injuries of the shoulder. Am J Sports Med 2005;33(7):1088–105.
[34] Wilkins KE. Epidemiology of shoulder injuries. In: Stanitski CL, DeLee JC, Drez D, editors, Pediatric and adolescent sports medicine. Philadelphia: W.B. Saunders; 1994. p. 175–82.
[35] Gainor BJ, Piotrowski G, Puhl J, et al. The throw: biomechanics and acute injury. Am J Sports Med 1980;8(2):114–8.
[36] Carson WG Jr, Gasser SI. Little Leaguer's shoulder. A report of 23 cases. Am J Sports Med 1998;26(4):575–80.
[37] Bright RW, Burstein AH, Elmore SM. Epiphyseal-plate cartilage. A biomechanical and histological analysis of failure modes. J Bone Joint Surg Am 1974;56(4):688–703.

[38] Jaramillo D, Hoffer FA. Cartilaginous epiphysis and growth plate: normal and abnormal MR imaging findings. AJR Am J Roentgenol 1992;158(5):1105–10.
[39] Jaramillo D, Hoffer FA, Shapiro F, et al. MR imaging of fractures of the growth plate. AJR Am J Roentgenol 1990;155(6):1261–5.
[40] Jaramillo D, Laor T, Zaleske DJ. Indirect trauma to the growth plate: results of MR imaging after epiphyseal and metaphyseal injury in rabbits. Radiology 1993;187(1):171–8.
[41] Jaramillo D, Shapiro F. Musculoskeletal trauma in children. Magn Reson Imaging Clin N Am 1998;6(3):521–36.
[42] Wasserlauf BL, Paletta GA Jr. Shoulder disorders in the skeletally immature throwing athlete. Orthop Clin North Am 2003;34(3):427–37.
[43] Itoi E, Tabata S. Rotator cuff tears in the adolescent. Orthopedics 1993;16(1):78–81.
[44] Tarkin IS, Morganti CM, Zillmer DA, et al. Rotator cuff tears in adolescent athletes. Am J Sports Med 2005;33(4):596–601.
[45] Jobe FW, Kvitne RS, Giangarra CE. Shoulder pain in the overhand or throwing athlete. The relationship of anterior instability and rotator cuff impingement. Orthop Rev 1989;18(9):963–75.
[46] Burk DL Jr, Karasick D, Kurtz AB, et al. Rotator cuff tears: prospective comparison of MR imaging with arthrography, sonography, and surgery. AJR Am J Roentgenol 1989;153(1):87–92.
[47] Quinn SF, Sheley RC, Demlow TA, et al. Rotator cuff tendon tears: evaluation with fat-suppressed MR imaging with arthroscopic correlation in 100 patients. Radiology 1995;195(2):497–500.
[48] Patten RM. Tears of the anterior portion of the rotator cuff (the subscapularis tendon): MR imaging findings. AJR Am J Roentgenol 1994;162(2):351–4.
[49] Needell SD, Zlatkin MB, Sher JS, et al. MR imaging of the rotator cuff: peritendinous and bone abnormalities in an asymptomatic population. AJR Am J Roentgenol 1996;166(4):863–7.
[50] Giaroli EL, Major NM, Higgins LD. MRI of internal impingement of the shoulder. AJR Am J Roentgenol 2005;185(4):925–9.
[51] Gugenheim JJ Jr, Stanley RF, Woods GW, et al. Little League survey: the Houston study. Am J Sports Med 1976;4(5):189–200.
[52] Rudzki JR, Paletta GA Jr. Juvenile and adolescent elbow injuries in sports. Clin Sports Med 2004;23(4):581–608.
[53] Woods GW, Tullos HS. Elbow instability and medial epicondyle fractures. Am J Sports Med 1977;5(1):23–30.
[54] Chambers HG, Wilkins KE. Apophyseal injuries of the distal humerus. In: Rockwood CA, Wilkins KE, Beaty JH, editors. Fractures in children. Philadelphia: Lippincott-Raven; 1996. p. 801–18.
[55] Brogdon BG, Crow NE. Little leaguer's elbow. Am J Roentgenol Radium Ther Nucl Med 1960;83:671–5.
[56] Kocher MS, Waters PM, Micheli LJ. Upper extremity injuries in the paediatric athlete. Sports Med 2000;30(2):117–35.
[57] Goldberg MJ. Gymnastic injuries. Orthop Clin North Am 1980;11(4):717–26.
[58] Hang DW, Chao CM, Hang YS. A clinical and roentgenographic study of Little League elbow. Am J Sports Med 2004;32(1):79–84.
[59] Mirowitz SA, London SL. Ulnar collateral ligament injury in baseball pitchers: MR imaging evaluation. Radiology 1992;185(2):573–6.
[60] Mulligan SA, Schwartz ML, Broussard MF, et al. Heterotopic calcification and tears of the ulnar collateral ligament: radiographic and MR imaging findings. AJR Am J Roentgenol 2000;175(4):1099–102.
[61] Sugimoto H, Ohsawa T. Ulnar collateral ligament in the growing elbow: MR imaging of normal development and throwing injuries. Radiology 1994;192(2):417–22.

[62] Timmerman LA, Schwartz ML, Andrews JR. Preoperative evaluation of the ulnar collateral ligament by magnetic resonance imaging and computed tomography arthrography. Evaluation in 25 baseball players with surgical confirmation. Am J Sports Med 1994;22(1): 26–31. [discussion: 32].

[63] Schwartz ML, al-Zahrani S, Morwessel RM, et al. Ulnar collateral ligament injury in the throwing athlete: evaluation with saline-enhanced MR arthrography. Radiology 1995;197(1):297–9.

[64] Kijowski R, De Smet AA. Magnetic resonance imaging findings in patients with medial epicondylitis. Skeletal Radiol 2005;34(4):196–202.

[65] Martin CE, Schweitzer ME. MR imaging of epicondylitis. Skeletal Radiol 1998;27(3): 133–8.

[66] Chung CB, Chew FS, Steinbach L. MR imaging of tendon abnormalities of the elbow. Magn Reson Imaging Clin N Am 2004;12(2):233–45. [vi.].

[67] Bordalo-Rodrigues M, Rosenberg ZS. MR imaging of entrapment neuropathies at the elbow. Magn Reson Imaging Clin N Am 2004;12(2):247–63. [vi.].

[68] Kobayashi K, Burton KJ, Rodner C, et al. Lateral compression injuries in the pediatric elbow: Panner's disease and osteochondritis dissecans of the capitellum. J Am Acad Orthop Surg 2004;12(4):246–54.

[69] Bradley JP, Petrie RS. Osteochondritis dissecans of the humeral capitellum. Diagnosis and treatment. Clin Sports Med 2001;20(3):565–90.

[70] Kijowski R, Tuite M, Sanford M. Magnetic resonance imaging of the elbow. Part I: normal anatomy, imaging technique, and osseous abnormalities. Skeletal Radiol 2004;33(12): 685–97.

[71] Stoane JM, Poplausky MR, Haller JO, et al. Panner's disease: X-ray, MR imaging findings and review of the literature. Comput Med Imaging Graph 1995;19(6):473–6.

[72] Haraldsson S. On osteochondrosis deformas juvenilis capituli humeri including investigation of intra-osseous vasculature in distal humerus. Acta Orthop Scand 1959;(Suppl 38): 1–232.

[73] Schenck RC Jr, Athanasiou KA, Constantinides G, et al. A biomechanical analysis of articular cartilage of the human elbow and a potential relationship to osteochondritis dissecans. Clin Orthop Relat Res 1994;299:305–12.

[74] Paes RA. Familial osteochondritis dissecans. Clin Radiol 1989;40(5):501–4.

[75] Takahara M, Ogino T, Takagi M, et al. Natural progression of osteochondritis dissecans of the humeral capitellum: initial observations. Radiology 2000;216(1):207–12.

[76] Takahara M, Ogino T, Fukushima S, et al. Nonoperative treatment of osteochondritis dissecans of the humeral capitellum. Am J Sports Med 1999;27(6):728–32.

[77] Kijowski R, De Smet AA. Radiography of the elbow for evaluation of patients with osteochondritis dissecans of the capitellum. Skeletal Radiol 2005;34(5):266–71.

[78] Takahara M, Ogino T, Tsuchida H, et al. Sonographic assessment of osteochondritis dissecans of the humeral capitellum. AJR Am J Roentgenol 2000;174(2):411–5.

[79] Takahara M, Shundo M, Kondo M, et al. Early detection of osteochondritis dissecans of the capitellum in young baseball players. Report of three cases. J Bone Joint Surg Am 1998;80(6):892–7.

[80] Bowen RE, Otsuka NY, Yoon ST, et al. Osteochondral lesions of the capitellum in pediatric patients: role of magnetic resonance imaging. J Pediatr Orthop 2001;21(3): 298–301.

[81] Takahara M, Ogino T, Sasaki I, et al. Long term outcome of osteochondritis dissecans of the humeral capitellum. Clin Orthop Relat Res 1999;363:108–15.

[82] Loredo R, Sanders TG. Imaging of osteochondral injuries. Clin Sports Med 2001;20(2): 249–78.

[83] Peiss J, Adam G, Casser R, et al. Gadopentetate-dimeglumine-enhanced MR imaging of osteonecrosis and osteochondritis dissecans of the elbow: initial experience. Skeletal Radiol 1995;24(1):17–20.

[84] Emery KH. Gadoliniuim enhanced MRI in juvenile osteochondritis dissecans (OCD) of the knee: Is it helpful for predicting the need for surgical therapy? Presented at the Annual Meeting, Society for Pediatric Radiology. San Francisco, May 7–10, 2003.
[85] Dubberley JH, Faber KJ, Patterson SD, et al. The detection of loose bodies in the elbow: the value of MRI and CT arthrography. J Bone Joint Surg Br 2005;87(5):684–6.
[86] Waldt S, Bruegel M, Ganter K, et al. Comparison of multislice CT arthrography and MR arthrography for the detection of articular cartilage lesions of the elbow. Eur Radiol 2005;15(4):784–91.
[87] Kramer J, Stiglbauer R, Engel A, et al. MR contrast arthrography (MRA) in osteochondrosis dissecans. J Comput Assist Tomogr 1992;16(2):254–60.
[88] Alt V, Gasnier J, Sicre G. Injuries of the scapholunate ligament in children. J Pediatr Orthop B 2004;13(5):326–9.
[89] Terry CL, Waters PM. Triangular fibrocartilage injuries in pediatric and adolescent patients. J Hand Surg [Am] 1998;23(4):626–34.
[90] Palmer AK. Triangular fibrocartilage complex lesions: a classification. J Hand Surg [Am] 1989;14(4):594–606.
[91] Haims AH, Schweitzer ME, Morrison WB, et al. Limitations of MR imaging in the diagnosis of peripheral tears of the triangular fibrocartilage of the wrist. AJR Am J Roentgenol 2002;178(2):419–22.
[92] Zanetti M, Bram J, Hodler J. Triangular fibrocartilage and intercarpal ligaments of the wrist: does MR arthrography improve standard MRI? J Magn Reson Imaging 1997;7(3):590–4.
[93] Greene MH, Hadied AM, LaMont RL. Scaphoid fractures in children. J Hand Surg [Am] 1984;9(4):536–41.
[94] Terry DW Jr, Ramin JE. The navicular fat stripe: a useful roentgen feature for evaluating wrist trauma. Am J Roentgenol Radium Ther Nucl Med 1975;124(1):25–8.
[95] Cook PA, Yu JS, Wiand W, et al. Suspected scaphoid fractures in skeletally immature patients: application of MRI. J Comput Assist Tomogr 1997;21(4):511–5.
[96] Chang CY, Shih C, Penn IW, et al. Wrist injuries in adolescent gymnasts of a Chinese opera school: radiographic survey. Radiology 1995;195(3):861–4.
[97] DiFiori JP, Puffer JC, Mandelbaum BR, et al. Distal radial growth plate injury and positive ulnar variance in nonelite gymnasts. Am J Sports Med 1997;25(6):763–8.
[98] Mandelbaum BR, Bartolozzi AR, Davis CA, et al. Wrist pain syndrome in the gymnast. Pathogenetic, diagnostic, and therapeutic considerations. Am J Sports Med 1989;17(3):305–17.
[99] Roy S, Caine D, Singer KM. Stress changes of the distal radial epiphysis in young gymnasts. A report of twenty-one cases and a review of the literature. Am J Sports Med 1985;13(5):301–8.
[100] Liebling MS, Berdon WE, Ruzal-Shapiro C, et al. Gymnast's wrist (pseudorickets growth plate abnormality) in adolescent athletes: findings on plain films and MR imaging. AJR Am J Roentgenol 1995;164(1):157–9.
[101] Shih C, Chang CY, Penn IW, et al. Chronically stressed wrists in adolescent gymnasts: MR imaging appearance. Radiology 1995;195(3):855–9.
[102] Laor T, Hartman AL, Jaramillo D. Local physeal widening on MR imaging: an incidental finding suggesting prior metaphyseal insult. Pediatr Radiol 1997;27(8):654–62.
[103] Mandelbaum BR, Nattiv A. Gymnastics. In: Reider B, editor. Sports medicine: the school-age athlete. Philadelphia: W.B. Saunders; 1996. p. 460.

Clin Sports Med 25 (2006) 569–590

CLINICS IN SPORTS MEDICINE

ELSEVIER
SAUNDERS

The Role of Ultrasound in the Evaluation of Sports Medicine Injuries of the Upper Extremity

Richard Kijowski, MD*, Arthur A. De Smet, MD

Division of Musculoskeletal Radiology, Department of Radiology, University of Wisconsin Clinical Science Center, 600 Highland Avenue, E3/311 CSC, Madison, WI 53792-3252, USA

The two major imaging modalities used for assessment of soft tissue injuries are ultrasound and MRI. Although ultrasound of the extremities is used only to a limited extent in the United States, it is widely used in many other countries for evaluation of extremity injuries.

This article first considers the advantages and disadvantages of MRI and ultrasound. Understanding these differences will help the reader understand the role of ultrasound as compared with MRI in evaluating upper extremity injuries. The uses of ultrasound for evaluating sports medicine injuries in specific regions of the upper extremity are then reviewed. Where the data are available, the reported accuracy of ultrasound is compared with MRI for each type of injury.

ADVANTAGES AND DISADVANTAGES OF MRI

The most obvious advantage of MRI is its ability to show all tissues of the extremity in multiple planes; thus the examination provides detailed evaluation of all the soft tissues, the bones, and the joints in a single study (Fig. 1). Although the correct MR pulse sequences must be obtained to optimize detection of pathology, the physician assessing the patient can readily determine whether the MRI examination is a complete study that fully delineates the region of interest.

The major disadvantages of MRI are its higher cost and longer examination time when compared with ultrasound. Most MRI examinations take 30 to 45 minutes to perform, whereas an ultrasound examination takes about 15 minutes. Charges for MRI and ultrasound examinations vary by region and imaging center; however, the Medicare global relative value units are 13.44 for an MRI of the lower extremity without intravenous (IV) contrast and 2.31 for an ultrasound of the lower extremity. In addition, MRI cannot be performed in patients who are claustrophobic or who have certain implanted devices such

*Corresponding author. *E-mail address*: r.kijowski@hosp.wisc.edu (R. Kijowski).

0278-5919/06/$ – see front matter
doi:10.1016/j.csm.2006.03.004

sportsmed.theclinics.com

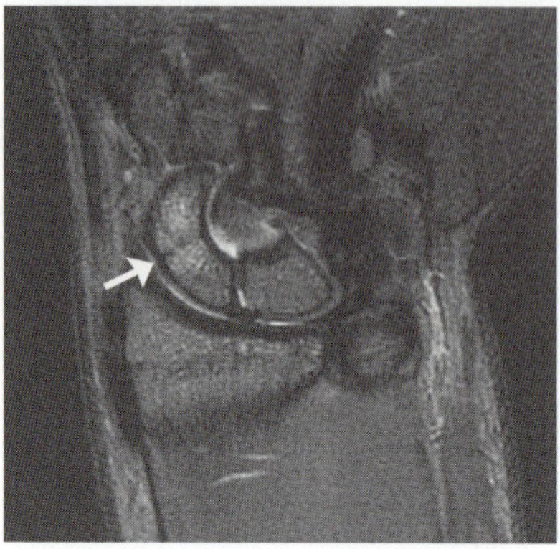

Fig. 1. Radiographically occult scaphoid fracture. Coronal fat-saturated, T2-weighted, fast spin-echo MR image of the wrist shows a low signal intensity fracture line (*arrow*) within the waist of the scaphoid that is surrounded by high signal intensity marrow edema. MRI offers complete assessment of all osseous, articular, and soft tissue structures, in contrast with ultrasound, which provides smaller field of view images primarily limited to the soft tissues.

as cardiac pacemakers. Furthermore, high-quality MRI examinations are difficult to obtain in obese patients and patients who have implanted metallic orthopedic hardware.

ADVANTAGES AND DISADVANTAGES OF ULTRASOUND

Ultrasound is superior to MRI in that it provides higher resolution imaging of superficial structures such as nerves and tendons (Fig. 2). Ultrasound can also be used to dynamically assess for tendon or nerve intermittent subluxation, and to determine the severity of a tendon, ligament, or muscle injury. Dynamic

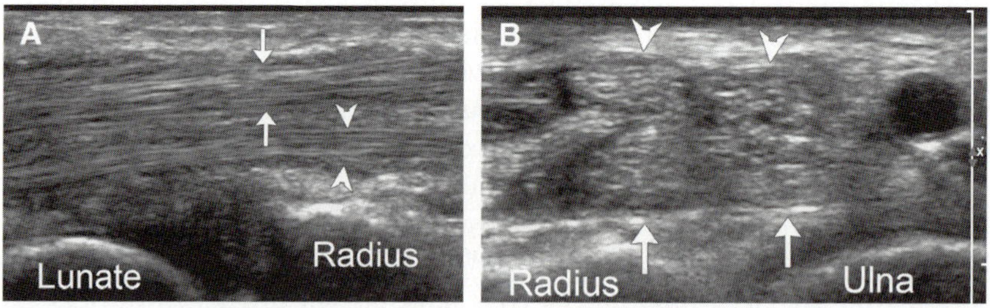

Fig. 2. Normal volar anatomy of the distal forearm. (*A*) Longitudinal ultrasound image of the volar forearm shows the superficialis (*arrows*) and profunda (*arrowheads*) flexor tendons. The tendons have the normal fibrillar pattern consisting of parallel echogenic white lines that represent the tendon fascicles. (*B*) Transverse ultrasound image of the volar wrist shows two superficialis (*arrowheads*) and two profunda (*arrows*) flexor tendons. Tendons have the fine mesh patterns of echogenic white dots and lines of normal tendons.

imaging is particularly useful in evaluating whether a tendon or ligament tear is partial or complete. It can also be useful in confirming a suspected intermittent fascial or muscle hernia. Ultrasound is also the preferred modality for imaging non-radiopaque foreign bodies, although this is not a typical sports medicine injury.

The major disadvantages of ultrasound are its limited field of view and lack of assessment of deep soft tissue structures and bones. Because only a small area of the extremity is visualized on a given image, the visualized pathology cannot be easily related to anatomical landmarks. In addition, ultrasound provides only limited evaluation of intra-articular structures. Finally, if the physician assessing the patient had not personally performed the examination, it is often difficult to determine if an adequate study has been performed.

GENERAL IMAGING APPEARANCE

Tendons and ligaments, being highly collagenized, are seen as a fibrillar pattern of parallel lines when imaged longitudinally (see Fig. 2A). Disruption of these fibrils indicates tendon degeneration or tear. When a tendon or ligament is visualized in cross section, its appearance on an ultrasound scan is that of a fine mesh of dense echogenic dots and short lines (see Fig. 2B). In contrast, only the fascial planes within muscles are echogenic. The muscle bundles themselves are hypoechoic. Ultrasound waves cannot pass through bones. Therefore, the surface of the bone is visualized as an echogenic structure with no internal detail (Fig. 3). A disruption in the echogenic outline of a bone is a sign of an acute fracture. There is increased transmission of ultrasound waves through relatively simple, serous-type fluid collections. As a result, a simple fluid collection will appear anechoic with no internal echoes, and there will be considerable increase in echoes within the soft tissue distal to the fluid.

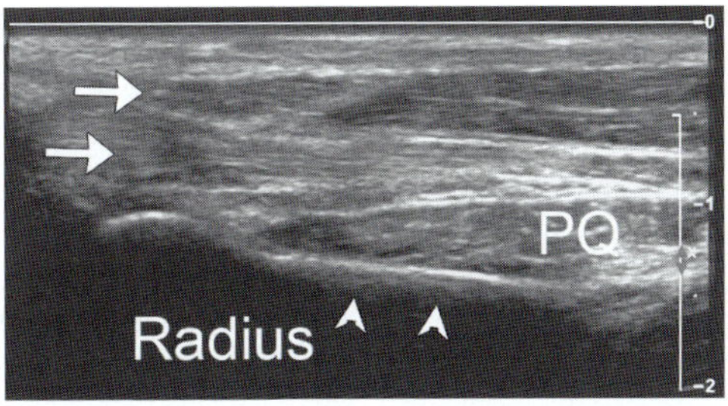

Fig. 3. Normal flexor tendons on the wrist. Longitudinal ultrasound image of the volar wrist shows the superficialis and profunda flexor tendons (*arrows*) and pronator quadratus muscle (PQ). Only the volar periosteal surface of the radius is seen as a continuous echogenic white line. The hazy echoes (*arrowheads*) are common artifacts seen in bones on ultrasound, and are secondary to reverberation of the sound waves off the cortex.

OPTIMAL USES FOR ULTRASOUND EXAMINATION OF SPORTS MEDICINE INJURIES

Ultrasound is best characterized as a targeted examination to confirm or exclude a suspected diagnosis. Many imagers who use ultrasound to assess for tendon or ligament pathology feel that ultrasound provides higher resolution and greater detail than MRI, especially in the small tendons of the distal extremities. The dynamic real-time nature of ultrasound during provocative maneuvers is ideal for assessing subluxing tendons and nerves and intermittent fascia hernias. The major limitation in using ultrasound remains the difficulty in performing the technique. In addition, although ultrasound provides excellent delineation of the superficial soft tissues, its accuracy in detecting pathology has been documented in only a limited number of conditions.

SONOGRAPHIC EVALUATION OF THE SHOULDER

Rotator Cuff Tendon

Ultrasound is an effective method for evaluating the rotator cuff tendons. On ultrasound, the normal rotator cuff tendons appear as an echogenic fibrillar structure with a convex outer border that is located between the humeral head and subacromial/subdeltoid bursa (Fig. 4) [1–3]. The sonographic finding of a partial-thickness rotator cuff tear is a focal hypoechoic area, or more commonly, a mixed hyperechoic and hypoechoic area within either the articular or bursal side of the tendon (Fig. 5) [1]. The main sonographic finding of a full-thickness rotator cuff tear is a focal anechoic or hypoechoic defect through the width of the tendon (Fig. 6). Occasionally, the overlying deltoid muscle, peribursal fat, and hypertrophied synovium within the subacromial bursa drop into the defect, which results in loss of the normal convex outer border of the rotator cuff tendon (Fig. 7). The loss of the normal convex outer border

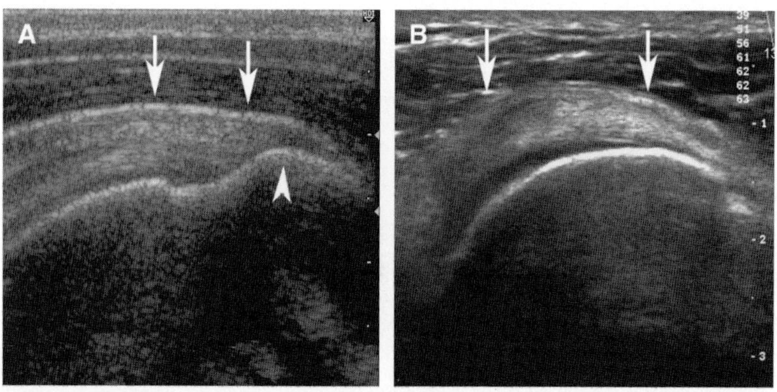

Fig. 4. Normal rotator cuff tendon. Longitudinal (*A*) and transverse (*B*) ultrasound images of the shoulder show the normal rotator cuff tendon (*arrows*) as an echogenic fibrillar structure with a convex outer border that attaches to the greater tuberosity of the proximal humerus (*arrowhead*).

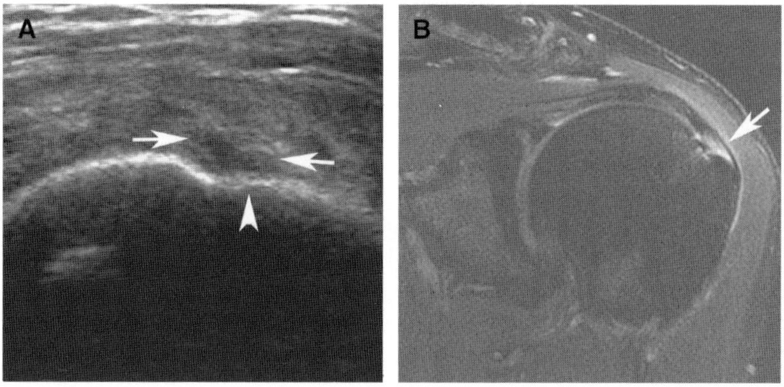

Fig. 5. Partial-thickness articular surface tear of the rotator cuff tear. (*A*) Longitudinal ultrasound image of the shoulder shows a focal hypoechoic area within the articular surface of the rotator cuff tendon (*arrows*) at its insertion site onto the greater tuberosity (*arrowhead*). (*B*) Corresponding coronal fat-suppressed, T2-weighted, fast spin-echo MR image of the shoulder shows a focal area of high signal intensity within the articular surface of the rotator cuff tendon (*arrow*) at its insertion site onto the greater tuberosity.

of the torn rotator tendon may only be visualized when firm pressure is applied with the transducer to displace the more superficially located structures from the defect within the tendon (Fig. 8) [2,3].

When using ultrasound to assess the integrity of the rotator cuff tendon, it is important to evaluate the adjacent structures of the shoulder for secondary findings of a rotator cuff tear. These secondary findings include cortical

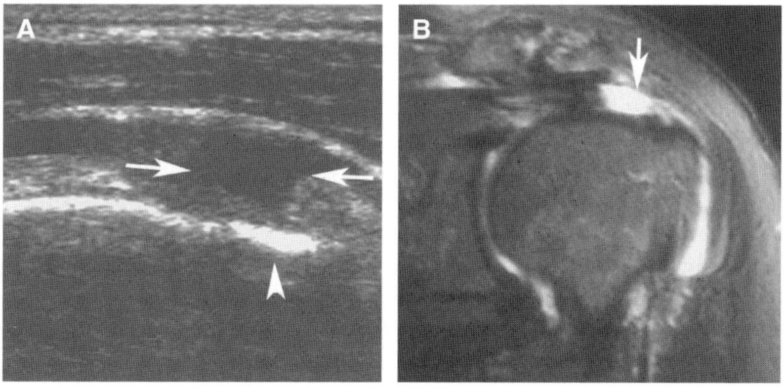

Fig. 6. Full-thickness tear of the rotator cuff tendon. (*A*) Longitudinal ultrasound image of the shoulder shows a focal anechoic defect through the width of the rotator cuff tendon (*arrows*) at its insertion site onto the greater tuberosity (*arrowhead*). (*B*) Corresponding coronal fat-suppressed, T2-weighted, fast spin-echo MR image of the shoulder shows a focal high signal intensity defect through the width of the rotator cuff tendon (*arrow*) at its insertion site onto the greater tuberosity.

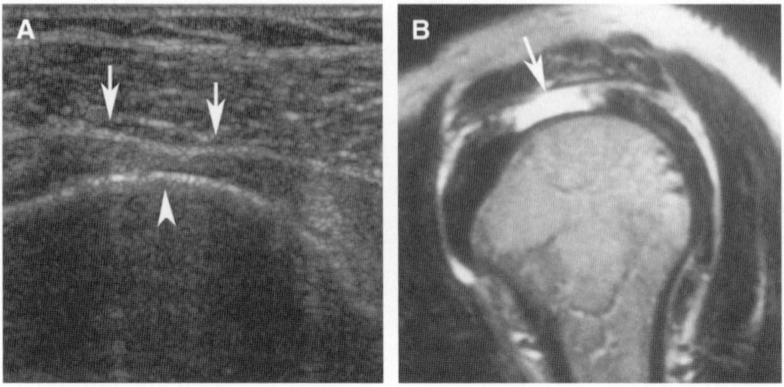

Fig. 7. Full-thickness tear of the rotator cuff tendon. (*A*) Transverse ultrasound image of the shoulder shows loss of the normal convex outer border of the rotator cuff tendon (*arrows*) at its insertion site onto the greater tuberosity (*arrowhead*). (*B*) Corresponding sagittal T2-weighted, spin-echo MR image of the shoulder shows a focal high signal intensity defect through the width of the rotator cuff tendon (*arrow*) at its insertion site onto the greater tuberosity.

irregularity of the greater tuberosity, fluid within the subacromial/subdeltoid bursa, fluid within the glenohumeral joint, and the cartilage interface sign [2,4–8]. The cartilage interface sign refers to the unusually prominent sonographic reflections from the interface between fluid within a defect in the rotator cuff tendon and the adjacent articular cartilage of the humeral head [2,8]. These secondary signs may be more useful for the diagnosis of a rotator cuff

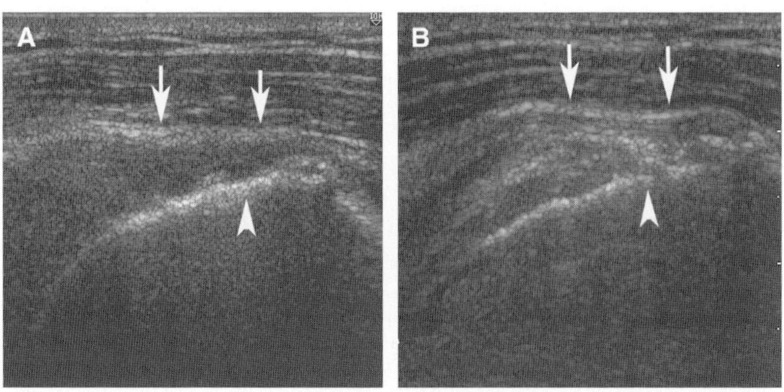

Fig. 8. Full-thickness tear of the rotator cuff tendon. (*A*) Longitudinal ultrasound image of the shoulder without compression shows subtle flattening of the normal convex outer border of the rotator cuff tendon (*arrows*) near its insertion site onto the greater tuberosity (*arrowhead*). (*B*) Longitudinal ultrasound image of the shoulder with compression shows concavity of the normal convex outer border of the rotator cuff tendon (*arrows*) near its insertion site onto the greater tuberosity (*arrowhead*).

tear than the primary finding of abnormal echogenicity and loss of the convex outer border of the rotator cuff tendon [9].

Multiple studies have investigated the ability of ultrasound to detect tears of the rotator cuff tendons, with a wide range in reported accuracy. Ultrasound for cuff tears has a reported sensitivity of 57% to 100% and specificity of 76% to 100% for the detection of full-thickness rotator cuff tears [10–19]. Ultrasound has a reported sensitivity of 41% to 93% and a specificity of 85% to 94% for the detection of partial-thickness rotator cuff tears [1,11,12,19]. The main difficulties in evaluating the rotator cuff tendon with ultrasound are distinguishing partial-thickness, articular surface tears from tendinopathy; and distinguishing high-grade, partial-thickness tears from full-thickness tears [20]. With the use of modern equipment, improved scanning technique, and refined diagnostic criteria, however, many centers with experienced musculoskeletal sonographers have reported sensitivities and specificities values exceeding 90% for the detection of both full-thickness and partial-thickness rotator cuff tears [1,11,18]. Ultrasound also has low interobserver variability in the detection and characterization of rotator cuff tears [21]. In addition, ultrasound can provide important information about the location, size, and degree of retraction of the torn rotator cuff tendon [11,13,22].

There has been much recent debate about what is best imaging modality for evaluating the rotator cuff tendon. A retrospective review of the literature [23], which included 38 cohort studies on ultrasound and 29 cohort studies on MRI, concluded that both imaging modalities are equally effective at detecting full-thickness rotator cuff tears. In addition, a recent prospective study on 71 consecutive patients who had surgically confirmed tears of the rotator cuff tendon [18] found that ultrasound and MRI were equally effective at identifying and determining the size of both full-thickness and partial-thickness tears. Thus, the decision regarding the most appropriate imaging modality for evaluating the rotator cuff tendon need not be based upon accuracy concerns. Instead, the decision should be based on other factors, such as the experience of the sonographer, patient tolerance, cost, and the need to evaluate the adjacent structures of the shoulder.

Ultrasound is faster, cheaper, and more comfortable for the patient than MRI. Ultrasound can also provide excellent evaluation of the rotator cuff tendon in obese and claustrophobic patients, and in patients who have certain metallic implanted devices; however, MRI provides a more global evaluation of the shoulder, and is superior to ultrasound at detecting abnormalities of the osseous and muscular structures, glenoid labrum, glenohumeral ligaments, and joint capsule. Perhaps the most important factor when choosing the best imaging modality for evaluating the rotator cuff tendon is the experience of the sonographer [24]. The identification and characterization of rotator cuff tears is one of the most challenging aspects of musculoskeletal ultrasound, and has a very steep learning curve. For this reason, most general radiologists and even most fellowship-trained musculoskeletal radiologists are more comfortable using MRI to evaluate the rotator cuff tendon.

Long Head of the Biceps Tendon

Ultrasound may also be used to evaluate the long head of the biceps tendon. The normal biceps tendon is an echogenic fibrillar structure that is visualized sonographically as it emerges from beneath the acromion and courses distally through the glenohumeral joint and into the bicipital groove of the proximal humerus (Fig. 9). The sonographic findings of tendinopathy and partial-thickness tear of the biceps tendon are similar, and include enlargement and decreased echogenicity of the tendon and fluid within the tendon sheath. Hypervascularity of the synovium within the tendon sheath may also be noted on Doppler ultrasound (Fig. 10). The most common sonographic finding of complete rupture of the biceps tendon is nonvisualization of the tendon within the bicipital groove; however, a completely ruptured biceps tendon that is attached by adhesions within the bicipital sheath may have a normal sonographic appearance within the bicipital groove. Furthermore, nonvisualization of the biceps tendon within the bicipital groove may also be secondary to tendon subluxation or dislocation. For this reason, it is important to evaluate the entire length of the biceps tendon, from where it emerges from beneath the acromion proximally to its musculotendinous junction distally. Displacement of the proximal biceps tendon anterior or medial to the lesser tuberosity indicates tendon subluxation or dislocation. Nonvisualization of the proximal biceps tendon, especially at the entrance to the bicipital groove, indicates complete tendon rupture [2,3,11,19].

Two preliminary studies have investigated the ability of ultrasound to evaluate the long head of the biceps tendon [11,19]. Ultrasound has a sensitivity of 63% to 100% and specificity of 100% for the detection of biceps tendon rupture, and a sensitivity of 75% to 83% and specificity of 100% for the detection of biceps tendon subluxation and dislocation; These preliminary studies included

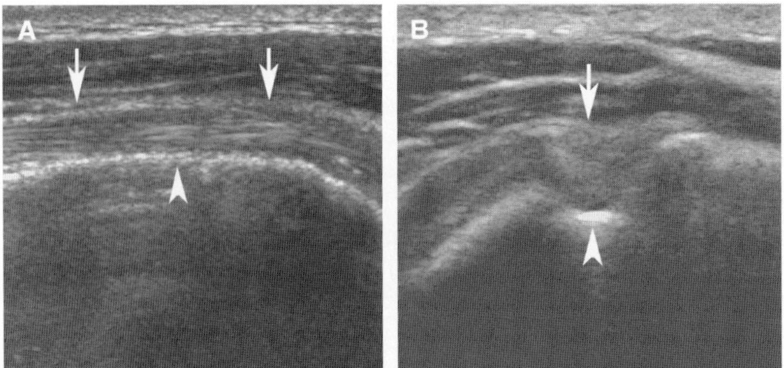

Fig. 9. Normal long head of the biceps tendon. Longitudinal (*A*) and transverse (*B*) ultrasound images of the shoulder shows the normal biceps tendon as an echogenic fibrillar structure (*arrows*) that is located within the bicipital groove of the proximal humerus. (*arrowheads*).

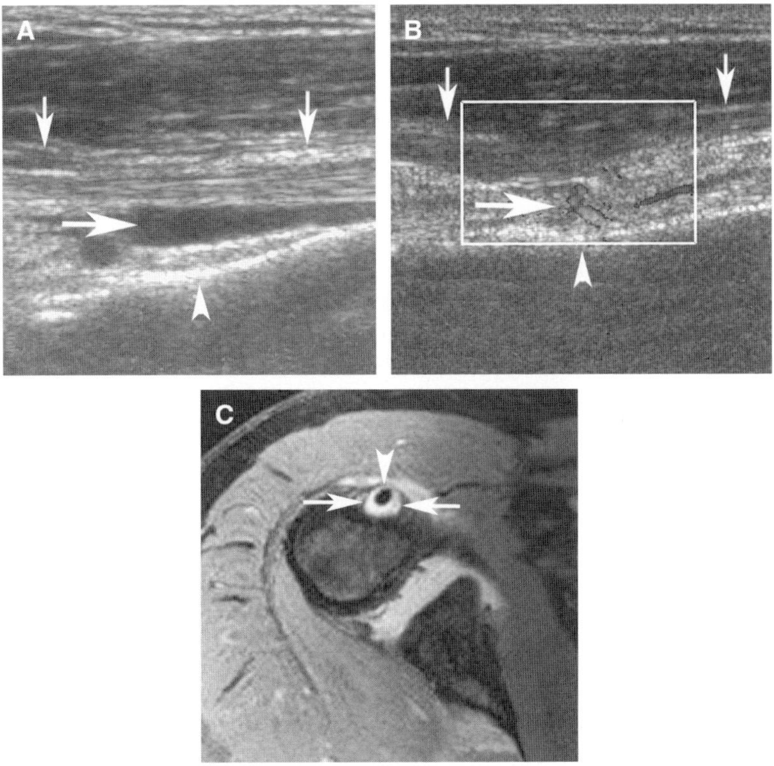

Fig. 10. Tendonopathy of the long head of the biceps tendon. (*A*) Longitudinal ultrasound image of the shoulder shows anechoic fluid (*large arrow*) within the synovial sheath surrounding the biceps tendon (*small arrows*) as the tendon passes through the bicipital groove (*arrowhead*). (*B*) Longitudinal Doppler ultrasound image of the shoulder shows increased vascularity (*large arrow*) of the synovial sheath surrounding the biceps tendon (*small arrows*) as the tendon passes through the bicipital groove (*arrowhead*). (*C*) Corresponding axial fat-suppressed, proton density-weighted, fast spin-echo MR image of the shoulder shows high signal intensity fluid (*arrows*) surrounding the biceps tendon (*arrowhead*).

only a small number of patients with surgical correlation, however. Multiple large clinical studies with surgical correlation have documented the accuracy of MRI for the detection of biceps tendon rupture and biceps tendon subluxation and dislocation [25,26]. Furthermore, many abnormalities of the biceps tendon involve the proximal intra-articular portion of the tendon, which is located beneath the acromion and is difficult to visualize on ultrasound [27]. In view of the lower sensitivity of ultrasound, MRI remains the best imaging modality for evaluating of the long head of the biceps tendon.

Glenohumeral Joint

Ultrasound may be used to evaluate limited portions of the glenoid labrum and humeral head in patients who have shoulder instability. The normal labrum appears as a triangular-shaped, homogenously hypoechoic structure that projects off of the glenoid rim. A thin (less than 2 mm) hypoechoic zone may be present at the base of the normal labrum [28]. The sonographic findings of a labral tear include absence or truncation of the labrum, abnormal labral motion during dynamic imaging, and an enlarged (greater than 2 mm) hypoechoic zone at the base of the labrum [29–31]. An associated Hill-Sachs deformity of the humeral head may also be identified using ultrasound, and appears as a wedge-shaped defect of the hyperechoic bony contour of the humeral head, at the site of attachment of the infraspinatus tendon [32–34].

Multiple preliminary studies have investigated the ability of ultrasound to evaluate patients who have shoulder instability [29–34]. Ultrasound has a sensitivity of 88% to 95% and specificity of 67% to 100% for the detection of labral tears, and a sensitivity of 91% to 100% and specificity of 89% to 100% for detection of Hill-Sachs deformities. These preliminary studies, however, included a relatively small number of patients with surgical correlation. Furthermore, all ultrasound examinations were performed by experienced musculoskeletal sonographers. Multiple large clinical studies with surgical correlation have documented the accuracy of MRI for the detection of labral tears and associated Hill-Sachs deformities [35–38]. In view of the limited visualization of intra-articular structures, MRI remains the best imaging modality for evaluating patients who have shoulder instability.

Acromioclavicular Joint

Ultrasound may be used to evaluate the acromioclavicular joint. Ultrasound may identify joint space widening, thickening of the joint capsule and adjacent ligaments, and intra-articular and subcutaneous hematomas in patients who have acromioclavicular joint separation [39]. Ultrasound can detect osteophytes, subchondral cysts, joint space narrowing, intra-articular fluid, and dystrophic calcification in patients who have osteoarthritis of the acromioclavicular joint [40]. Ultrasound may also identify irregular cortical erosions within the distal clavicle, joint space widening, intra-articular fluid, and soft tissue swelling in patients who have post-traumatic osteolysis of the distal clavicle [41].

Subacromial-Subdeltoid Bursa

Ultrasound may be used to evaluate the subacromial/subdeltoid bursa. The normal subacromial-subdeltoid bursa appears as a thin hypoechoic stripe that is separated from the underlying rotator cuff tendon and overlying deltoid muscle by a thin layer of echogenic peribursal fat. Fluid within the subacromial/subdeltoid bursa tends to accumulate along the lateral edge of the greater tuberosity of the proximal humerus, which produces a typical anechoic "teardrop" appearance on longitudinal ultrasound images. When fluid is identified within the subacromial/subdeltoid bursa, it is important to closely evaluate the adjacent rotator cuff tendon for evidence of a full-thickness tear; however, fluid may also be present within the subacromial/subdeltoid bursa in patients who have infectious and inflammatory bursitis (Fig. 11), and in patients who have shoulder impingement syndrome [42]. One important sonographic finding in

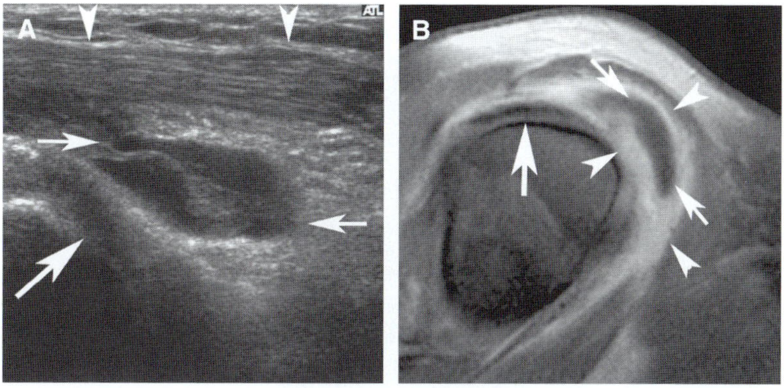

Fig. 11. Septic subacromial/subdeltoid bursitis. (*A*) Longitudinal ultrasound image of the shoulder shows anechoic fluid within the subacromial/subdeltoid bursa (*small arrows*). Note the overlying deltoid muscle (*arrowheads*) and the underlying rotator cuff tendon (*large arrow*). (*B*) Corresponding coronal post-contrast, fat-suppressed, T1-weighted, spin-echo MR image of the shoulder shows low signal intensity fluid within the subacromial/subdeltoid bursa (*small arrows*). Note the high signal intensity enhancing synovium (*arrowheads*) within the subacromial bursa, and the underlying low signal intensity rotator cuff tendon (*large arrow*).

patients who have impingement syndrome is gradual distension of the subacromial/subdeltoid bursa and pooling of fluid within the lateral subdeltoid portion of the bursal system with elevation of the arm [43].

SONOGRAPHIC EVALUATION OF THE ELBOW

Ulnar Collateral Ligament

Ultrasound may be used to evaluate the ulnar collateral ligament. The normal anterior bundle of the ulnar collateral ligament appears as an echogenic fibrillar structure that arises from the medial epicondyle and courses distally to insert onto the base of the coronoid process of the proximal ulna (Fig. 12) [44]. Ultrasound may be useful at identifying acute partial-thickness and full-thickness tears of the ulnar collateral ligament, and chronic ligamentous injuries secondary to repetitive microtrauma. The sonographic findings of an acute partial-thickness tear of the ulnar collateral ligament include diffuse thickening and decreased echogenicity of the ligament, and focal hypoechoic areas within the ligament (Fig. 13) [44,45]. The sonographic findings of an acute full-thickness tear of the ulnar collateral ligament include an anechoic or hypoechoic fluid-filled gap within the ligament, and nonvisualization of the ligament (Fig. 14) [44,45]. The sonographic findings of chronic injury to the ulnar collateral ligament secondary to repetitive microtrauma include diffuse thickening of the ligament, intraligamentous calcification, and focal hypoechoic areas within the ligament [46]. In patients who have both acute and chronic ulnar collateral ligament injuries, dynamic imaging may demonstrate ligamentous laxity with asymmetric widening of the medial joint space with valgus stress [46–48].

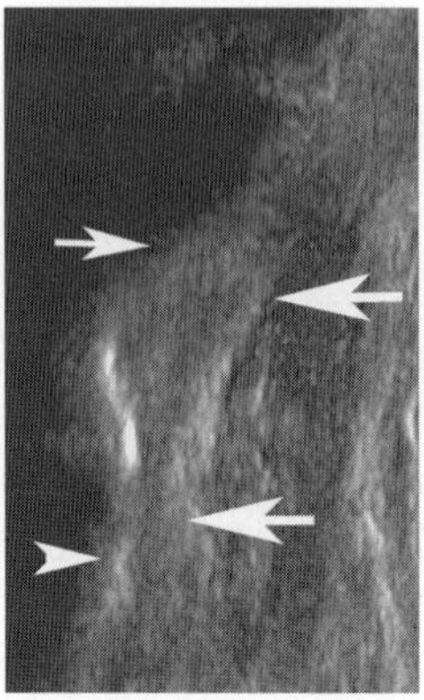

Fig. 12. Normal ulnar collateral ligament. Longitudinal ultrasound image of the medial elbow shows the normal ulnar collateral ligament as an echogenic fibrillar structure (*large arrows*) coursing between the medial epicondyle of the distal humerus (*small arrow*) and the base of the coronoid process of the proximal ulna (*arrowhead*).

Clinical studies with surgical correlation that document the accuracy of ultrasound for the detection of ulnar collateral ligament tears have yet to be performed. In contrast, multiple clinical studies with surgical correlation have shown that MRI can accurately detect full-thickness and partial-thickness tears of the ulnar collateral ligament [49–52]. Until studies are reported with surgical correlation of sonographic findings, MRI, especially with intra-articular

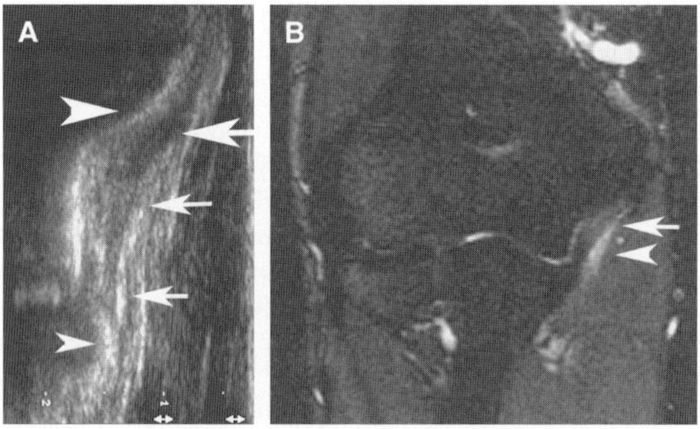

Fig. 13. Partial-thickness tear of the proximal ulnar collateral ligament. (*A*) Longitudinal ultrasound image of the medial elbow shows a focal hypoechoic area within the superficial surface of the proximal ulnar collateral ligament (*large arrow*) near its origin from the medial epicondyle (*large arrowhead*). The more distal ulnar collateral ligament (*small arrows*), which attaches to the base of the coronoid process (*small arrowhead*), appears normal. (*B*) Corresponding coronal fat-suppressed, T2-weighted, fast spin-echo MR image of the elbow shows diffuse high signal intensity within the intact proximal ulnar collateral ligament (*arrow*) and high signal intensity edema within the adjacent soft tissue (*arrowhead*).

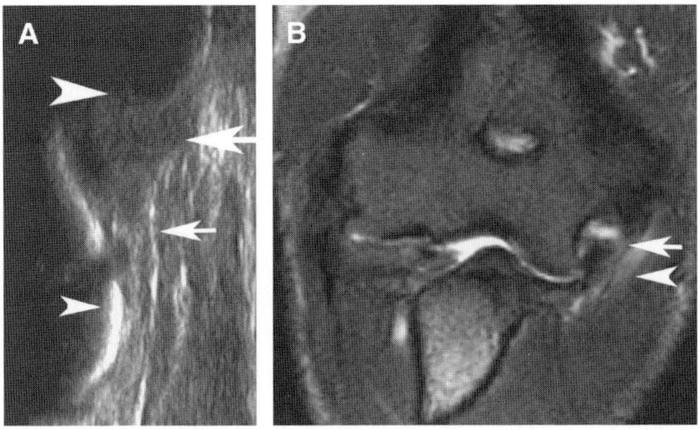

Fig. 14. Full-thickness tear of the proximal ulnar collateral ligament. (*A*) Longitudinal ultrasound image of the medial elbow shows a focal hypoechoic defect through the width of the proximal ulnar collateral ligament (*large arrow*) near its origin from the medial epicondyle (*large arrowhead*). The more distal ulnar collateral ligament (*small arrow*), which attaches to the base of the coronoid process (*small arrowhead*), appears normal. (*B*) Corresponding coronal fat-suppressed, proton density-weighted, fast spin-echo MR image of the elbow shows a focal high signal intensity defect through the width of the proximal ulnar collateral ligament (*arrow*) and high signal intensity edema within the adjacent soft tissue (*arrowhead*).

contrast, should be considered the best imaging modality for evaluating the ulnar collateral ligament.

Distal Biceps and Triceps Tendon

Ultrasound may be used to evaluate the distal biceps tendon. The normal biceps tendon appears as an echogenic fibrillar structure that courses distally through the antecubital fossa to insert onto the radial tuberosity. The sonographic findings of tendinopathy and a partial-thickness tear of the biceps tendon are similar, and include tendon thickening or thinning, decreased echogenicity of the tendon, and peritendinous fluid. The sonographic findings of a full-thickness biceps tendon tear include complete absence of the distal biceps tendon at the radial tuberosity, an anechoic fluid-filled gap within the tendon, a heterogeneous mass within the antecubital fossa, and peritendinous fluid. The degree of retraction of a torn biceps tendon may be assessed on longitudinal ultrasound images [53–55].

Ultrasound may be also used to evaluate the distal triceps tendon. The normal triceps tendon appears as an echogenic fibrillar structure that courses distally to insert onto the olecranon process of the proximal ulna. The sonographic findings of a triceps tendon tear include complete absence of the distal triceps tendon at the olecranon process, an anechoic fluid-filled gap within the tendon, and peritendinous fluid. The degree of retraction of a torn triceps tendon may be assessed on longitudinal ultrasound images. In patients who have a torn but nonretracted triceps tendon, dynamic imaging during elbow flexion and extension may be helpful in distinguishing a partial-thickness tear, in which residual fibers remain attached to the olecranon process, from a full-thickness tear [56,57].

Clinical studies with surgical correlation that document the accuracy of ultrasound for the detection of biceps and triceps tendon tears have yet to be performed. Multiple clinical studies with surgical correlation have shown that MRI can accurately detect full-thickness and partial-thickness tears of the biceps tendon and triceps tendon [58–62]. Until studies are reported with surgical correlation of sonographic findings, MRI, should be considered the best imaging modality for evaluating patients who have distal biceps and triceps tendon injuries.

Elbow-Common Extensor Tendon

Ultrasound may be used to evaluate the common extensor tendon. The normal common extensor tendon appears as an echogenic fibrillar structure that arises from the lateral epicondyle and courses distally to blend in with the extensor carpi radialis brevis and extensor digitorum muscles (Fig. 15). The sonographic findings of lateral epicondylitis include tendon thickening, intratendinous calcification, diffuse heterogeneous echotexture of the tendon with loss of the normal fibrillar pattern, focal hypoechoic areas within the tendon, peritendinous edema, and cortical irregularity of the lateral epicondyle. Anechoic areas within the common extensor tendon may be seen in patients who have severe lateral epicondylitis, and are thought to represent partial-thickness tendon tears (Fig. 16) [63–65].

Many large clinical studies have documented the usefulness of ultrasound for evaluating patients who have lateral epicondylitis. Ultrasound can confirm the presence of lateral epicondylitis and can provide information about the severity of the disease process. Ultrasound has a sensitivity of 64% to 88% for the detection of lateral epicondylitis; however, the main disadvantage of using

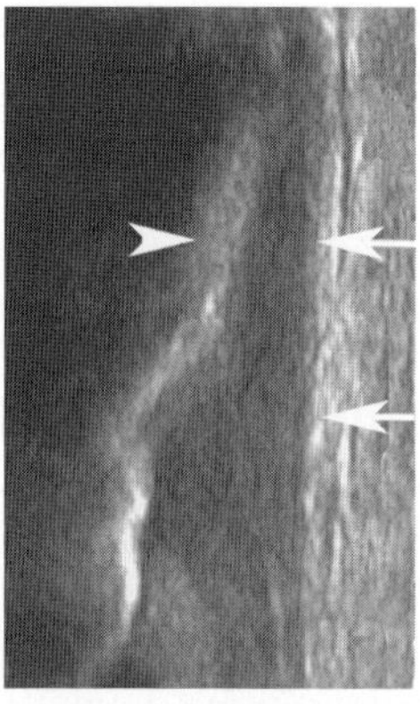

Fig. 15. Normal common extensor tendon. Longitudinal ultrasound image of the lateral elbow shows the normal common extensor tendon as an echogenic fibrillar structure (*arrows*) originating from the lateral epicondyle of the distal humerus (*arrowhead*).

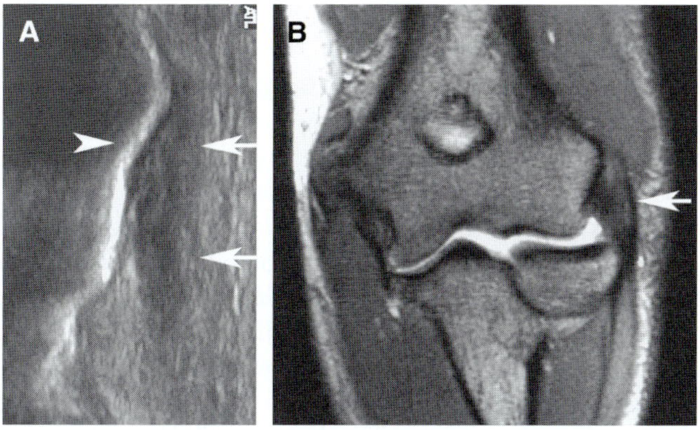

Fig. 16. Lateral epicondylitis. (*A*) Longitudinal ultrasound image of the lateral elbow shows a focal hypoechoic area within the common extensor tendon (*arrows*), near its origin from the lateral epicondyle (*arrowhead*). (*B*) Corresponding coronal fat-suppressed, proton density-weighted, fast spin-echo MR image of the elbow shows diffuse high signal intensity within a thickened common extensor tendon (*arrow*).

ultrasound for the diagnosis of patients who have lateral epicondylitis is its poor specificity, which is as low as 36% in some studies [63–65]. Multiple clinical studies with surgical correlation have shown that MRI can be accurately used to diagnose patients who have lateral epicondylitis [66–68]. Furthermore, MRI was found to be more sensitive and specific than ultrasound for the detection of lateral epicondylitis in a prospective study comparing both imaging modalities [65]. In light of the reported lower sensitivity and specificity of ultrasound, MRI remains the best imaging modality for evaluating the common extensor tendon in patients who have lateral elbow pain.

SONOGRAPHIC EVALUATION OF THE WRIST AND HAND

Ligaments of the Wrist and Hand

Ultrasound may be used to evaluate the intrinsic ligaments of the wrist. The scapholunate and lunotriquetral ligaments are well-visualized on ultrasound and appear as echogenic fibrillar structures connecting the proximal carpal bones [69,70]. The sonographic findings of a torn scapholunate or lunotriquetral ligament include loss of the normal echogenic appearance of the ligament, disruption or absence of the ligament, or the presence of fluid interposed between the proximal carpal bones [56,69]. In a small preliminary study using arthrography as the reference standard [56], ultrasound was found to have a sensitivity of 100% for the detection of scapholunate ligament tears, and a sensitivity of 25% for the detection of lunotriquetral ligament tears. Although this preliminary study is encouraging, MRI remains the imaging modality of choice for evaluating the intrinsic ligaments of the wrist [71–73].

Ultrasound may be used to evaluate the ulnar collateral ligament of the thumb. The normal ulnar collateral ligament appears as homogenous, hypoechoic, bandlike structure extending from the metacarpal head to the base of the proximal phalanx. The sonographic findings of a partial-thickness tear and a nondisplaced, full-thickness tear of the ulnar collateral ligament are identical, and include thickening and heterogeneously increased echogenicity of the ligament. The sonographic findings of a displaced, full-thickness tear of the ulnar collateral ligament include nonvisualization of the ligament and identification of a hyperechoic lesion (Stener's lesion), with a surrounding hypoechoic halo lying on the dorsal aspect of the adductor pollicis muscle [74–77].

Multiple clinical studies with surgical correlation have documented the ability of both ultrasound and MRI to identify full-thickness and partial-thickness tears of the ulnar collateral ligament of the thumb, and to distinguish between displaced and nondisplaced full-thickness tears [75–84]. In a prospective study comparing both imaging modalities [78], however, MRI was found to be more sensitive and specific than ultrasound for differentiating displaced and nondisplaced full-thickness ligament tears. Because ultrasound is less expensive than MRI, it may be considered as a good alternative to MRI at institutions with highly experienced musculoskeletal sonographers.

Triangular Fibrocartilage Complex

Ultrasound may be used to evaluate the triangular fibrocartilage complex of the wrist. The normal triangular fibrocartilage complex appears as a homogenous echogenic, triangular structure that is located distal to the ulna and deep to the extensor carpi ulnaris tendon. The sonographic findings of a tear of the triangular fibrocartilage complex include loss of the normal homogenously echogenic appearance and triangular shape of the structure, absence of portion of the structure, and focal or linear areas of decreased echogenicity within the structure. In a small preliminary study using arthrography as the reference standard [56], ultrasound was found to have 64% sensitivity for the detection of tears of the triangular fibrocartilage complex. Although this preliminary study is encouraging, MRI remains the imaging modality of choice for evaluating of the triangular fibrocartilage complex of the wrist [85–87].

Tendons of the Wrist and Hand

Ultrasound may be used to evaluate the flexor and extensor tendons of the wrist and hand. The normal flexor and extensor tendons appear as homogenous echogenic, fibrillar structures that are surrounded by a thin, barely discernible hypoechoic synovial sheath (Fig. 17). The sonographic findings of tendinopathy include tendon thickening, diffuse or focal areas of decreased echogenicity within the tendon, and anechoic fluid within the tendon sheath. The sonographic findings of partial-thickness tendon tear include a focal anechoic or hypoechoic cleft within the tendon, and anechoic fluid within the tendon sheath (Fig. 18). The sonographic findings of a full-thickness tendon tear include nonvisualization of the tendon at the site of rupture, and anechoic fluid or heterogeneous hyperechoic hematoma within the tendon sheath that separates the retracted edges of the torn tendon [88–90].

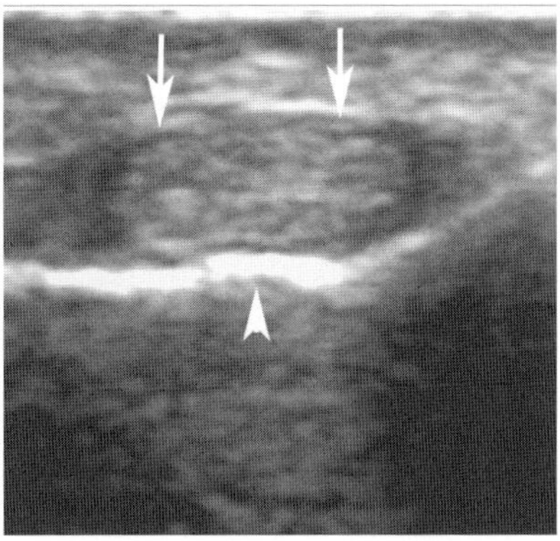

Fig. 17. Normal extensor carpi ulnaris tendon. Transverse ultrasound image of the ulnar aspect of the wrist shows the normal extensor carpi ulnaris tendon (*arrows*) as an echogenic fibrillar structure that is located within the ulnar styloid groove (*arrowhead*).

Clinical studies with surgical correlation that document the accuracy of ultrasound for the detection of flexor and extensor tendon injuries have yet to be performed. Multiple clinical studies with surgical correlation have shown that MRI can accurately detect acute and chronic injuries of the flexor and extensor tendons [91–96]. Until studies are reported with surgical correlation of sonographic findings, MRI should be considered the best imaging modality for evaluating patients who have abnormalities of the flexor and extensor tendons of the wrist and hand.

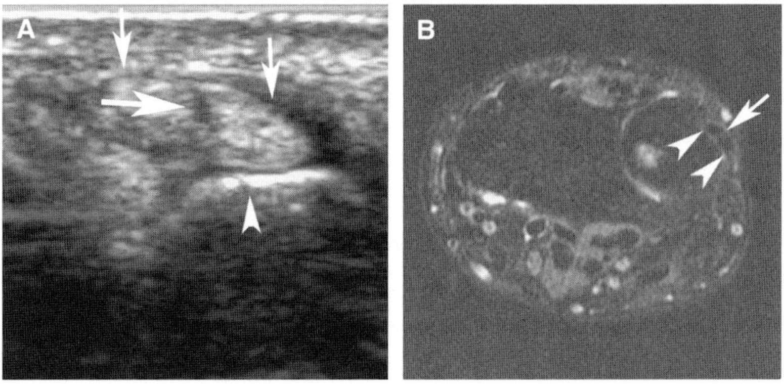

Fig. 18. Tear of the extensor carpi ulnaris tendon. (*A)* Transverse ultrasound image of the ulnar aspect of the wrist shows a focal hypoechoic defect (*large arrow*) within the extensor carpi ulnaris tendon (*small arrows*) that is located within the ulnar styloid groove (*arrowheads*). (*B*) Corresponding axial fat-suppressed, T2-weighted, fast spin-echo MR image of the wrist shows an intermediate signal intensity defect (*arrow*) splitting the extensor carpi ulnaris tendon into two separate low signal intensity fragments (*arrowheads*).

SUMMARY

Ultrasound examination of the extremities is a rapidly growing area for the evaluation of sports medicine injuries. It is likely that in coming years, further studies with surgical correlation will document the accuracy of ultrasound. The authors suspect that MRI will be found to be the most accurate method for the assessment of some injuries, whereas ultrasound will have an accuracy comparable to MRI for the assessment of many other injuries, as has been documented for rotator cuff tears. The most important point to remember when considering whether to use ultrasound, however, is that it is best used as a focused examination for specific conditions. The skill of the sonographer will always be important in view of the steep learning curve in examining many types of sports medicine injuries.

References

[1] van Holsbeeck MT, Kolowich PA, Eyler WR, et al. US depiction of partial-thickness tear of the rotator cuff. Radiology 1995;197(2):443–6.

[2] Teefey SA, Middleton WD, Yamaguchi K. Shoulder sonography. State of the art. Radiol Clin North Am 1999;37(4):767–85.

[3] Bianchi S, Martinoli C, Abdelwahab IF. Ultrasound of tendon tears. Part 1: general considerations and upper extremity. Skeletal Radiol 2005;34:500–12.

[4] Wohlwend JR, van Holsbeeck M, Craig J, et al. The association between irregular greater tuberosities and rotator cuff tears: a sonographic study. AJR Am J Roentgenol 1998;171(1):229–33.

[5] Huang LF, Rubin DA, Britton CA. Greater tuberosity changes as revealed by radiography: lack of clinical usefulness in patients with rotator cuff disease. AJR Am J Roentgenol 1999;172(5):1381–8.

[6] Hollister MS, Mack LA, Patten RM, et al. Association of sonographically detected subacromial/subdeltoid bursal effusion and intraarticular fluid with rotator cuff tear. AJR Am J Roentgenol 1995;165(3):605–8.

[7] Arslan G, Apaydin A, Kabaalioglu A, et al. Sonographically detected subacromial/subdeltoid bursal effusion and biceps tendon sheath fluid: reliable signs of rotator cuff tear? J Clin Ultrasound 1999;27(6):335–9.

[8] van Holsbeeck M, Introcaso JH, Kolowich PA. Sonography of tendons: patterns of disease. Instr Course Lect 1994;43:475–81.

[9] Jacobson JA, Lancaster S, Prasad A, et al. Full-thickness and partial-thickness supraspinatus tendon tears: value of US signs in diagnosis. Radiology 2004;230(1):234–42.

[10] Crass JR, Craig EV, Feinberg SB. Ultrasonography of rotator cuff tears: a review of 500 diagnostic studies. J Clin Ultrasound 1988;16(5):313–27.

[11] Teefey SA, Hasan SA, Middleton WD, et al. Ultrasonography of the rotator cuff. A comparison of ultrasonographic and arthroscopic findings in one hundred consecutive cases. J Bone Joint Surg Am 2000;82(4):498–504.

[12] Brenneke SL, Morgan CJ. Evaluation of ultrasonography as a diagnostic technique in the assessment of rotator cuff tendon tears. Am J Sports Med 1992;20(3):287–9.

[13] Wiener SN, Seitz WH Jr. Sonography of the shoulder in patients with tears of the rotator cuff: accuracy and value for selecting surgical options. AJR Am J Roentgenol 1993;160(1):103–7.

[14] Paavolainen P, Ahovuo J. Ultrasonography and arthrography in the diagnosis of tears of the rotator cuff. J Bone Joint Surg Am 1994;76(3):335–40.

[15] Hodler J, Fretz CJ, Terrier F, et al. Rotator cuff tears: correlation of sonographic and surgical findings. Radiology 1988;169(3):791–4.

[16] Mack LA, Matsen FA 3rd, Kilcoyne RF, et al. US evaluation of the rotator cuff. Radiology 1985;157(1):205–9.
[17] Brandt TD, Cardone BW, Grant TH, et al. Rotator cuff sonography: a reassessment. Radiology 1989;173(2):323–7.
[18] Teefey SA, Rubin DA, Middleton WD, et al. Detection and quantification of rotator cuff tears. Comparison of ultrasonographic, magnetic resonance imaging, and arthroscopic findings in seventy-one consecutive cases. J Bone Joint Surg Am 2004;86-A(4):708–16.
[19] Read JW, Perko M. Shoulder ultrasound: diagnostic accuracy for impingement syndrome, rotator cuff tear, and biceps tendon pathology. J Shoulder Elbow Surg 1998;7(3):264–71.
[20] Teefey SA, Middleton WD, Payne WT, et al. Detection and measurement of rotator cuff tears with sonography: analysis of diagnostic errors. AJR Am J Roentgenol 2005;184(6): 1768–73.
[21] Middleton WD, Teefey SA, Yamaguchi K. Sonography of the rotator cuff: analysis of interobserver variability. AJR Am J Roentgenol 2004;183(5):1465–8.
[22] Kluger R, Mayrhofer R, Kroner A, et al. Sonographic versus magnetic resonance arthrographic evaluation of full-thickness rotator cuff tears in millimeters. J Shoulder Elbow Surg 2003;12(2):110–6.
[23] Dinnes J, Loveman E, McIntyre L, et al. The effectiveness of diagnostic tests for the assessment of shoulder pain due to soft tissue disorders: a systematic review. Health Technol Assess 2003;7(29):iii.
[24] Chang CY, Wang SF, Chiou HJ, et al. Comparison of shoulder ultrasound and MR imaging in diagnosing full-thickness rotator cuff tears. Clin Imaging 2002;26(1):50–4.
[25] Beall DP, Williamson EE, Ly JQ, et al. Association of biceps tendon tears with rotator cuff abnormalities: degree of correlation with tears of the anterior and superior portions of the rotator cuff. AJR Am J Roentgenol 2003;180(3):633–9.
[26] Mohtadi NG, Vellet AD, Clark ML, et al. A prospective, double-blind comparison of magnetic resonance imaging and arthroscopy in the evaluation of patients presenting with shoulder pain. J Shoulder Elbow Surg 2004;13(3):258–65.
[27] Zanetti M, Pfirrmann CW. [Biceps tendon disorders: ultrasound, MR imaging and MR arthrography]. Radiologe 2004;44(6):591–6. [in German].
[28] Schydlowsky P, Strandberg C, Galatius S, et al. Ultrasonographic examination of the glenoid labrum of healthy volunteers. Eur J Ultrasound 1998;8(2):85–9.
[29] Schydlowsky P, Strandberg C, Galbo H, et al. The value of ultrasonography in the diagnosis of labral lesions in patients with anterior shoulder dislocation. Eur J Ultrasound 1998;8(2): 107–13.
[30] Hammar MV, Wintzell GB, Astrom KG, et al. Role of US in the preoperative evaluation of patients with anterior shoulder instability. Radiology 2001;219(1):29–34.
[31] Taljanovic MS, Carlson KL, Kuhn JE, et al. Sonography of the glenoid labrum: a cadaveric study with arthroscopic correlation. AJR Am J Roentgenol 2000;174(6):1717–22.
[32] Farin PU, Kaukanen E, Jaroma H, et al. Hill-Sachs lesion: sonographic detection. Skeletal Radiol 1996;25(6):559–62.
[33] Pancione L, Gatti G, Mecozzi B. Diagnosis of Hill-Sachs lesion of the shoulder. Comparison between ultrasonography and arthro-CT. Acta Radiol 1997;38:523–6.
[34] Cicak N, Bilic R, Delimar D. Hill-Sachs lesion in recurrent shoulder dislocation: sonographic detection. J Ultrasound Med 1998;17(9):557–60.
[35] Flannigan B, Kursunoglu-Brahme S, Snyder S, et al. MR arthrography of the shoulder: comparison with conventional MR imaging. AJR Am J Roentgenol 1990;155(4):829–32.
[36] Palmer WE, Caslowitz PL. Anterior shoulder instability: diagnostic criteria determined from prospective analysis of 121 MR arthrograms. Radiology 1995;197(3):819–25.
[37] Chandnani VP, Yeager TD, DeBerardino T, et al. Glenoid labral tears: prospective evaluation with MRI imaging, MR arthrography, and CT arthrography. AJR Am J Roentgenol 1993;161(6):1229–35.

[38] Chandnani VP, Gagliardi JA, Murnane TG, et al. Glenohumeral ligaments and shoulder capsular mechanism: evaluation with MR arthrography. Radiology 1995;196(1):27–32.
[39] Martinoli C, Bianchi S, Prato N, et al. US of the shoulder: non-rotator cuff disorders. Radiographics 2003;23(2):381–401.
[40] Blankstein A, Ganel A, Givon U, et al. Ultrasonography as a diagnostic modality in acromioclavicular joint pathologies. Isr Med Assoc J 2005;7(1):28–30.
[41] Yu YS, Dardani M, Fischer RA. MR observations of postraumatic osteolysis of the distal clavicle after traumatic separation of the acromioclavicular joint. J Comput Assist Tomogr 2000;24(1):159–64.
[42] van Holsbeeck M, Strouse PJ. Sonography of the shoulder: evaluation of the subacromial-subdeltoid bursa. AJR Am J Roentgenol 1993;160(3):561–4.
[43] Farin PU, Jaroma H, Harju A, et al. Shoulder impingement syndrome: sonographic evaluation. Radiology 1990;176(3):845–9.
[44] Jacobson JA, Propeck T, Jamadar DA, et al. US of the anterior bundle of the ulnar collateral ligament: findings in five cadaver elbows with MR arthrographic and anatomic comparison—initial observations. Radiology 2003;227(2):561–6.
[45] Miller TT, Adler RS, Friedman L. Sonography of injury of the ulnar collateral ligament of the elbow-initial experience. Skeletal Radiol 2004;33(7):386–91.
[46] Nazarian LN, McShane JM, Ciccotti MG, et al. Dynamic US of the anterior band of the ulnar collateral ligament of the elbow in asymptomatic major league baseball pitchers. Radiology 2003;227(1):149–54.
[47] De Smet AA, Winter TC, Best TM, et al. Dynamic sonography with valgus stress to assess elbow ulnar collateral ligament injury in baseball pitchers. Skeletal Radiol 2002;31(11):671–6.
[48] Sasaki J, Takahara M, Ogino T, et al. Ultrasonographic assessment of the ulnar collateral ligament and medial elbow laxity in college baseball players. J Bone Joint Surg Am 2002;84-A(4):525–31.
[49] Nakanishi K, Masatomi T, Ochi T, et al. MR arthrography of elbow: evaluation of the ulnar collateral ligament of elbow. Skeletal Radiol 1996;25(7):629–34.
[50] Mirowitz SA, London SL. Ulnar collateral ligament injury in baseball pitchers: MR imaging evaluation. Radiology 1992;185(2):573–6.
[51] Timmerman LA, Schwartz ML, Andrews JR. Preoperative evaluation of the ulnar collateral ligament by magnetic resonance imaging and computed tomography arthrography. Evaluation in 25 baseball players with surgical confirmation. Am J Sports Med 1994;22(1):26–31. [discussion: 32].
[52] Schwartz ML, al-Zahrani S, Morwessel RM, et al. Ulnar collateral ligament injury in the throwing athlete: evaluation with saline-enhanced MR arthrography. Radiology 1995;197(1):297–9.
[53] Belli P, Costantini M, Mirk P, et al. Sonographic diagnosis of distal biceps tendon rupture: a prospective study of 25 cases. J Ultrasound Med 2001;20(6):587–95.
[54] Miller TT, Adler RS. Sonography of tears of the distal biceps tendon. AJR Am J Roentgenol 2000;175(4):1081–6.
[55] Finlay K, Ferri M, Friedman L. Ultrasound of the elbow. Skeletal Radiol 2004;33(2):63–79.
[56] Finlay K, Lee R, Friedman L. Ultrasound of intrinsic wrist ligament and triangular fibrocartilage injuries. Skeletal Radiol 2004;33(2):85–90.
[57] Kaempffe FA, Lerner RM. Ultrasound diagnosis of triceps tendon rupture. A report of 2 cases. Clin Orthop Relat Res 1996;332:138–42.
[58] Gaines ST, Durbin RA, Marsalka DS. The use of magnetic resonance imaging in the diagnosis of triceps tendon ruptures. Contemp Orthop 1990;20(6):607–11.
[59] Tiger E, Mayer DP, Glazer R. Complete avulsion of the triceps tendon: MRI diagnosis. Comput Med Imaging Graph 1993;17(1):51–4.
[60] Williams BD, Schweitzer ME, Weishaupt D, et al. Partial tears of the distal biceps tendon: MR appearance and associated clinical findings. Skeletal Radiol 2001;30(10):560–4.

[61] Fitzgerald SW, Curry DR, Erickson SJ, et al. Distal biceps tendon injury: MR imaging diagnosis. Radiology 1994;191(1):203–6.
[62] Falchook FS, Zlatkin MB, Erbacher GE, et al. Rupture of the distal biceps tendon: evaluation with MR imaging. Radiology 1994;190(3):659–63.
[63] Connell D, Burke F, Coombes P, et al. Sonographic examination of lateral epicondylitis. AJR Am J Roentgenol 2001;176(3):777–82.
[64] Levin D, Nazarian LN, Miller TT, et al. Lateral epicondylitis of the elbow: US findings. Radiology 2005;237(1):230–4.
[65] Miller TT, Shapiro MA, Schultz E, et al. Comparison of sonography and MRI for diagnosing epicondylitis. J Clin Ultrasound 2002;30(4):193–202.
[66] Martin CE, Schweitzer ME. MR imaging of epicondylitis. Skeletal Radiol 1998;27(3):133–8.
[67] Aoki M, Wada T, Isogai S, et al. Magnetic resonance imaging findings of refractory tennis elbows and their relationship to surgical treatment. J Shoulder Elbow Surg 2005;14(2):172–7.
[68] Potter HG, Hannafin JA, Morwessel RM, et al. Lateral epicondylitis: correlation of MR imaging, surgical, and histopathologic findings. Radiology 1995;196(1):43–6.
[69] Jacobson JA, Oh E, Propeck T, et al. Sonography of the scapholunate ligament in four cadaveric wrists: correlation with MR arthrography and anatomy. [see comment]. AJR Am J Roentgenol 2002;179(2):523–7.
[70] Boutry N, Lapeque F, Masi L, et al. Ultrasonographic evaluation of normal extrinsic and intrinsic carpal ligaments: preliminary experience. Skeletal Radiol 2005;34:513–21.
[71] Scheck RJ, Kubitzek C, Hierner R, et al. The scapholunate interosseous ligament in MR arthrography of the wrist: correlation with non-enhanced MRI and wrist arthroscopy. Skeletal Radiol 1997;26(5):263–71.
[72] Schweitzer ME, Brahme SK, Hodler J, et al. Chronic wrist pain: spin-echo and short tau inversion recovery MR imaging and conventional and MR arthrography [erratum appears in Radiology 1992;184(2):583]. Radiology 1992;182(1):205–11.
[73] Totterman SM, Miller R, Wasserman B, et al. Intrinsic and extrinsic carpal ligaments: evaluation by three-dimensional Fourier transform MR imaging. AJR Am J Roentgenol 1993;160(1):117–23.
[74] Hergan K, Mittler C. Sonography of the injured ulnar collateral ligament of the thumb. J Bone Joint Surg Br 1995;77(1):77–83.
[75] Bronstein AJ, Koniuch MP, von Holsbeeck M. Ultrasonographic detection of thumb ulnar collateral ligament injuries: a cadaveric study. J Hand Surg [Am] 1994;19(2):304–12.
[76] O'Callaghan BI, Kohut G, Hoogewoud HM. Gamekeeper thumb: identification of the Stener lesion with US. Radiology 1994;192(2):477–80.
[77] Noszian IM, Dinkhauser LM, Orthner E, et al. Ulnar collateral ligament: differentiation of displaced and nondisplaced tears with US. Radiology 1995;194(1):61–3.
[78] Hergan K, Mittler C, Oser W. Ulnar collateral ligament: differentiation of displaced and nondisplaced tears with US and MR imaging. Radiology 1995;194(1):65–71.
[79] Hinke DH, Erickson SJ, Chamoy L, et al. Ulnar collateral ligament of the thumb: MR findings in cadavers, volunteers, and patients with ligamentous injury (gamekeeper's thumb). AJR Am J Roentgenol 1994;163(6):1431–4.
[80] Harper MT, Chandnani VP, Spaeth J, et al. Gamekeeper thumb: diagnosis of ulnar collateral ligament injury using magnetic resonance imaging, magnetic resonance arthrography and stress radiography. J Magn Reson Imaging 1996;6(2):322–8.
[81] Ahn JM, Sartoris DJ, Kang HS, et al. Gamekeeper thumb: comparison of MR arthrography with conventional arthrography and MR imaging in cadavers. Radiology 1998;206(3):737–44.
[82] Plancher KD, Ho CP, Cofield SS, et al. Role of MR imaging in the management of "skier's thumb" injuries. Magn Reson Imaging Clin N Am 1999;7(1):73–84.

[83] Lohman M, Vasenius J, Kivisaari A, et al. MR imaging in chronic rupture of the ulnar collateral ligament of the thumb. Acta Radiol 2001;42(1):10–4.
[84] Romano WM, Garvin G, Bhayana D, et al. The spectrum of ulnar collateral ligament injuries as viewed on magnetic resonance imaging of the metacarpophalangeal joint of the thumb. Can Assoc Radiol J 2003;54(4):243–8.
[85] Potter HG, Asnis-Ernberg L, Weiland AJ, et al. The utility of high-resolution magnetic resonance imaging in the evaluation of the triangular fibrocartilage complex of the wrist. J Bone Joint Surg Am 1997;79(11):1675–84.
[86] Haims AH, Schweitzer ME, Morrison WB, et al. Internal derangement of the wrist: indirect MR arthrography versus unenhanced MR imaging. Radiology 2003;227(3):701–7.
[87] Haims AH, Schweitzer ME, Morrison WB, et al. Limitations of MR imaging in the diagnosis of peripheral tears of the triangular fibrocartilage of the wrist. AJR Am J Roentgenol 2002;178(2):419–22.
[88] Daenen B, Houben G, Bauduin E, et al. Sonography in wrist tendon pathology. J Clin Ultrasound 2004;32(9):462–9.
[89] Teefey SA, Middleton WD, Boyer MI. Sonography of the hand and wrist. Semin Ultrasound CT MR 2000;21(3):192–204.
[90] Bianchi S, Martinoli C, Abdelwahab IF. High-frequency ultrasound examination of the wrist and hand. Skeletal Radiol 1999;28(3):121–9.
[91] Drape JL, Tardif-Chastenet de Gery S, Silbermann-Hoffman O, et al. Closed ruptures of the flexor digitorum tendons: MRI evaluation. Skeletal Radiol 1998;27(11):617–24.
[92] Scott JR, Cobby M, Taggart I. Magnetic resonance imaging of acute tendon injury in the finger. J Hand Surg [Br] 1995;20(3):286–8.
[93] Rubin DA, Kneeland JB, Kitay GS, et al. Flexor tendon tears in the hand: use of MR imaging to diagnose degree of injury in a cadaver model. AJR Am J Roentgenol 1996;166(3): 615–20.
[94] Drape JL, Dubert T, Silbermann O, et al. Acute trauma of the extensor hood of the metacarpophalangeal joint: MR imaging evaluation. Radiology 1994;192(2):469–76.
[95] Valeri G, Ferrara C, Ercolani P, et al. Tendon involvement in rheumatoid arthritis of the wrist: MRI findings. Skeletal Radiol 2001;30(3):138–43.
[96] Glajchen N, Schweitzer M. MRI features in de Quervain's tenosynovitis of the wrist. Skeletal Radiol 1996;25(1):63–5.

ELSEVIER SAUNDERS

Clin Sports Med 25 (2006) 591–606

CLINICS IN SPORTS MEDICINE

Low Field MRI: A Review of the Literature and Our Experience in Upper Extremity Imaging

Shaya Ghazinoor, MD*, John V. Crues III, MD

Radnet Management, 1516 Cotner Avenue, Santa Monica, CA 90024, USA

Since its introduction to medical imaging in the early 1980s, MRI has become essential in diagnosis and treatment of musculoskeletal conditions. Most imaging in the United States is performed on high-field whole-body scanners (>1.0 T). Imaging on low (<0.5 T) and medium (0.5–1.0 T) field strengths using small, low-cost, easily installed scanners in physicians' offices or imaging centers has gained increasing popularity. These scanners can be useful in imaging the upper extremity from the shoulder to the fingers. In this review, we provide an overview of the different extremity scanners available and their advantages and disadvantages, a brief review of the literature regarding their use, and a discussion of our experience in using the low-field extremity scanners in evaluating the upper extremity.

Extremity scanners are designed to provide MRI of the arms and legs using small magnets to limit construction and installation costs. Today there are more than 400 extremity scanners operating in referring physicians' offices in the United States. In other countries, such as Japan, there are a proportional number of low-field and high-field MRI scanners, with a large number of middle-field scanners [1]. Currently, there are four commercially available extremity scanners that are approved by the Food and Drug Administration [2]. Three image at 0.2 T, at which permanent magnets are cost-effective, and the fourth, the OrthoOne ONI scanner, operates at 1.0 T using a superconducting magnet. The ONI scanner is not reviewed in this paper because it is a high-field scanner.

The Applause 0.2 T portable scanner is manufactured by MagneVu and until recently was distributed by General Electric (GE) Medical Systems (Fig. 1). It is the least expensive and most restrictive of the extremity scanners, with a compact design that does not require magnetic field or radiofrequency shielding. A local surface coil is built into the scanner, optimizing the signal-to-noise ratio and placing the acquisition field of view in a fixed position close to the magnet face. It is the only scanner that images in a nonuniform field,

*Corresponding author. *E-mail address*: sghazinoor@yahoo.com (S. Ghazinoor).

0278-5919/06/$ – see front matter
doi:10.1016/j.csm.2006.03.001

sportsmed.theclinics.com

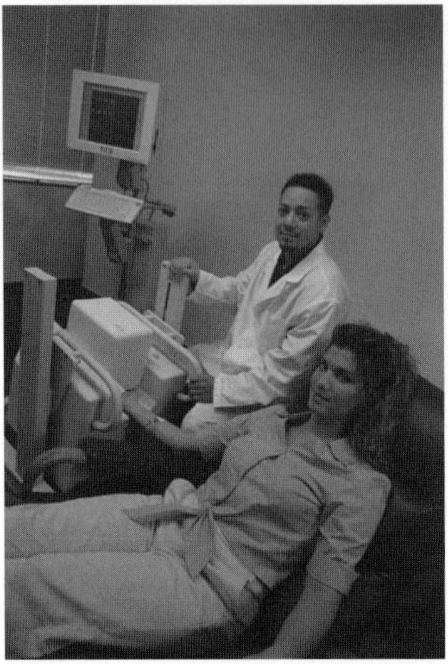

Fig. 1. The MagneVu extremity scanner's open design allows patients to be scanned in sitting or recumbent postions. (Courtesy of O. Troum, MD, Santa Monica, CA.)

significantly increasing the imaging time, because the phase-encoding gradient needs to be applied in two dimensions. To decrease imaging time, therefore, the imaging volume is restricted. Current applications for the Applause include foot, wrist, and hand imaging for the detection and characterization of bone erosions in inflammatory arthropathies (Table 1) [3].

The C-scan, manufactured by the Esaote Company in Italy and distributed by GE, operates at a uniform 0.2 T and uses a permanent magnet that does not need magnetic shielding (Fig. 2). Radiofrequency shielding is supplied by flexible material placed around the aperture of the magnet. This magnet is not portable like the Applause scanner. It is designed to image the extremities from the elbows to the fingers and the knees to the toes. The 12 cm three-dimensional (3D) field of view of this device allows imaging of entire joints with accuracy typical of full-body scanners at similar field strength [4]. This scanner has a confined imaging space and cannot be used for scanning the shoulders and hips. This space limitation also forces the ankle to be scanned in plantarflexion, instead of the usual dorsiflexed position in which the ankles are scanned on whole-body scanners. The anatomy in this position maybe confusing for the radiologist who is unfamiliar with viewing images in plantarflexion until adequate experience is gained.

The E-scan 0.2 T MRI is also manufactured by Esaote and marketed by GE (Fig. 3). This scanner is designed with open access to the imaging volume,

Table 1
Applause imaging protocols

Series	Weighting	Anatomic centering
Hand for rheumatoid arthritis		
1	T1	2nd and 3rd MCP
2	STIR	2nd and 3rd MCP
3	T1	Medial margin lunate
4	STIR	Medial margin lunate
Foot for rheumatoid arthritis		
1	T1	2nd and 3rd MTP
2	STIR	2nd and 3rd MTP

All sequences are performed using a 3D Fourier transform spin-echo technique. The field of view is 7 cm in distal to proximal length, 5 cm in medial to lateral length, and 1 cm in anteroposterior dimension. Sixteen contiguous slices are obtained and displayed in the coronal plane of the hand and axial plane of the foot.

Abbreviations: MCP, metacarpophalangeal; MTP, metatarsophalangeal.

Data from Edelman RR, Hesselink JR, Zlatkin MB, et al. Clinical magnetic resonance imaging. 3rd edition. Philadelphia: Saunders-Elsevier; 2005.

allowing examination of not only the distal extremities but also the shoulder and the hip. The permanent magnet poles are located above and below the table, making this a vertical-field scanner with magic-angle artifacts similar to those seen on whole-body scanners. The table rotates around the magnetic pole, which helps with patient positioning.

The main advantages of the extremity scanners compared with the whole-body high-field scanners are lower purchase and maintenance costs, low

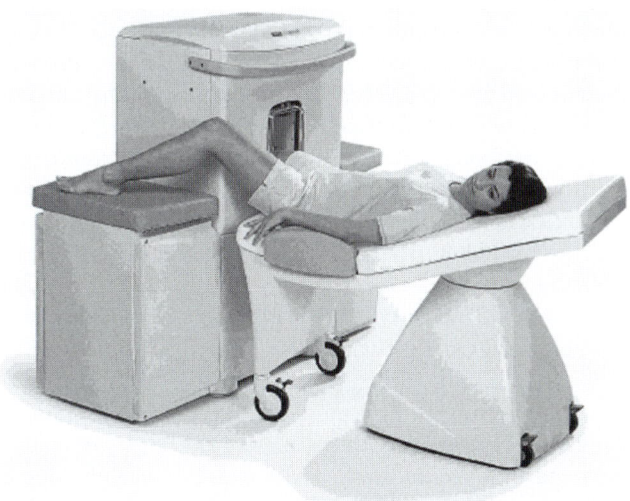

Fig. 2. The Esaote C-scan has a compact design. (Courtesy of Hologic, Inc., Bedford, MA; with permission.)

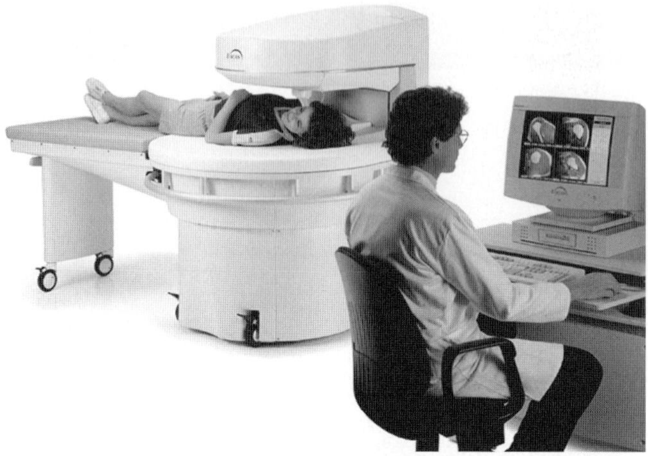

Fig. 3. The Esaote E-scan has an open design allowing imaging of the hip and shoulder in addition to other joints. (Courtesy of Hologic, Inc., Bedford, MA; with permission.)

weight, ease of installation in a limited space, and faster patient diagnosis in the in-office setting. In numerous musculoskeletal injuries, such as subchondral bone injuries that are occult on plain films, delay in diagnosis causing a delay in treatment can be detrimental. Another advantage of extremity scanners is that they are tolerated better by claustrophobic patients and children, who may otherwise require sedation.

The main disadvantage of low-field scanners is the concern of poor-quality images secondary to a worsening signal-to-noise ratio (SNR) compared with the whole-body high-field scanners. In general, the SNR, contrast, and resolution increase with field strength. The literature states that to compensate for the decreased SNR in low-field scanners, the voxel volume or acquisition time needs to be increased. Longer acquisition times lead to an increased risk for patient motion causing poor quality images. Increasing voxel volume by increasing the slice thickness or the field of view makes the detection of signal abnormalities more difficult secondary to worsening spatial resolution. Additional factors, such as radiofrequency penetration, radiative loss, optimized pulse sequences, and coil sensitivity, also play significant roles in the theoretic SNR benefit at high field strengths [5].

Care must be taken not to make up for the poor SNR inherent at 0.2 T with voxel dimensions too large to provide adequate spatial resolution for evaluation of the joints. At our practice, therefore, we do not sacrifice the spatial resolution (ie, increase the slice thickness and field of view) for an increase in SNR (see recommended protocols in Tables 2 and 3). In addition, we do not increase acquisition time, which would lead to a longer scan time and increase the risk for motion artifact. For example, our routine shoulder MRI on an extremity scanner is performed at a field of view of 14 to 16 cm, with a slice thickness

Table 2
Imaging protocols for the Esaote C-scan

Pulse sequence	Contrast	Plane	TR (ms)	No.of slices	Gap (mm)	Thickness (mm)	TE (ms)	TI (ms)	FOV (mm)	Matrix	Acquisitions	Time (min)
Elbow												
SE	T1	Axial	620	18	0.4	4.0	18	—	140	192 × 192	3	5:59
SE	T2	Axial	3000	13	1.0	5.0	100	—	140	192 × 160	1	8:06
SE	T1	Coronal	600	13	0.4	4.0	24	—	140	192 × 192	3	5:49
STIR		Coronal	900	10	0.8	4.0	16	75	140	192 × 160	2	4:51
SE	T1	Sagittal	580	15	0.4	4.0	18	—	140	192 × 192	4	7:28
Wrist or hand												
SE	T1	Axial	550	16	0.4	4.0	18	—	120	192 × 160	4	5:55
SE	T1	Coronal	500	12	0.4	4.0	20	—	120	192 × 176	4	5:55
STIR		Coronal	1150	12	0.4	4.0	24	—	140	192 × 160	2	6:10
GRE	TE	Coronal	540	12	0.4	3.5	16	Flip angle 45	130	192 × 176	4	6:23
SE	T1	Sagittal	690	18	0.4	4.0	20	—	120	192 × 192	3	6:40
SE	T2	Axial	3000	16	0.4	4.0	90	—	120	192 × 160	1	8:06

Abbreviations: FOV, field of view; GRE, gradient echo; SE, spin echo; STIR, short-T1 inversion recovery; TE, echo time; TI, inversion time; TR, repetition time.

Data from Edelman RR, Hesselink JR, Zlatkin MB, et al. Clinical magnetic resonance imaging. 3rd edition. Philadelphia: Saunders-Elsevier; 2005.

Table 3
Imaging protocols for the Esaote E-scan

Pulse sequence	Contrast	Plane	TR (ms)	No. of slices	Gap (mm)	Thickness (mm)	TE (ms)	TI (ms)	FOV (mm)	Matrix	Acquisitions
Shoulder											
SE	T1	Coronal	580	12	0.5	5	24	—	140	192 × 160	2
SE	T2	Coronal	2400	12	0.5	5	80	—	140	192 × 160	1
GRE	T2	Axial	630	14	0.5	5	74	75	140	192 × 160	2
SE	T1	Axial	680	14	0.5	5	24	—	140	192 × 160	2
SE	T2	Sagittal	2400	12	0.5	5	80	—	140	192 × 160	1
STIR		Coronal	1850	12	0.5	5	24	80	140	192 × 128	2
Elbow											
SE	T1	Axial	400	18	1.0	4	24	—	130	192 × 152	2
SE	T2	Axial	870	18	1.0	4	80	—	130	192 × 152	1
STIR		Axial	1700	18	1.0	4	25	70	150	192 × 152	2
SE	T1	Coronal	680	14	1.0	4	24	—	150	192 × 160	2
STIR		Coronal	1410	14	1.0	4	24	75	160	192 × 160	2
GRE-3D	TE	Coronal	50	52	0.0	1.2	16	Flip angle 40	160	192 × 192	1
SE	T1	Sagittal	900	18	1.0	4.0	26	—	120	162 × 160	2
Wrist or hand											
SE	T1	Axial	770	15	0.5	4.0	24	—	110	192 × 160	2
STIR		Axial	1450	15	0.5	4.0	25	70	130	162 × 160	2
SE	T1	Coronal	560	12	0.5	3.5	24	—	130	192 × 160	2
STIR		Coronal	1100	12	0.5	3.5	24	75	130	192 × 128	2
GRE-3D	T1	Coronal	32	52	0	2.5	16	Flip angle 40	110	192 × 176	1
SE	T1	Sagittal	510	15	0.5	43.5	18	—	110	192 × 160	2
SE	T2	Axial	2400	15	0.5	4.0	90	—	120	192 × 160	1

Abbreviations: FOV, field of view; GRE, gradient echo; SE, spin echo; STIR, short-T1 inversion recovery; TE, echo time; TI, inversion time; TR; repetition time.

Data from Edelman RR, Hesselink JR, Zlatkin MB, et al. Clinical magnetic resonance imaging. 3rd edition. Philadelphia: Saunders-Elsevier; 2005.

of 4 to 5 mm, using two acquisitions. We find that although images are subjectively noisier compared with high-field images, they are still of diagnostic quality. We touch on this point further when we discuss a review of the literature comparing high- and low-field MRI of the upper extremity.

For musculoskeletal MRI, the contrast-to-noise ratio (CNR) is a clinically relevant parameter because it determines the extent to which adjacent structures can be distinguished from one another [4]. The CNR, unlike the SNR, is independent of field strength and more dependent on imaging parameters. CNR is not sacrificed, therefore, on the lower-field extremity scanners.

The other major disadvantage of low-field scanners is that there is less spectral separation between water and fat, thus restricting the ability to perform frequency-selective fat suppression. Fat suppression is an invaluable technique in musculoskeletal imaging because it is used to demonstrate bone marrow pathology. It also is used to increase the contrast between gadolinium-enhanced tissue and the adjacent fat. An alternative method to suppress fat signal, which can be preformed by low-field scanners, is the short-T1 inversion recovery (STIR) sequence. STIR images are extremely useful for demonstrating bone marrow edema. The major disadvantage is incompatibility with gadolinium enhancement; therefore, magnetic resonance (MR) arthrograms and contrast-enhanced studies are of poorer diagnostic value on low-field scanners, because at low field the intrinsic contrast of gadolinium is less [6]. In addition, the inability to perform T1-weighted images with fat saturation also decreases the intrinsic contrast needed for diagnostic accuracy with intra-articular or intravenous contrast enhanced studies.

A major pitfall in the use of extremity scanners is the potential for suboptimal image quality and loss of quality control by radiologists. Lawsuits already have made their way through United States courts for alleged losses because of poor quality control. Treating physicians and their office managers are not trained in MRI quality control. We believe that the radiologist should be responsible for establishing imaging protocols, determining appropriate indications as determined by American College of Radiology guidelines, and supervising technologists. Most important of all, it should be the responsibility of the radiologist as the professional component of the imaging team to supervise quality control.

Given that the use of extremity scanners by orthopedic surgeons has increased, it is important to analyze the available clinical data comparing the diagnostic performance of low-field scanners compared with high-field scanners.

In 1999, Merl and colleagues [7] performed a prospective study evaluating 122 patients with suspected disease of the shoulder joint. These patients were scanned in both low- and high-field MRI scanners. Results were confirmed operatively in 78 patients. After taking into account the 95% confidence interval, no difference was found between the different strength scanners in the diagnosis of impingement, rotator cuff lesions, or labral lesions.

In 2000, Tung and coworkers [8] found that sensitivity and specificity in the diagnosis of superior labrum anterior posterior (SLAP) tears were 95% and 63% on high-field scanners ($n = 46$) and 64% and 79% on low-field scanners (n = 21). The study was limited in that a fat-suppressed sequence was performed on the high-field studies, whereas no comparable technique (STIR) was performed on the low field. In addition, the spatial resolution was sacrificed on the low-field studies.

In 2001, Shellock and colleagues [9] retrospectively compared the surgical findings of 47 patients who had undergone open or arthroscopic shoulder surgery with their MRI performed using a 0.2 Tesla scanner. They found that the sensitivity and specificity for rotator cuff tears (n = 29) were 89% and 100%, and for labral lesions (n = 9) they were 89% and 95% respectively. These results compared favorably with those values published in the literature for high-field MRI systems. There were three false negative studies associated with partial tears of the rotator cuff. There was one false negative study associated with a type I SLAP tear. In addition, two false positive studies had diagnosed ill-defined tears of the labrum that were found to be normal on surgery. In this study, spatial resolution was not sacrificed and the authors used a slice thickness of 5 mm (with the exception of a 7-mm slice thickness on the STIR sequence) and a field of view of 14 to 16 cm.

In 2003, Magee and coworkers [10] prospectively studied 40 patients who had MRI of the shoulder on both 0.2 T and 1.5 T scanners. Twenty-eight of these patients underwent arthroscopy. Of the 40 studies, nine of the interpretations performed from the low-field images changed after reviewing the high-field images. Three labral tears and two SLAP tears were depicted definitively on the high-field images and not on the low-field images. In addition, in 4 patients the interpreters had difficulty deciding between partial and full-thickness rotator cuff tears, whereas high field allowed more definitive interpretation. Three of these were small focal full-thickness tears with no retraction, and one was a larger full-thickness tear with 3 cm retraction. Fibrosis in the area of tear had prevented it from showing increased signal and made it difficult for the interpreters to visualize the retracted free edge on the low-field study. All nine of the labral and rotator cuff tears were confirmed at arthroscopy. This study is significant in that in 9 out of 40 patients the high field strength interpretation altered clinical

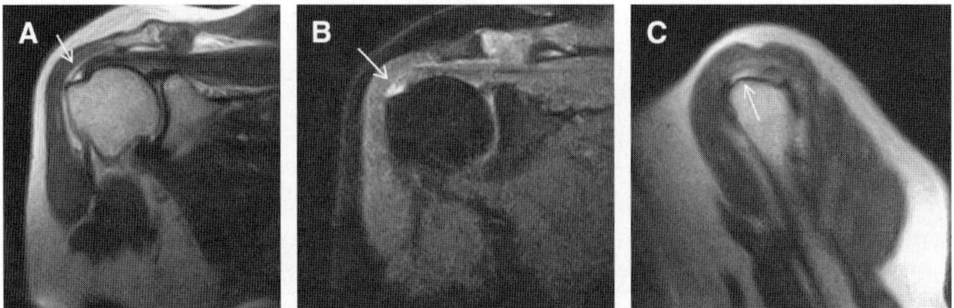

Fig. 4. Coronal T2 (*A*), coronal STIR (*B*), and sagittal T2 (*C*) images demonstrate a focal full-thickness rotator cuff tear at the distal insertion of the supraspinatus tendon.

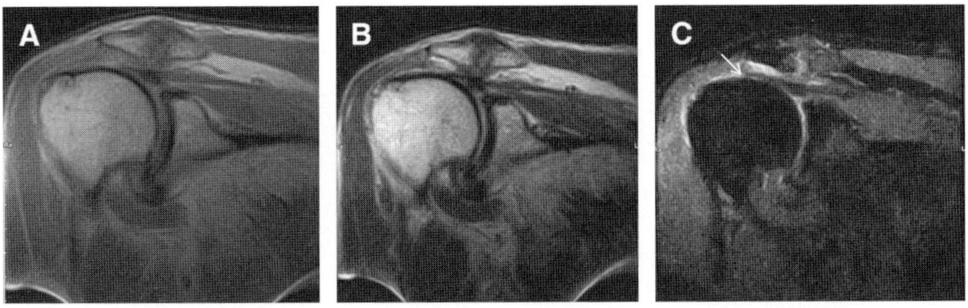

Fig. 5. (*A*) Coronal T1-weighted and (*B*) T2-weighted images demonstrate a high-riding shoulder but fail to demonstrate the increased T2 signal seen with full-thickness rotator cuff tears, likely secondary to granulation tissue formation. The coronal STIR (*C*) sequence, however, nicely demonstrates the signal abnormality attributable to a full-thickness rotator cuff tear with retraction of the distal tendon (*arrow*).

treatment as surgery was performed to address the findings not seen on the low-field images. The main limitation of this study was that the low-field images were performed using a field of view of 20 cm to maintain adequate SNR, causing a significant reduction in spatial resolution. This need not be done in low-field imaging, because the sacrifice in spatial resolution is a diagnostic hindrance that outweighs the benefits gained from improved SNR.

In 2004, Zlatkin and colleagues [11] performed a retrospective study involving 160 patients comparing low-field shoulder MRI findings to surgical findings. They found that the sensitivity and specificity for rotator cuff tears (n = 131) were 90% and 93%, respectively. For labral tears (n = 60) the sensitivity and specificity were 55% and 100%. Prior investigations using medium- and high-field MRI systems to identify labral tears reported sensitivities ranging from 44% to 95% [5,12,13].

In summary, a handful of studies have been performed comparing high-field versus low-field MRI of the shoulder. Most have demonstrated no significant

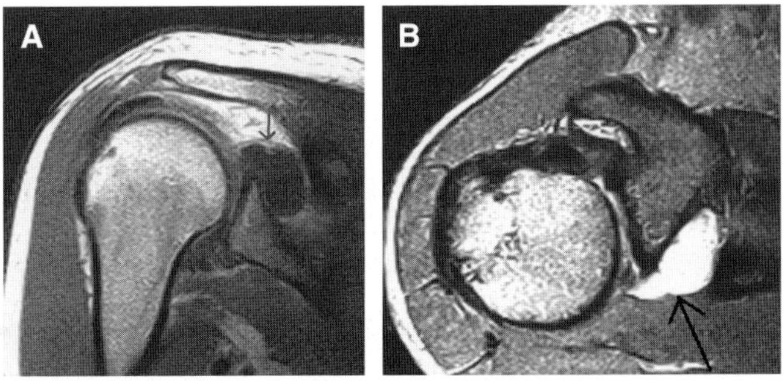

Fig. 6. (*A*) Coronal T1-weighted and (*B*) axial gradient-echo–weighted images nicely demonstrate a low T1/high T2 signal intensity fluid collection located just adjacent to the superior labrum (*arrows*).

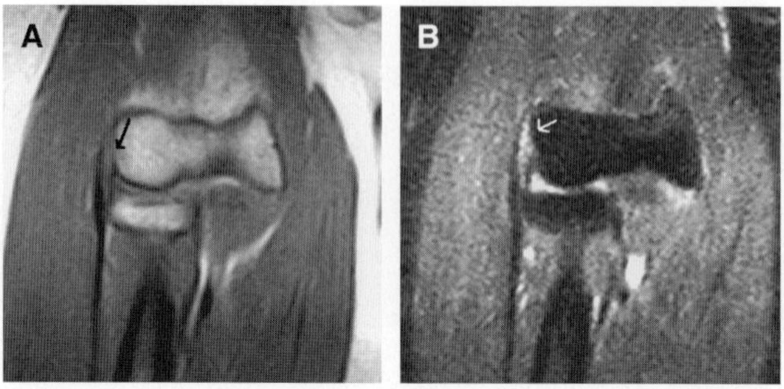

Fig. 7. (*A*) Coronal T1-weighted and (*B*) STIR-weighted images show high signal intensity at the insertion of the common extensor tendon consistent with tendinosis or lateral epicondylitis.

difference in sensitivity and specificity in detection of rotator cuff and labral lesions. Although it is true that high-field MRI systems provide nicer images that are more pleasing to the eye, only one of the above studies demonstrated a relevant therapeutic difference between imaging at low and high field strength. In the study performed by Magee and colleagues [10], 9 out of 40 patients demonstrated findings on the high-field study not seen on the low-field study, which lead to a significant change in patient management. Their investigation was limited in that the low-field studies were performed with decreased spatial resolution, thus limiting the ability to see abnormalities secondary to volume averaging.

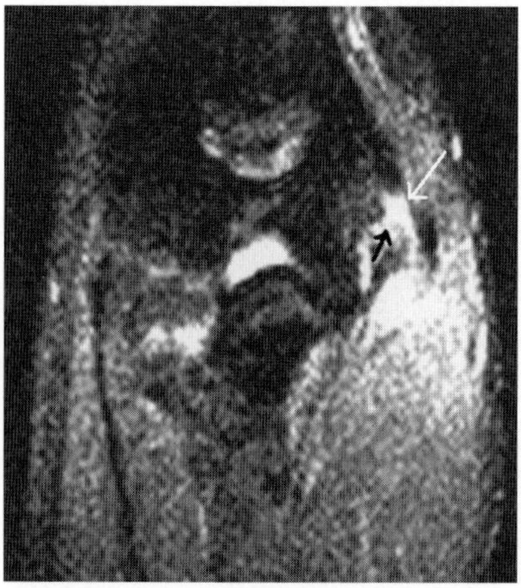

Fig. 8. Fluid signal intensity is seen at the proximal insertion of the ulnar collateral ligament (*black arrow*) on this coronal STIR image of the elbow. There is also a partial tear of the flexor tendon (*white arrow*).

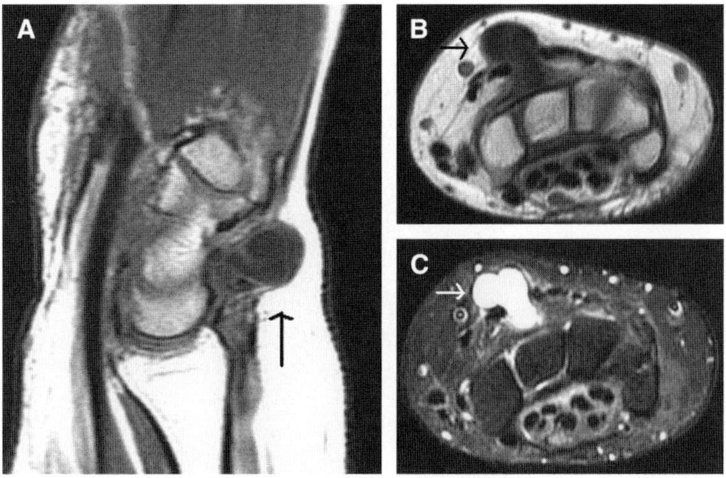

Fig. 9. (*A,B*) Sagittal and axial T1-weighted and (*C*) axial STIR-weighted images demonstrate a lobulated fluid collection (*black and white arrows*) along the dorsal surface of the hands consistent with a ganglion cyst.

In our subjective experience reading hundreds of low-field shoulder MRI scans, rotator cuff pathology is seen well (Fig. 4). In the beginning, an inexperienced reader of low-field studies may have difficulty in the identification of chronic full-thickness rotator cuff tears secondary to scar and granulation tissue

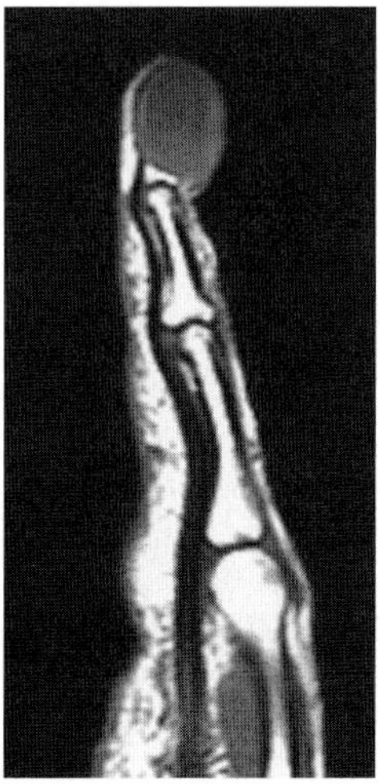

Fig. 10. Sagittal T1 image of the index finger demonstrates an intermediate signal intensity, well-defined, expansile, intramedullary lesion within the distal phalanx pathologically proven to be a glomus tumor.

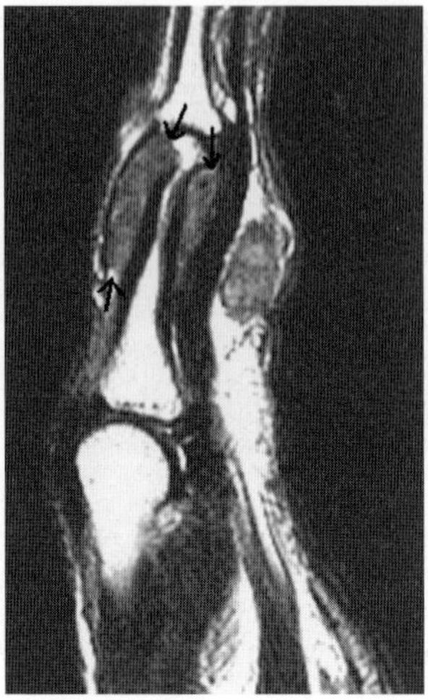

Fig. 11. Soft tissue intensity is seen surrounding the proximal middle phalanx beneath the flexor and extensor tendons of the finger (*black arrows*) worrisome for a giant cell tumor of the tendon sheath.

formation and the lack of increased T2 signal. This pathology should be evident on the STIR sequences, however, as should the secondary findings of a high-riding humeral head and tendon retraction (Fig. 5). Paralabral cysts can be identified easily on low-field studies (Fig. 6). The diagnosis of labral tears, on the other hand, is limited with low-field imaging as compared with high-field imaging secondary to the inferior SNR. Often pathology can be suggested but the increased noise makes a definitive diagnosis difficult. Many studies have demonstrated the superior diagnostic accuracy of intra-articular

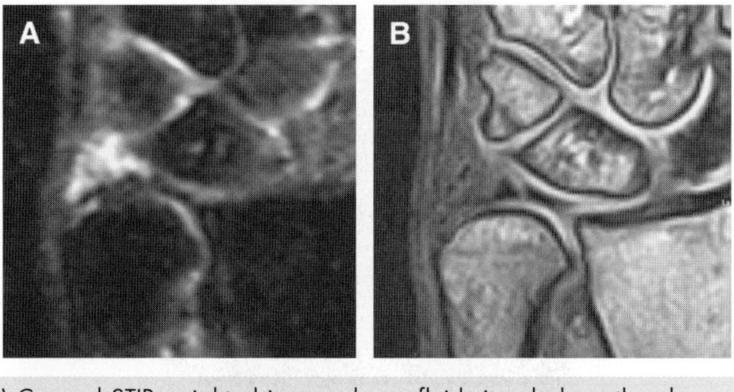

Fig. 12. (*A*) Coronal STIR-weighted image shows fluid signal along the ulnar aspect of the triangular fibrocartilage (TFCC) with a suggestion of fluid extending across the more central portion of the TFCC. (*B*) The high-resolution coronal gradient-echo–weighted images clearly demonstrate fluid signal traversing the TFCC consistent with a focal tear.

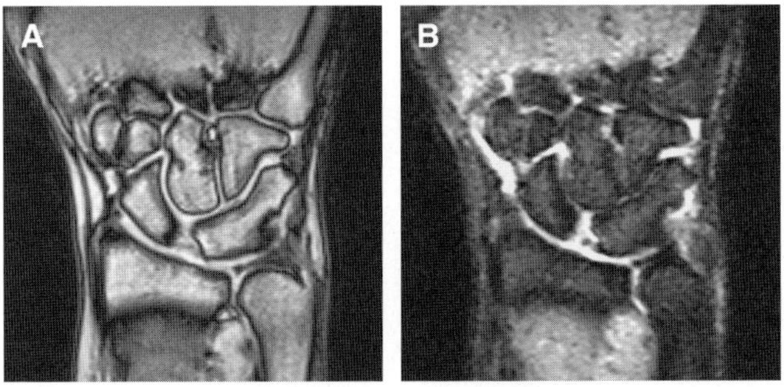

Fig. 13. (*A*) High-resolution coronal gradient-echo–weighted image demonstrates widening of the scapholunate space. (*B*) Coronal STIR nicely demonstrates fluid signal at the radial attachment of the scapholunate ligament consistent with a tear. Incidentally, there is fusion of the lunate and triquetrum.

gadolinium for labral pathology [14–16]. MR arthrography is of poor diagnostic value on low-field scanners secondary to the suboptimal contrast of gadolinium and the inability to perform fat-saturated T1-weighted images. High-field scanners clearly have a diagnostic superiority over low-field scanners in the diagnosis of labral tears.

Elbow imaging using the extremity scanner has been of great diagnostic value also. We have found the extremity scanner useful in the diagnosis of multiple conditions of the elbow, including lateral or medial epicondylitis (Fig. 7), biceps tendon injuries, ligament pathology (Fig. 8), and evaluation of fractures.

We have had extensive experience reading hundreds of wrist and hand MRI scans using the E-scan. We find the images to be of superb diagnostic quality. We commonly diagnose soft tissue and bony masses, such as ganglion cysts (Fig. 9), glomus tumors of the finger (Fig. 10), and giant cell tumors of the tendon sheath (Fig. 11). The low-field scanners also are of superb diagnostic value

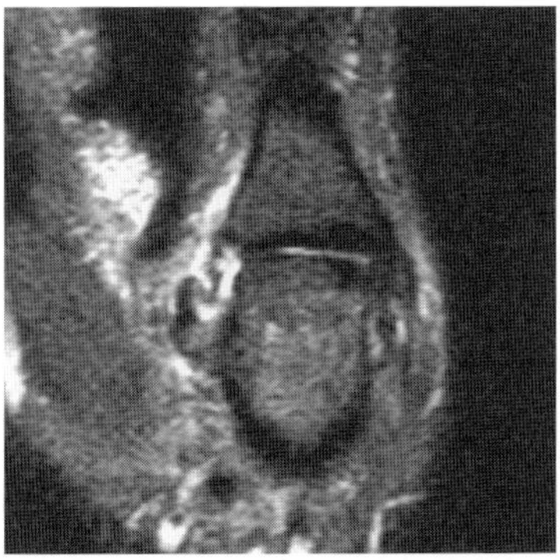

Fig. 14. Coronal STIR image of the thumb demonstrates a wavy, retracted ulnar collateral ligament, which has been avulsed from its attachment to the base of the proximal phalanx.

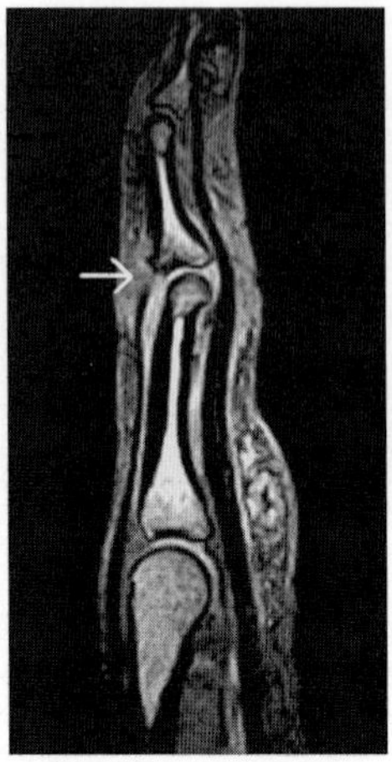

Fig. 15. Sagittal gradient-echo–weighted image demonstrates a focal tear of the central slip of the extensor tendon at its distal attachment into the base of the middle phalanx.

in pathology that is more difficult to visualize, such as triangular fibrocartilage tears (Fig. 12), intracarpal ligament tears (Fig. 13), tears of the ulnar collateral ligament (ie, gamekeeper's thumb) (Fig. 14), and tears of the tendons of the fingers (Fig. 15). It also is useful in evaluation of the flexor and extensor tendons of the wrist (Fig. 16).

A special area of research interest in the use of low-field MRI has been the evaluation of scaphoid fractures (Fig. 17). Byrdie and Raby [17] evaluated 195 patients with clinically suspected, radiographically occult scaphoid fractures. They underwent limited MRI examination (consisting of coronal T1 and STIR images) on a 0.2 T extremity scanner. A total of 50.8% were normal, 19% had scaphoid fractures, 14.4% had distal radial fracture, 10.3% had bone contusions, and 4.5% had other carpal bone fractures. Breitenseher [18] compared the diagnostic capabilities of a 0.2 T extremity scanner and a 1.0 T

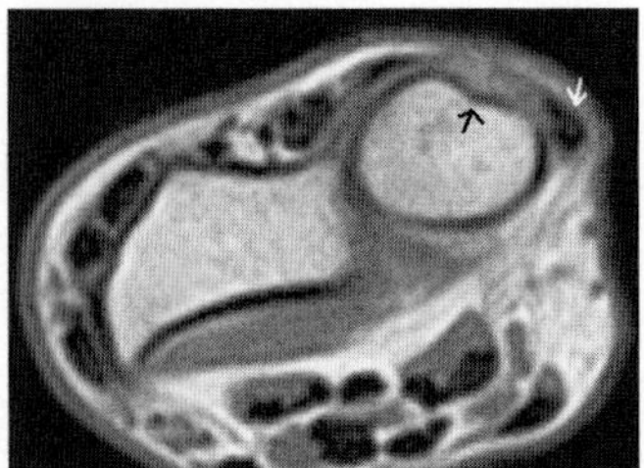

Fig. 16. T1 axial image of the wrist demonstrates subluxation of the extensor carpi ulnaris tendon (*white arrow*) from its normal position in the ulnar groove (*black arrow*), indicating disruption of the ECU tendon sheath.

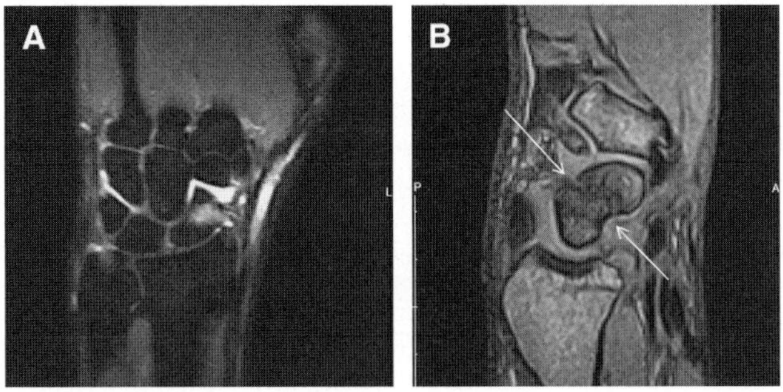

Fig. 17. Coronal T2 image (*A*) demonstrates focal increased signal within the scaphoid waist with a suggestion of cortical disruption along the ulnar aspect of the waist. The cortical step-off is confirmed on the sagittal high-resolution gradient-echo–weighted image (*B, yellow arrows*).

body scanner in scaphoid fractures and concluded that there was no difference in fracture detection between the two systems. MRI in this clinical scenario allows a definitive diagnosis to be made, having a significant impact on patient management.

There is no debate that high-field MRI images are of better quality compared with low-field images; however, this does not necessarily translate into greater diagnostic power. Our subjective experience is in concordance with many studies demonstrating the high diagnostic value in the use of low-field scanners in musculoskeletal pathology. In general, the experience and training of the reader is likely to impact the interpretation of these images. MRI performed on extremity scanners would be performed best by musculoskeletal-trained radiologists with experience reading on low-field systems, working closely with referring orthopedic surgeons.

References

[1] Hayshi N, Watananbe Y, Masumoto T, et al. Utilization of low-field MR scanners. Magn Reson Med Sci 2004;3(1):27–38.

[2] Crues JV. Extremity scanners. In: Edelman RR, Hesselink JR, Zlatkin MB, et al, editors. Clinical magnetic resonance imaging, 3rd edition. Philadelphia: Elsevier; 2005. p. 3649–67.

[3] Crues JV, Shellock FG, Dardashti S, et al. Identification of wrist and metacarpophalangeal joint erosions using a portable-MR system compared to conventional X-ray. J Rheumatol 2004;31(4):676–85.

[4] Peterfy CG, Roberts T, Genant HK. Dedicated extremity MR imaging: an emerging technology. Radiol Clin North Am 1997;33:1–20.

[5] Maubon AJ, Ferru J, Berger V, et al. Effect of field strength on MR images: comparison of the same subject at 0.5, 1.0, and 1.5 T. Radiographics 1999;19(4):1057–67.

[6] Desai NK, Runge VM. Contrast use at low field: A review. Top Magn Reson Imaging 2003;14(5):360–4.

[7] Merl T, Scholz M, Gerhardt P, et al. Results of a prospective multicenter study for evaluation of the diagnostic quality of an open whole-body low-filed MRI unit: a comparison with high-filed MRI measured by the applicable gold standard. Eur J Radiol 1999;30:43–53.

[8] Tung GA, Entzian D, Green A, et al. High-field and low-field MR imaging of superior glenoid labral tears and associated tendon injuries. AJR 2000;174:1107–14.

[9] Shellock FG, Bert JM, Fritts HM, et al. Evaluation of the rotator cuff and glenoid labrum using a 0.2 tesla extremity magnetic resonance (MR) system: MR results compared to surgical findings. J Magn Reson Imaging 2001;14:763–70.
[10] Magee T, Shapiro M, Williams D. Comparison of high-field-strength versus low-field-strength MRI of the shoulder. AJR Am J Roentgenol 2003;181:1211–5.
[11] Zlatkin MB, Hoffman C, Shellock FG. Assessment of the rotator cuff and glenoid labrum using an extremity MR system: MR results compared to surgical findings form a multi-center study. J Magn Reson Imaging 2004;19:623–31.
[12] Garneau RA, Renfrew DL, Moore TE, et al. Glenoid labrum: evaluation with MR imaging. Radiology 1991;179:519–22.
[13] Monu J, Pope TL Jr, Chabon SJ, et al. MR diagnosis of superior labrum-anterior to posterior (SLAP) injuries of the glenoid: value of routine imaging without intraarticular injection of contrast material. AJR Am J Roentgenol 1994;163:1425–9.
[14] Palmer WE, Brown JH, Rosenthal DJ. Labral-ligamentous complex of the shoulder: evaluation with MR arthrography. Radiology 1994;190:645–51.
[15] Chandnani VP, Yeager TD, DeBerardino T, et al. Glenoid labral tears: prospective evaluation with MR imaging, MR arthrography and CT arthrography. AJR Am J Roentgenol 1993;161:1229–35.
[16] Flannigan B, Kursunoglu-Brahme S, Snyder S, et al. MR arthrography of the shoulder: comparison with conventional MR imaging. AJR Am J Roentgenol 1990;155:829–32.
[17] Brydie A, Raby N. Early MRI in the management of clinical scaphoid fracture. Br J Radiol 2003;76:296–300.
[18] Breitenseher MJ, Trattnig S, Gabler C, et al. MRI in radiologically occult scaphoid fractures: initial experiences with 1.0 Tesla (whole body middle-field equipment) versus 0.2 Tesla (dedicated low-field equipment). Radiologe 1997;37:812–8.

Clin Sports Med 25 (2006) 607–611

CLINICS IN SPORTS MEDICINE

INDEX

Note: Page numbers of article titles are in **boldface** type.

0278-5919/06/$ – see front matter
doi:10.1016/S0278-5919(06)00058-5

sportsmed.theclinics.com

N

O

P

Q

R